Genetic Testing for Rare Diseases

Genetic Testing for Rare Diseases

Editor

José Millán

MDPI • Basel • Beijing • Wuhan • Barcelona • Belgrade • Manchester • Tokyo • Cluj • Tianjin

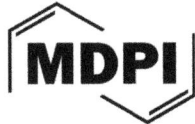

Editor
José Millán
Molecular, Cellular and
Genomics Biomedicine
Health Research Institute La Fe
Valencia
Spain

Editorial Office
MDPI
St. Alban-Anlage 66
4052 Basel, Switzerland

This is a reprint of articles from the Special Issue published online in the open access journal *Diagnostics* (ISSN 2075-4418) (available at: www.mdpi.com/journal/diagnostics/special_issues/Genetic_Rare_Diseases).

For citation purposes, cite each article independently as indicated on the article page online and as indicated below:

LastName, A.A.; LastName, B.B.; LastName, C.C. Article Title. *Journal Name* **Year**, *Volume Number*, Page Range.

ISBN 978-3-0365-3728-3 (Hbk)
ISBN 978-3-0365-3727-6 (PDF)

© 2022 by the authors. Articles in this book are Open Access and distributed under the Creative Commons Attribution (CC BY) license, which allows users to download, copy and build upon published articles, as long as the author and publisher are properly credited, which ensures maximum dissemination and a wider impact of our publications.

The book as a whole is distributed by MDPI under the terms and conditions of the Creative Commons license CC BY-NC-ND.

Contents

Preface to "Genetic Testing for Rare Diseases" vii

José M. Millán and Gema García-García
Genetic Testing for Rare Diseases
Reprinted from: *Diagnostics* **2022**, *12*, 809, doi:10.3390/diagnostics12040809 1

Luke Mansard, Christel Vaché, Julie Bianchi, Corinne Baudoin, Isabelle Perthus and Bertrand Isidor et al.
Identification of the First Single *GSDME* Exon 8 Structural Variants Associated with Autosomal Dominant Hearing Loss
Reprinted from: *Diagnostics* **2022**, *12*, 207, doi:10.3390/diagnostics12010207 5

Valeriia Yu. Danilchenko, Marina V. Zytsar, Ekaterina A. Maslova, Marita S. Bady-Khoo, Nikolay A. Barashkov and Igor V. Morozov et al.
Different Rates of the *SLC26A4*-Related Hearing Loss in Two Indigenous Peoples of Southern Siberia (Russia)
Reprinted from: *Diagnostics* **2021**, *11*, 2378, doi:10.3390/diagnostics11122378 13

Camille Cenni, Luke Mansard, Catherine Blanchet, David Baux, Christel Vaché and Corinne Baudoin et al.
When Familial Hearing Loss Means Genetic Heterogeneity: A Model Case Report
Reprinted from: *Diagnostics* **2021**, *11*, 1636, doi:10.3390/diagnostics11091636 29

Nassim Boutouchent, Julie Bourilhon, Bénédicte Sudrié-Arnaud, Antoine Bonnevalle, Lucie Guyant-Maréchal and Cécile Acquaviva et al.
An Atypical Case of Head Tremor and Extensive White Matter in an Adult Female Caused by 3-Hydroxy-3-methylglutaryl-CoA Lyase Deficiency
Reprinted from: *Diagnostics* **2021**, *11*, 1561, doi:10.3390/diagnostics11091561 35

Agnieszka Lecka-Ambroziak, Marta Wysocka-Mincewicz, Katarzyna Doleżal-Ołtarzewska, Agata Zygmunt-Górska, Teresa Żak and Anna Noczyńska et al.
Correlation of Genotype and Perinatal Period, Time of Diagnosis and Anthropometric Data before Commencement of Recombinant Human Growth Hormone Treatment in Polish Patients with Prader–Willi Syndrome
Reprinted from: *Diagnostics* **2021**, *11*, 798, doi:10.3390/diagnostics11050798 41

Andrea Barp, Lorena Mosca and Valeria Ada Sansone
Facilitations and Hurdles of Genetic Testing in Neuromuscular Disorders
Reprinted from: *Diagnostics* **2021**, *11*, 701, doi:10.3390/diagnostics11040701 53

Bénédicte Sudrié-Arnaud, Sarah Snanoudj, Ivana Dabaj, Hélène Dranguet, Lenaig Abily-Donval and Axel Lebas et al.
Next-Generation Molecular Investigations in Lysosomal Diseases: Clinical Integration of a Comprehensive Targeted Panel
Reprinted from: *Diagnostics* **2021**, *11*, 294, doi:10.3390/diagnostics11020294 71

Deborah A. Sival, Martinica Garofalo, Rick Brandsma, Tom A. Bokkers, Marloes van den Berg and Tom J. de Koning et al.
Early Onset Ataxia with Comorbid Dystonia: Clinical, Anatomical and Biological Pathway Analysis Expose Shared Pathophysiology
Reprinted from: *Diagnostics* **2020**, *10*, 997, doi:10.3390/diagnostics10120997 81

Eu Gene Park, Eun-Jung Kim, Eun-Jee Kim, Hyun-Young Kim, Sun-Hee Kim and Aram Yang
Coexistence of Growth Hormone Deficiency and Pituitary Microadenoma in a Child with Unique Mosaic Turner Syndrome: A Case Report and Literature Review
Reprinted from: *Diagnostics* **2020**, *10*, 783, doi:10.3390/diagnostics10100783 . . . . **99**

Yasmin Tatour and Tamar Ben-Yosef
Syndromic Inherited Retinal Diseases: Genetic, Clinical and Diagnostic Aspects
Reprinted from: *Diagnostics* **2020**, *10*, 779, doi:10.3390/diagnostics10100779 . . . . **107**

Sara Álvaro-Sánchez, Irene Abreu-Rodríguez, Anna Abulí, Clara Serra-Juhé and Maria del Carmen Garrido-Navas
Current Status of Genetic Counselling for Rare Diseases in Spain
Reprinted from: *Diagnostics* **2021**, *11*, 2320, doi:10.3390/diagnostics11122320 . . . . **123**

Preface to "Genetic Testing for Rare Diseases"

Rare diseases, or orphan diseases, are those that individually affect a small number of patients, but taken together, affect over 300 million people worldwide. They are characterized by their etiological, diagnostic and evolutionary complexity, and important morbi-mortality, with high levels of disability that entail and hinder the development of a normal vital project, not only in those who suffers them, but also their families; therefore, a comprehensive social health approach is necessary to address this problem.

It is estimated that there are currently between 6000 and 8000 different rare diseases, affecting between 6% and 8% of the global population at some point of their life. These are people who need multiple social and health resources, which require a variety of healthcare and health care settings and medical specialties.

It is estimated that 80% of rare diseases are genetic. Thus, genetic testing is mandatory for the confirmation of clinical diagnostics and ensuring correct genetic counseling.

In this Special Issue, we present several examples of the complexity of genetic diagnosis for most of these diseases and the consequences that genetic testing implies for genetic counseling.

José Millán
Editor

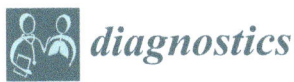

Editorial

Genetic Testing for Rare Diseases

José M. Millán [1,2,*] and Gema García-García [1,2]

1. Instituto de Investigación Sanitaria La Fe, Molecular, Cellular and Genomics Biomedicine, 46026 Valencia, Spain; gema.gegargar@gmail.com
2. Centro de Investigación Biomédica en Red de Enfermedades Raras (CIBERER), 28029 Madrid, Spain
* Correspondence: millan_jos@gva.es

The term rare disease was coined in the 1970s to refer to diseases that have a low prevalence. However, the definition varies among countries. The European Commission defines a rare disease as a disease that affects less than 5 in 10,000 people. In the US, a global number of cases is used (less than 200,000 cases for the entire country) [1]. Other countries use a more restrictive definition, such as less than 4 cases per 10,000 in Japan or even less than 2 cases per 10,000 in other countries [2].

Beyond the prevalence, the definition of a rare disease must include other issues, such as chronic and severe disorders that usually have an early onset but can begin in adulthood; diseases that can affect every organ or even different organs; diseases that are not well-understood and lack information about them; diseases that do not have a treatment or only a treatment that is not very effective.

It is estimated that there are 6000–8000 diseases included in this denomination [1]. They are tremendously heterogeneous, and about 80% are genetic (often monogenic) [3].

Even though a single rare disease affects only a few patients, the high number of rare diseases means they affect about 3.5–6% of all people globally, which is between 263 and 446 million people [4].

In summary, the definition of the term rare disease, besides the prevalence, must see them as a wide and varied group of disorders that each affect a small number of persons, which are chronic and disabling and have a high rate of morbi-mortality, with scarce and limited therapeutical resources [5].

The absence of a diagnosis (or perhaps a correct diagnosis) can have serious consequences for the patients and their relatives. Additionally, the heterogeneity of national capabilities regarding genetic testing (and changing technologies for such testing) may impact the access to diagnosis. The diagnosis of some rare diseases may delay even five years.

Delays in the diagnosis may cause further aggravation of the disease, inadequate treatments, lack of treatments or support, and the possibility of recurrence in the family as most rare diseases are genetic and the absence of diagnosis has prevented successful genetic counseling [6].

In this sense, the International Rare Diseases Research Consortium, IRDiRC, has marked as a key objective to improve the time of diagnosis and the accessibility to it. A new general vision was adopted for the period 2017–2027: "To make it possible for all people suffering from a rare disease to receive an accurate diagnosis, care and available therapy within one year of seeking medical assistance." [7].

To turn this vision into a reality, three new goals were agreed upon:

Goal 1: All patients coming to medical attention with a suspected rare disease will be diagnosed within one year if their disorder is known in the medical literature; all currently undiagnosable individuals will enter a globally coordinated diagnostic and research pipeline;

Goal 2: A total of 1000 new therapies for rare diseases will be approved, the majority of which will focus on diseases without approved options;

Citation: Millán, J.M.; García-García, G. Genetic Testing for Rare Diseases. *Diagnostics* **2022**, *12*, 809. https://doi.org/10.3390/diagnostics12040809

Received: 15 March 2022
Accepted: 23 March 2022
Published: 25 March 2022

Publisher's Note: MDPI stays neutral with regard to jurisdictional claims in published maps and institutional affiliations.

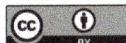

Copyright: © 2022 by the authors. Licensee MDPI, Basel, Switzerland. This article is an open access article distributed under the terms and conditions of the Creative Commons Attribution (CC BY) license (https://creativecommons.org/licenses/by/4.0/).

Goal 3: Methodologies will be developed to assess the impact of diagnoses and therapies on rare disease patients.

An increment of medical products for rare diseases based on gene therapy can be foreseen. Spinal muscular atrophy is a good example of how gene therapy can change the nature of a devastating disease. The good prognosis of SMA with early administration of the available medical products recently approved by the FDA and EMA has boosted the implementation of SMA newborn screening in several countries [8,9].

However, there are other examples of gene-based therapeutical approaches approved by medical agencies or in clinical trials.

All the information mentioned above makes the (as earlier as possible) genetic diagnoses of rare diseases essential to apply these therapies to the right patients.

In this Special Issue, there are several interesting examples of genetic diagnosis of rare diseases that affect different organs and tissues.

Boutouchent et al. [10] describe a case report of an atypical late-onset patient with 3-Hydroxy-3-methylglutaryl-CoA Lyase Deficiency (HMGLD). A 54-year-old female was suspicious of HMGLD, although this disease usually has its onset in the first few months of life. They sequenced the HMGCL gene and found two variants, one of them previously described as pathogenic and the other one was not reported before but was predicted to skip the exon 1. These variants would explain the disease. The late onset of the disease, in this case, led to it being undiagnosed for years, and the integrative interpretation of imaging, biochemical, and molecular findings enabled the authors to reach the diagnosis of this treatable condition.

The genetic diagnosis allows correct genetic counseling. This is key for patients to plan their professional lives and to choose among the different reproductive options. Álvaro-Sánchez et al. [11] evaluate the current situation in which rare disease patients receive genetic services in Spain. The Spanish laws state that genetic counselling is mandatory before and after the genetic test, but, surprisingly, there is a lack of recognition in Spain of Clinical Genetics as a healthcare specialty). They provide a comprehensive review of the number of centers (public and private) and their distribution among the different regions. They conclude that the lack of specialty makes it difficult to implement genetic counselling in Spain and that the Clinical Genetics specialty urgently needs to be recognized to provide a multidisciplinary service to patients with rare diseases.

Danilchenko et al. [12] reported the prevalence of SLC26A4 among patients with hearing impairment in two different South Siberian populations: Tuvinians and Altaians. With this and a previous study, they were able to uncover the genetic causes of hearing loss in 50.5% and 34.5% of Tuvinian and Altaian patients, respectively, expanding the landscape of the genetics underlying the hearing loss in two understudied populations.

An additional case report concerning hearing loss is reported by Cenni et al. [13]. They report a large family in which thrombocytopenia, post-lingual hearing loss, and congenital hearing loss coexist. After a hearing loss panel sequencing and whole-exome sequencing, they found a pathogenic variant in MHY9 that explains the thrombocytopenia, a mutation in MYO7A that explains the post-lingual hearing loss and a de novo mutation in a child responsible for the congenital hearing loss. This family illustrates not only the issue of the coexistence of several rare diseases in a single family but also the presence of several mutated genes for a single medical condition (in this case, hearing loss) genetically heterogeneous.

Sival et al. [14] conducted a comprehensive multidisciplinary study on 80 patients with Early adult Onset Ataxia (EOA) with and without dystonic comorbidity. They found that comorbid dystonia is present in the majority of the EOA patients. They found mutations in genes involved in pathways, such as energy depletion and signal transduction in the cortical–basal–ganglia–pontine–cerebellar network.

Another manuscript about the genetics in hearing impairment in this Special Issue is the one by Mansard et al. [15]. Their study of two unrelated families with autosomal dominant non-syndromic hearing loss identified for the first time one copy number variant in the exon 8 of the *GSDME* gene in each family. They remark the importance of a comprehensive analysis of copy number variants for genetic diagnosis.

Barp et al. [16] conducted a review about the complexity of the molecular diagnosis of neuromuscular disorders, including gene panels sequencing, whole-exome sequencing, and whole-genome sequencing. They highlight the importance of clinical diagnoses in order to target the appropriate technique and candidate genes according to the suspected clinical entity and the challenge that supposes the pathogenic nature of a high number of variants of unknown significance that are found with the use of next-generation sequencing.

Lecka-Ambroziak et al. [17] reported a genotype–phenotype correlation in a cohort of 147 Polish patients with Prader-Willi syndrome, stratifying them according to the genetic defect that causes the disease and the importance of the time of diagnosis before the commencement of the recombinant human growth hormone treatment.

Park and colleagues [18] report a case of a 13-year-old female with mosaic Turner syndrome and complete growth hormone deficiency and pituitary microadenoma. They also make an excellent review of the literature and compare all the cases of Turner syndrome and growth hormone deficiency and of Turner syndrome and pituitary microadenoma reported to date.

Sudrié-Arnaud et al. [19] designed a custom gene panel sequencing including 51 genes responsible for lysosomal disorders and validated it in 21 well-characterized patients. The bioinformatic pipelines used were also validated to detect single nucleotide variants, copy number variants and indels. Furthermore, they validated the panel in five new cases.

Finally, Tatur and Ben-Yosef [20] review the clinical entities and genetics of over 80 syndromic inherited retinal dystrophies, highlighting the percentage of organs/tissues involved in these syndromes apart of the retina.

In summary, this Special Issue shows a wide variety of rare diseases and the great advances that next-generation sequencing has supposed genetically diagnosing them.

Author Contributions: Conception and design, J.M.M. and G.G.-G.; writing: J.M.M. and G.G.-G. All authors have read and agreed to the published version of the manuscript.

Funding: This research received no external funding.

Conflicts of Interest: The authors declare conflict of interest for this article.

References

1. Tong, N. Priority Diseases and Reasons for Inclusion. In *Priority Medicines for Europe and the World 2013 Update*; World Health Organization: Geneva, Switzerland, 2013.
2. Hayashi, S.; Umeda, T. 35 years of Japanese policy on rare diseases. *Lancet* **2008**, *372*, 889–890. [CrossRef]
3. Klimova, B.; Storek, M.; Valis, M.; Kuca, K. Global View on Rare Diseases: A Mini Review. *Curr. Med. Chem.* **2017**, *24*, 3153–3158. [CrossRef] [PubMed]
4. Nguengang Wakap, S.; Lambert, D.M.; Olry, A.; Rodwell, C.; Gueydan, C.; Lanneau, V.; Murphy, D.; Le Cam, Y.; Rath, A. Estimating cumulative point prevalence of rare diseases: Analysis of the Orphanet database. *Eur. J. Human Genet.* **2020**, *28*, 165–173. [CrossRef] [PubMed]
5. Danese, E.; Lippi, G. Rare diseases: The paradox of an emerging challenge. *Ann. Trans. Med.* **2018**, *6*, 329. [CrossRef] [PubMed]
6. De Vries, E.; Fransen, L.; van den Aker, M.; Meijboom, B.R. Preventing gatekeeping delays in the diagnosis of rare diseases. *Br. J. Gen. Pract.* **2018**, *68*, 145–146. [CrossRef] [PubMed]
7. International Rare Diseases Research Consortium. Available online: https://irdirc.org (accessed on 14 March 2022).
8. Amaral, M.D. Precision medicine for rare diseases: The times they are A-Changin'. *Curr. Opin. Pharmacol.* **2022**, *63*, 102201. [CrossRef] [PubMed]
9. Jablonka, S.; Hennlein, L.; Sendtner, M. Therapy development for spinal muscular atrophy: Perspectives for muscular dystrophies and neurodegenerative disorders. *Neurol. Res. Pract.* **2022**, *4*, 2. [CrossRef] [PubMed]
10. Boutouchent, N.; Bourilhon, J.; Sudrié-Arnaud, B.; Bonnevalle, A.; Guyant-Maréchal, L.; Acquaviva, C.; Dujardin-Ippolito, L.; Bekri, S.; Dabaj, I.; Tebani, A. An Atypical Case of Head Tremor and Extensive White Matter in an Adult Female Caused by 3-Hydroxy-3-methylglutaryl-CoA Lyase Deficiency. *Diagnostics* **2021**, *11*, 1561. [CrossRef] [PubMed]
11. Álvaro-Sánchez, S.; Abreu-Rodríguez, I.; Abulí, A.; Clara Serra-Juhe, C.; Garrido-Navas, M.C. Current Status of Genetic Counselling for Rare Diseases in Spain. *Diagnostics* **2021**, *11*, 2320. [CrossRef]

12. Danilchenko, V.Y.; Zytsar, M.V.; Maslova, E.A.; Bady-Khoo, M.S.; Barashkov, N.A.; Morozov, I.V.; Bondar, A.A.; Posukh, O.L. Different Rates of the SLC26A4-Related Hearing Loss in Two Indigenous Peoples of Southern Siberia (Russia). *Diagnostics* 2021, *11*, 2378. [CrossRef] [PubMed]
13. Cenni, C.; Mansard, L.; Blanchet, C.; Baux, D.; Vaché, C.; Baudoin, C.; Moclyn, M.; Faugère, V.; Mondain, M.; Jeziorski, E.; et al. When Familial Hearing Loss Means Genetic Heterogeneity: A Model Case Report. *Diagnostics* 2021, *11*, 1636. [CrossRef] [PubMed]
14. Sival, D.A.; Garofalo, M.; Brandsma, R.; Bokkers, T.A.; van den Berg, M.; de Koning, T.J.; Tijssen, M.A.J.; Verbeek, D.S. Early Onset Ataxia with Comorbid Dystonia: Clinical, Anatomical and Biological Pathway Analysis Expose Shared Pathophysiology. *Diagnostics* 2020, *10*, 997. [CrossRef] [PubMed]
15. Mansard, L.; Vaché, C.; Bianchi, J.; Baudoin, C.; Perthus, I.; Isidor, B.; Blanchet, C.; Baux, D.; Koenig, M.; Kalatzis, V.; et al. Identification of the First Single GSDME Exon 8 Structural Variants Associated with Autosomal Dominant Hearing Loss. *Diagnostics* 2022, *12*, 207. [CrossRef] [PubMed]
16. Barp, A.; Mosca, L.; Sansone, V.A. Facilitations and Hurdles of Genetic Testing in Neuromuscular Disorders. *Diagnostics* 2021, *11*, 701. [CrossRef] [PubMed]
17. Lecka-Ambroziak, A.; Wysocka-Mincewicz, M.; Katarzyna Doleżal-Ołtarzewska, K.; Zygmunt-Górska, A.; Żak, T.; Noczyńska, A.; Birkholz-Walerzak, D.; Stawerska, R.; Hilczer, M.; Obara-Moszyńska, M.; et al. The Polish Coordination Group for rhGH Treatment. Correlation of Genotype and Perinatal Period, Time of Diagnosis and Anthropometric Data before Commencement of Recombinant Human Growth Hormone Treatment in Polish Patients with Prader–Willi Syndrome. *Diagnostics* 2021, *11*, 798. [CrossRef] [PubMed]
18. Park, E.G.; Kim, E.J.; Kim, E.J.; Kim, H.J.; Sun-Hee Kim, S.H.; Yang, A. Coexistence of Growth Hormone Deficiency and Pituitary Microadenoma in a Child with Unique Mosaic Turner Syndrome: A Case Report and Literature Review. *Diagnostics* 2020, *10*, 783. [CrossRef] [PubMed]
19. Sudrié-Arnaud, B.; Snanoudj, S.; Dabaj, I.; Dranguet, H.; Abily-Donval, L.; Lebas, A.; Vezain, M.; Héron, B.; Marie, I.; Marc Duval-Arnould, M.; et al. Next-Generation Molecular Investigations in Lysosomal Diseases: Clinical Integration of a Comprehensive Targeted Panel. *Diagnostics* 2021, *11*, 294. [CrossRef] [PubMed]
20. Tatour, Y.; Ben-Yosef, T. Syndromic Inherited Retinal Diseases: Genetic, Clinical and Diagnostic Aspects. *Diagnostics* 2020, *10*, 779. [CrossRef] [PubMed]

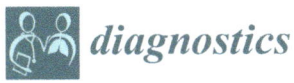

Case Report

Identification of the First Single *GSDME* Exon 8 Structural Variants Associated with Autosomal Dominant Hearing Loss

Luke Mansard [1], Christel Vaché [1,2,*], Julie Bianchi [1], Corinne Baudoin [1], Isabelle Perthus [3], Bertrand Isidor [4], Catherine Blanchet [5], David Baux [1,2], Michel Koenig [1], Vasiliki Kalatzis [2] and Anne-Françoise Roux [1,2]

1. Molecular Genetics Laboratory, Univ Montpellier, CHU Montpellier, 34000 Montpellier, France; l-mansard@chu-montpellier.fr (L.M.); j-bianchi@chu-montpellier.fr (J.B.); corinne.baudoin@inserm.fr (C.B.); david.baux@inserm.fr (D.B.); michel.koenig@inserm.fr (M.K.); anne-francoise.roux@inserm.fr (A.-F.R.)
2. Institute for Neurosciences of Montpellier (INM), Univ Montpellier, Inserm, 34000 Montpellier, France; vasiliki.kalatzis@inserm.fr
3. Department of Clinical Genetics, Reference Center for Rare Diseases, University Hospital of Clermont-Ferrand, 63000 Clermont-Ferrand, France; iperthus@chu-clermontferrand.fr
4. Department of Medical Genetics, CHU Nantes, 44000 Nantes, France; Bertrand.ISIDOR@chu-nantes.fr
5. National Reference Centre for Inherited Sensory Diseases, Otolaryngology Department, Univ Montpellier, CHU Montpellier, 34000 Montpellier, France; c-blanchet@chu-montpellier.fr
* Correspondence: christel.vache@inserm.fr

Abstract: *GSDME*, also known as *DFNA5*, is a gene implicated in autosomal dominant nonsyndromic hearing loss (ADNSHL), affecting, at first, the high frequencies with a subsequent progression over all frequencies. To date, all the *GSDME* pathogenic variants associated with deafness lead to skipping of exon 8. In two families with apparent ADNSHL, massively parallel sequencing (MPS) integrating a coverage-based method for detection of copy number variations (CNVs) was applied, and it identified the first two causal *GSDME* structural variants affecting exon 8. The deleterious impact of the c.991-60_1095del variant, which includes the acceptor splice site sequence of exon 8, was confirmed by the study of the proband's transcripts. The second mutational event is a complex rearrangement that deletes almost all of the exon 8 sequence. This study increases the mutational spectrum of the *GSDME* gene and highlights the crucial importance of MPS data for the detection of *GSDME* exon 8 deletions, even though the identification of a causal single-exon CNV by MPS analysis is still challenging.

Keywords: *GSDME*; *DFNA5*; hearing loss; single-exon CNV

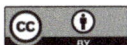

1. Introduction

The Gasdermin E gene (*GSDME*), also called deafness autosomal dominant 5 (*DFNA5*), located on chromosome 7p15, contains 10 exons and encodes the 496-amino acid Gasdermin-E protein. This protein, which is a member of the Gasdermin superfamily, displays a necrotic-inducing N-terminal domain (GSDME-N, amino acids 1 to 270) self-inhibited by a C-terminal domain (GSDME-C, amino acids 271 to 496) [1]. When the connection between these two domains is cleaved by the apoptotic protease caspase-3 or the killer cell granzyme B (GzmB), the released GSDME-N chain participates in the cell death pathway by forming pores in the plasma and mitochondrial membranes [2,3].

GSDME is considered as a potential tumor suppressor gene (for review, see [4]), and downregulation or suppression of its necrotic function has been observed in several cancers [3]. Gain-of-function pathogenic variants in *GSDME* have also been reported, but they all lead to exon 8 skipping at the mRNA level and result in autosomal, dominant, progressive, sensorineural and nonsyndromic DFNA5 hearing loss (OMIM #600994). These variations are located in the flanking sequences of exon 8 or within the exon itself. They alter the splice consensus sequences [5–12], impact the polypyrimidine tract [13] or disturb regulatory elements [10,14]. This out-of-frame exon 8 skipping results in the production of a C-terminally truncated, constitutively active necrotic protein (Figure A1).

In this article, we describe the molecular analysis of two unrelated families suffering from progressive nonsyndromic hearing loss with an apparent dominant inheritance, and the identification of two copy number variations (CNVs) affecting the single *GSDME* exon 8 as the causal variants.

2. Materials and Methods

2.1. Clinical Report of the Families

2.1.1. Family S2426

Family S2426 was a large French family with five generations, including sixteen members affected by nonsyndromic hearing loss (NSHL) with a dominant pattern of inheritance (Figure 1A). Family history reported post-lingual bilateral progressive hearing loss with an assumed onset in the first or second decade of life in all affected individuals. Superimposed audiograms (pure-tone audiometry at 250, 500, 1000, 2000 and 4000 Hz) from eight of the affected members (III:4, III:5, III:6, III:7, III:8, IV:6, V:1 and V:2) performed at different ages (59, 51, 31, 49, 51, 19, 4 and 9 years, respectively) confirmed progressive moderate to profound hearing loss that initially affected the high frequencies (downward-sloping curve) and then progressed across all frequencies (Figure 1B). The proband referred for molecular testing was a 55-year-old woman (IV:4) suffering from progressive hearing loss detected when she was 6 years old. Clinical examination of all available affected individuals of this family was otherwise unremarkable.

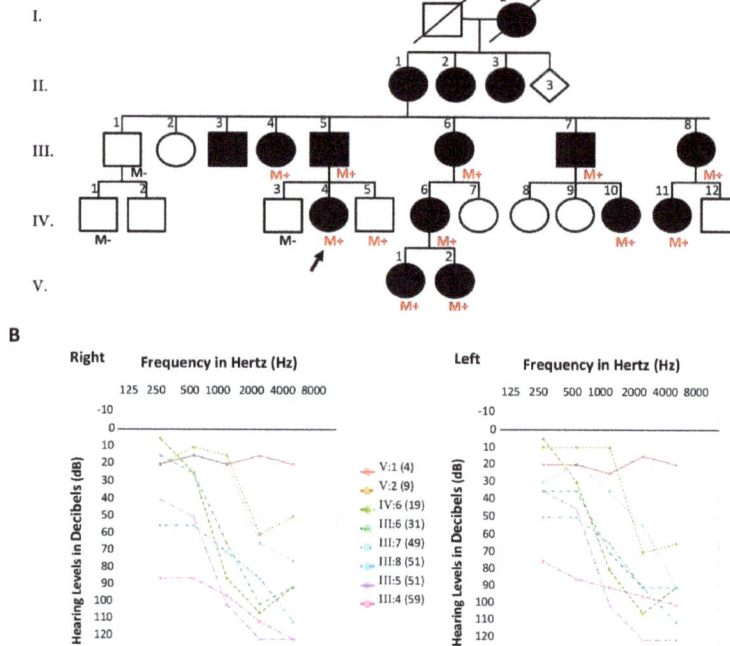

Figure 1. Family S2426. (**A**) Pedigree of the family. Filled symbols denote affected individuals. The proband referred for molecular testing is indicated by a black arrow. M+ (red font): presence of the *GSDME* deletion, M− (black font): absence of the *GSDME* deletion. (**B**) Superimposed pure-tone audiograms of eight affected individuals. The numbers in parentheses indicate the subject's age at the audiometric testing. Left chart: right ear, right chart: left ear.

2.1.2. Family S2106

Based on information obtained from the proband II:3, his family was composed of at least two generations including more than ten members presenting with NSHL. A likely autosomal dominant inheritance pattern of the disease was suspected (Figure 2A), although no precise clinical data on other affected members could be obtained. The hearing impairment of the proband (II:3) was diagnosed when he was 6 years old, and physical examination did not find any evidence of a syndromic disease. His deafness was progressive, and available data from an audiometric assessment at the age of 30 years old (Figure 2B) identified bilateral asymmetrical hearing loss with downward-sloping curves. These audiograms revealed pure-tone averages (PTAs) of 57.5 db HL and 72.5 db HL for the right and left ears, respectively. Due to substantial PTA differences across the right and left ears, and in accordance with the 02/1bis recommendation of the International Bureau for Audiophonology (BIAP; https://www.biap.org/ (accessed on 8 December 2021)), a PTA of 62 db HL was retained, corresponding to moderate group 2 hearing loss.

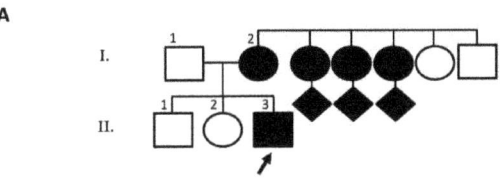

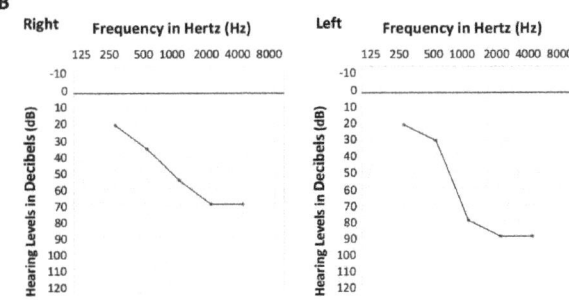

Figure 2. Family S2106. (**A**) Pedigree of the family. Filled symbols denote affected individuals. The proband referred for molecular testing is indicated by a black arrow. (**B**) Pure-tone audiogram of the patient at the age of 30 years old. Left chart: right ear, right chart: left ear.

2.2. DNA Analysis

Genomic DNA from the 15 participating family members from family S2426 and the proband from family S2106 was isolated from peripheral blood samples using standard procedures. The DNA of the two probands was analyzed by massively parallel sequencing (MPS) using a hearing loss gene panel on an Illumina MiniSeq sequencer (Illumina, San Diego, CA, USA). The screened genes and the complete workflow used to identify pathogenic alterations have already been described [15]. This molecular diagnosis strategy included a copy number estimation of each region by a depth of coverage- based method using the MobiCNV algorithm (https://github.com/mobidic/MobiCNV (accessed on 23 November 2021)), which was completed by a direct visualization of the sequenced reads with the open source Integrative Genomics Viewer (IGV) software (v2.7.2) [16].

Validation and familial segregation (when possible) of the *GSDME* variations were conducted by PCR-Sanger sequencing using the BigDye Terminator v3.1 cycle sequencing kit (Applied Biosystems, Courtaboeuf, France) on an Applied Biosytems® 3500Dx Genetic Analyzer (Applied Biosystems). PCRs were performed with the forward primer 5′-GAGGAATTTCCATCCATTTGC-3′ combined with the reverse primer 5′-CACAGTGTGGG

AATGATCTGG-3' for S2426, and the forward primer 5'-CCCGTCAGTGAAATGTAGCC-3' paired with the reverse primer 5'-CTCTGTGTCCCCAGAAGCA-3' for S2106.

2.3. RNA Analysis

The functional consequence of the *GSDME* variant identified in family S2426 was investigated by RNA analysis. Total RNA was isolated from whole blood collected in PAXgeneTM Blood RNA Tubes using the Nucleo Spin® RNA II isolation kit (Macherey-Nagel, Düren, Germany). Reverse transcription was performed using the SuperScriptTM III Reverse Transcriptase (Invitrogen, Carlsbad, CA, USA) and oligo (dT) primers, according to the manufacturer's instructions. PCRs were then carried out with *GSDME*-specific primers (forward: 5'-CACAGTGTGGGAATGATCTGG-3', reverse: 5'-TTCAGGGGAGTCAAGGTTGG-3'), and amplicons were Sanger sequenced.

2.4. Variant Description

The nomenclature of the variants follows the Human Genome Variation Society (HGVS) recommendations v20.05 (http://varnomen.hgvs.org/ (accessed on 23 November 2021)) [17], with nucleotide +1 corresponding to the A of the ATG initiation codon in the *GSDME* reference sequence NM_004403.2; NG_011593.1. The two *GSDME* variants have been added to the Leiden Open Variation Database Global Variome Shared Instance (LOVD GVShared, https://databases.lovd.nl/shared/variants/DFNA5 (accessed on 17 December 2021)) and classified in accordance with the adapted ACMG/AMP guidelines for variant interpretation in the context of hearing loss [18].

Several DNA variation databases, including the Human Gene Mutation Database (HGMD® Professional 2020.3; https://portal.biobase-international.com), the Genome Aggregation Database (gnomAD) (https://gnomad.broadinstitute.org/), the Single Nucleotide Polymorphism Database (dbSNP) (https://www.ncbi.nlm.nih.gov/snp/), the Clinical Variation Database (ClinVar) (https://www.ncbi.nlm.nih.gov/clinvar/), the Deafness Variation Database (DVD) (https://deafnessvariationdatabase.org/) and the LOVD GVShared, were accessed on 8 December 2021.

3. Results

3.1. Family S2426

Analyses of the MPS data obtained from proband IV:4, using the MobiCNV algorithm, pointed out a depth of coverage decrease in the *GSDME* gene compatible with a potential exon 8 deletion in the heterozygous state. Visualization of the sequenced reads with the IGV tool confirmed this CNV and identified the breakpoints of the deletion (Figure 3A). The presence of this c.991-60_1095del variant was validated by Sanger sequencing in the proband's DNA (Figure 3B), and flanking microhomologies of 2 bp were observed (Figure 3C).

However, as the deletion encompassed the splice acceptor consensus sequence of the exon, complementary RNA analysis was conducted to investigate its effect on splicing. The amplification of exons 7 to 10 of control cDNA led to the production of a 441 bp fragment. By contrast, the amplification of the patient's cDNA identified an additional and predominant 248 bp fragment, supporting a splice defect (Figure 4A). Sanger sequencing of the RT-PCR products confirmed the presence of transcripts lacking the 193 bp of the *GSDME* exon 8 (r.991_1183del) in the patient (Figure 4B).

Familial segregation of the deletion was performed on available members of the family. All tested members with bilateral progressive NSHL ($n = 10$) were heterozygous carriers of the deletion c.991-60_1095del (Figure 1A). A 13-year-old boy (IV:5), who had normal hearing to date, was also a carrier. The deletion was not detected in three additional members who had normal audition (III:1, IV:1 and IV:3).

This variant was absent from all the interrogated databases. In accordance with the ACMG/AMP hearing loss guidelines, it was considered as a class V pathogenic variant.

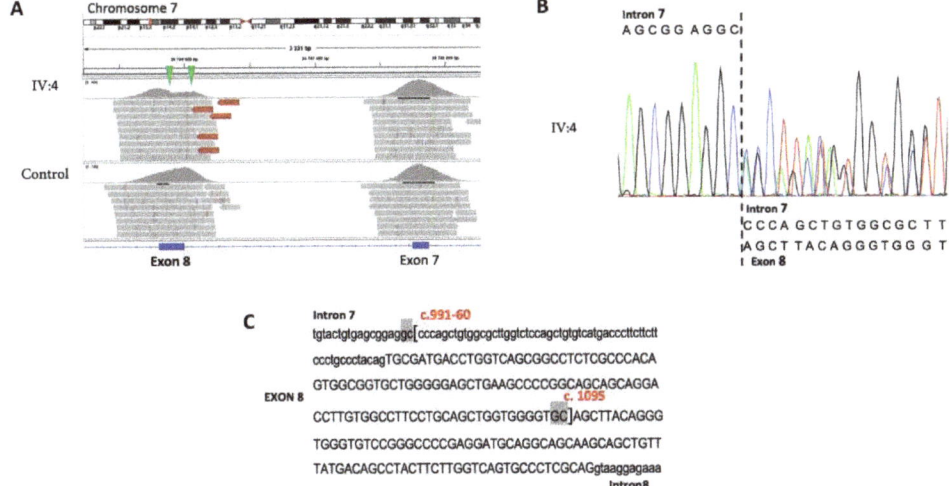

Figure 3. Identification and validation of the *GSDME* deletion in the proband IV:4. (**A**) Integrative genomics viewer screenshot focused on the *GSDME* exons 8 and 9. The sequence reads from the proband and a control are shown. Green arrowheads indicate the position of the deletion. (**B**) Sequence chromatogram of the c.991-60_1095del variant. (**C**) Sequence context of the deletion. The brackets indicate the 5′ and 3′ breakpoints of the deletion. The 2 bp flanking microhomologies are highlighted in gray.

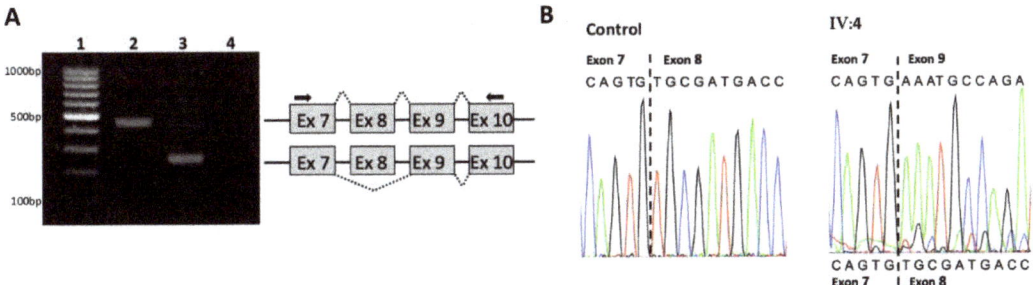

Figure 4. (**A**) RNA analysis of the c.991-60_1095del variant. (**A**) Agarose gel electrophoresis of the RT-PCR products from a control (lane 2) and the proband IV:4 (line 3). Lane 1: molecular weight markers, lane 4: control PCR reaction without template. A schematic representation of the spliced products is included. The position of the primers used for the amplification is shown by arrows. (**B**) Sanger sequencing electropherograms of the RT-PCR products for the control and the patient.

3.2. Family S2106

Molecular analysis of the proband II:3 by MPS identified the well-known class IV c.101T > C; p.(Met34Thr) *GJB2* variant and a single *GSDME* exon 8 deletion, both in the heterozygous state. Visual inspection of the reads, using the IGV tool, showed that the deletion breakpoints were not located in the 600 bp of the *GSDME* exon 8 target region. In order to validate this CNV and define its boundaries, a *GSDME* exon 7–exon 9 PCR was performed on the patient's DNA. The PCR conditions employed in this study allowed a specific amplification of the mutated allele, and Sanger sequencing revealed a complex rearrangement (Figure 5).

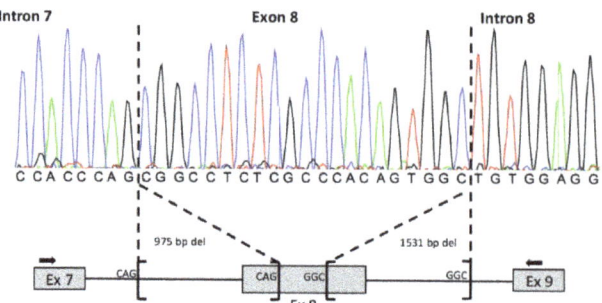

Figure 5. Sanger validation of the *GSDME* exon 8 deletion in the proband II:3. At the top: sequence chromatogram focused on the breakpoints of the deletions. At the bottom: schematic representation of the complex rearrangement. The position of the primers used for the amplification is shown by arrows. The 3 bp flanking microhomologies are indicated.

This structural variant was composed of two deletions of 975 and 1531 bp, leading to the loss of the 17 first and 155 last bps of exon 8, respectively. Flanking microhomologies of 3 bp were detected for each deletion (Figure 5). According to the HGVS recommendations, this mutational event was described as c.[990+793_1007del; 1029_1183+1376del]. It was not reported in all the consulted databases and was classified as a class V pathogenic variant in accordance with the ACMG/AMP hearing loss guidelines.

4. Discussion and Conclusions

We described the molecular diagnostic investigations of two unrelated families suffering from hearing loss, which led to the identification of two pathogenic *GSDME* CNVs. Except for the proband II:3 of family S2106, who presented asymmetrical audiograms, all affected individuals exhibited a typical DFNA5 phenotype with post-lingual, bilateral, symmetric, predominantly high-frequency hearing loss. Asymmetrical hearing loss has previously been described in a DFNA5 patient [19], but there was no explanation for this atypical phenotype. Patient IV:5 of family S2426 was a 13-year-old boy carrying the familial *GSDME* deletion without any sign of hearing loss. As the onset of DFNA5-related hearing loss has been shown to occur between 0 and 50 years of life [5,13], an audiometric follow-up will be offered to this patient. In addition, as already described [11], intrafamilial variability in the age of onset can be noted. As an example, patient IV:5 is asymptomatic at the age of 13 years, whereas V:2 displayed HL in the high frequencies at the age of 9 years.

In the context of molecular genetic testing, gene panel sequencing using MPS is a powerful strategy to identify causal variants, including single-nucleotide variants, insertions, deletions or CNVs in patients referred for NSHL [20–22]. Custom computational tools have been successfully used to detect CNVs in hearing gene panels [15,21,23], but detection of true single-exon or partial exon deletions is still challenging. Due to a notable false positive rate, these single-exon CNVs are often not considered in routine MPS data analysis. Here, we identified two pathogenic single *GSDME* exon 8 CNVs, highlighting the crucial importance of carefully checking the read depth of this specific exon.

Deletions correspond to the second largest class of pathogenic variants recorded in the ClinVar database [24]. Furthermore, approximately 57% of them are flanked by microhomologies [25] that are hallmarks of the microhomology-mediated end joining (MMEJ) repair mechanism involved in re-ligation of DNA ends caused by double-strand breaks. In this study, the two described *GSDME* mutational events were also deletions flanked by microhomologies of 2 or 3 bp, demonstrating the implication of the MMEJ pathway.

As *GSDME* transcripts are expressed in whole blood, functional analysis was performed on the cDNA of proband IV:4 of the S2426 family in order to characterize the splice defect generated by the c.991-60_1095del variant. As expected, this deletion, in accordance with all previously described DFNA5-related pathogenic variations, led to exon 8 skipping and resulted in the translation of a truncated necrotic protein due to the loss of its GSDME-C domain.

In conclusion, we report here the two first single *GSDME* exon 8 CNVs implicated in DFNA5. These findings enrich the mutational spectrum of this gene and pinpoint the importance of accurate exploration of single-exon CNVs in a diagnostic service.

Author Contributions: Conceptualization, A.-F.R.; software, D.B.; formal analysis, J.B., C.B. (Corinne Baudoin) and C.V.; clinical investigation, I.P. and B.I.; resources, C.B. (Catherine Blanchet); data curation, A.-F.R. and C.V.; writing—original draft preparation, L.M. and C.V.; writing—review and editing, A.-F.R., V.K., C.B. (Catherine Blanchet) and M.K.; supervision, A.-F.R. All authors have read and agreed to the published version of the manuscript.

Funding: This research received no external funding.

Institutional Review Board Statement: This study was conducted according to the guidelines of the Declaration of Helsinki and in accordance with the French law on bioethics: "loi de bioéthique", revised 7 July 2011, number 2011-814. The experimental protocol was approved by the Montpellier University Hospital (CHU Montpellier) as part of the molecular diagnostic activity. The authorization number given by the Agence Régionale de la Santé (ARS) is LR/2013-N°190.

Informed Consent Statement: Informed consent was obtained from all subjects involved in the study.

Data Availability Statement: All data are contained within the article. The variants, individuals and phenotypes described in this manuscript are available in the LOVD GVShared, Individual ID numbers #00396953 and #00396959.

Acknowledgments: The authors would like to acknowledge all participants involved in this study for their collaboration.

Conflicts of Interest: The authors declare no conflict of interest.

Appendix A

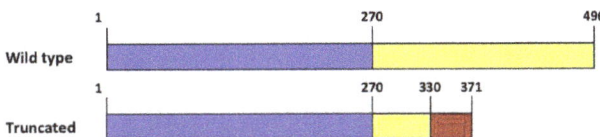

Figure A1. Schematic representation of the wild-type and truncated Gasdermin-E proteins. The necrotic N-terminal domain is represented in blue, and the C-terminal domain in yellow. The aberrant 41-amino acid tail of the truncated protein is represented in red.

References

1. Op de Beeck, K.; Van Camp, G.; Thys, S.; Cools, N.; Callebaut, I.; Vrijens, K.; Van Nassauw, L.; Van Tendeloo, V.F.I.; Timmermans, J.P.; Van Laer, L. The DFNA5 Gene, Responsible for Hearing Loss and Involved in Cancer, Encodes a Novel Apoptosis-Inducing Protein. *Eur. J. Hum. Genet.* **2011**, *19*, 965–973. [CrossRef] [PubMed]
2. Rogers, C.; Fernandes-Alnemri, T.; Mayes, L.; Alnemri, D.; Cingolani, G.; Alnemri, E.S. Cleavage of DFNA5 by Caspase-3 during Apoptosis Mediates Progression to Secondary Necrotic/Pyroptotic Cell Death. *Nat. Commun.* **2017**, *8*, 14128. [CrossRef] [PubMed]
3. Zhang, Z.; Zhang, Y.; Xia, S.; Kong, Q.; Li, S.; Liu, X.; Junqueira, C.; Meza-Sosa, K.F.; Mok, T.M.Y.; Ansara, J.; et al. Gasdermin E Suppresses Tumour Growth by Activating Anti-Tumour Immunity. *Nature* **2020**, *579*, 415–420. [CrossRef] [PubMed]
4. De Schutter, E.; Croes, L.; Ibrahim, J.; Pauwels, P.; Op de Beeck, K.; Vandenabeele, P.; Van Camp, G. GSDME and Its Role in Cancer: From behind the Scenes to the Front of the Stage. *Int. J. Cancer* **2021**, *148*, 2872–2883. [CrossRef] [PubMed]
5. Bischoff, A.M.L.C.; Luijendijk, M.W.J.; Huygen, P.L.M.; van Duijnhoven, G.; De Leenheer, E.M.R.; Oudesluijs, G.G.; Van Laer, L.; Cremers, F.P.M.; Cremers, C.W.R.J.; Kremer, H. A Novel Mutation Identified in the DFNA5 Gene in a Dutch Family: A Clinical and Genetic Evaluation. *Audiol. Neurootol.* **2004**, *9*, 34–46. [CrossRef] [PubMed]
6. Cheng, J.; Han, D.Y.; Dai, P.; Sun, H.J.; Tao, R.; Sun, Q.; Yan, D.; Qin, W.; Wang, H.Y.; Ouyang, X.M.; et al. A Novel DFNA5 Mutation, IVS8+4 A>G, in the Splice Donor Site of Intron 8 Causes Late-Onset Non-Syndromic Hearing Loss in a Chinese Family. *Clin. Genet.* **2007**, *72*, 471–477. [CrossRef]
7. Chai, Y.; Chen, D.; Wang, X.; Wu, H.; Yang, T. A Novel Splice Site Mutation in DFNA5 Causes Late-Onset Progressive Non-Syndromic Hearing Loss in a Chinese Family. *Int. J. Pediatr. Otorhinolaryngol.* **2014**, *78*, 1265–1268. [CrossRef]

8. Li-Yang, M.-N.; Shen, X.-F.; Wei, Q.-J.; Yao, J.; Lu, Y.-J.; Cao, X.; Xing, G.-Q. IVS8+1 DelG, a Novel Splice Site Mutation Causing DFNA5 Deafness in a Chinese Family. *Chin. Med. J. (Engl.)* **2015**, *128*, 2510–2515. [CrossRef]
9. Chen, S.; Dong, C.; Wang, Q.; Zhong, Z.; Qi, Y.; Ke, X.; Liu, Y. Targeted Next-Generation Sequencing Successfully Detects Causative Genes in Chinese Patients with Hereditary Hearing Loss. *Genet. Test. Mol. Biomark.* **2016**, *20*, 660–665. [CrossRef]
10. Booth, K.T.; Azaiez, H.; Kahrizi, K.; Wang, D.; Zhang, Y.; Frees, K.; Nishimura, C.; Najmabadi, H.; Smith, R.J. Exonic Mutations and Exon Skipping: Lessons Learned from DFNA5. *Hum. Mutat.* **2018**, *39*, 433–440. [CrossRef]
11. Wang, H.; Guan, J.; Guan, L.; Yang, J.; Wu, K.; Lin, Q.; Xiong, W.; Lan, L.; Zhao, C.; Xie, L.; et al. Further Evidence for "Gain-of-Function" Mechanism of DFNA5 Related Hearing Loss. *Sci. Rep.* **2018**, *8*, 8424. [CrossRef]
12. Yuan, Y.; Li, Q.; Su, Y.; Lin, Q.; Gao, X.; Liu, H.; Huang, S.; Kang, D.; Todd, N.W.; Mattox, D.; et al. Comprehensive Genetic Testing of Chinese SNHL Patients and Variants Interpretation Using ACMG Guidelines and Ethnically Matched Normal Controls. *Eur. J. Hum. Genet.* **2020**, *28*, 231–243. [CrossRef]
13. Yu, C.; Meng, X.; Zhang, S.; Zhao, G.; Hu, L.; Kong, X. A 3-Nucleotide Deletion in the Polypyrimidine Tract of Intron 7 of the DFNA5 Gene Causes Nonsyndromic Hearing Impairment in a Chinese Family. *Genomics* **2003**, *82*, 575–579. [CrossRef]
14. Van Laer, L.; Huizing, E.H.; Verstreken, M.; van Zuijlen, D.; Wauters, J.G.; Bossuyt, P.J.; Van de Heyning, P.; McGuirt, W.T.; Smith, R.J.; Willems, P.J.; et al. Nonsyndromic Hearing Impairment Is Associated with a Mutation in DFNA5. *Nat. Genet.* **1998**, *20*, 194–197. [CrossRef]
15. Baux, D.; Vaché, C.; Blanchet, C.; Willems, M.; Baudoin, C.; Moclyn, M.; Faugère, V.; Touraine, R.; Isidor, B.; Dupin-Deguine, D.; et al. Combined Genetic Approaches Yield a 48% Diagnostic Rate in a Large Cohort of French Hearing-Impaired Patients. *Sci. Rep.* **2017**, *7*, 16783. [CrossRef]
16. Thorvaldsdóttir, H.; Robinson, J.T.; Mesirov, J.P. Integrative Genomics Viewer (IGV): High-Performance Genomics Data Visualization and Exploration. *Brief. Bioinform.* **2013**, *14*, 178–192. [CrossRef]
17. den Dunnen, J.T.; Dalgleish, R.; Maglott, D.R.; Hart, R.K.; Greenblatt, M.S.; McGowan-Jordan, J.; Roux, A.-F.; Smith, T.; Antonarakis, S.E.; Taschner, P.E.M. HGVS Recommendations for the Description of Sequence Variants: 2016 Update. *Hum. Mutat.* **2016**, *37*, 564–569. [CrossRef] [PubMed]
18. Oza, A.M.; DiStefano, M.T.; Hemphill, S.E.; Cushman, B.J.; Grant, A.R.; Siegert, R.K.; Shen, J.; Chapin, A.; Boczek, N.J.; Schimmenti, L.A.; et al. Expert Specification of the ACMG/AMP Variant Interpretation Guidelines for Genetic Hearing Loss. *Hum. Mutat.* **2018**, *39*, 1593–1613. [CrossRef] [PubMed]
19. Park, H.J.; Cho, H.J.; Baek, J.I.; Ben-Yosef, T.; Kwon, T.J.; Griffith, A.J.; Kim, U.-K. Evidence for a Founder Mutation Causing DFNA5 Hearing Loss in East Asians. *J. Hum. Genet.* **2010**, *55*, 59–62. [CrossRef]
20. Cabanillas, R.; Diñeiro, M.; Cifuentes, G.A.; Castillo, D.; Pruneda, P.C.; Álvarez, R.; Sánchez-Durán, N.; Capín, R.; Plasencia, A.; Viejo-Díaz, M.; et al. Comprehensive Genomic Diagnosis of Non-Syndromic and Syndromic Hereditary Hearing Loss in Spanish Patients. *BMC Med. Genom.* **2018**, *11*, 58. [CrossRef] [PubMed]
21. Butz, M.; McDonald, A.; Lundquist, P.A.; Meyer, M.; Harrington, S.; Kester, S.; Stein, M.I.; Mistry, N.A.; Zimmerman Zuckerman, E.; Niu, Z.; et al. Development and Validation of a Next-Generation Sequencing Panel for Syndromic and Nonsyndromic Hearing Loss. *J. Appl. Lab. Med.* **2020**, *5*, 467–479. [CrossRef]
22. Abu Rayyan, A.; Kamal, L.; Casadei, S.; Brownstein, Z.; Zahdeh, F.; Shahin, H.; Canavati, C.; Dweik, D.; Jaraysa, T.; Rabie, G.; et al. Genomic Analysis of Inherited Hearing Loss in the Palestinian Population. *Proc. Natl. Acad. Sci. USA* **2020**, *117*, 20070–20076. [CrossRef] [PubMed]
23. Tropitzsch, A.; Schade-Mann, T.; Gamerdinger, P.; Dofek, S.; Schulte, B.; Schulze, M.; Battke, F.; Fehr, S.; Biskup, S.; Heyd, A.; et al. Diagnostic Yield of Targeted Hearing Loss Gene Panel Sequencing in a Large German Cohort With a Balanced Age Distribution from a Single Diagnostic Center: An Eight-Year Study. *Ear Hear.* **2021**. [CrossRef]
24. Rees, H.A.; Liu, D.R. Base Editing: Precision Chemistry on the Genome and Transcriptome of Living Cells. *Nat. Rev. Genet.* **2018**, *19*, 770–788. [CrossRef] [PubMed]
25. Grajcarek, J.; Monlong, J.; Nishinaka-Arai, Y.; Nakamura, M.; Nagai, M.; Matsuo, S.; Lougheed, D.; Sakurai, H.; Saito, M.K.; Bourque, G.; et al. Genome-Wide Microhomologies Enable Precise Template-Free Editing of Biologically Relevant Deletion Mutations. *Nat. Commun.* **2019**, *10*, 4856. [CrossRef] [PubMed]

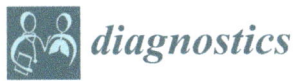

Article

Different Rates of the *SLC26A4*-Related Hearing Loss in Two Indigenous Peoples of Southern Siberia (Russia)

Valeriia Yu. Danilchenko [1,2], Marina V. Zytsar [1], Ekaterina A. Maslova [1,2], Marita S. Bady-Khoo [3], Nikolay A. Barashkov [4,5], Igor V. Morozov [2,6], Alexander A. Bondar [6] and Olga L. Posukh [1,2,*]

1. Federal Research Center Institute of Cytology and Genetics, Siberian Branch of the Russian Academy of Sciences, 630090 Novosibirsk, Russia; danilchenko_valeri@mail.ru (V.Y.D.); zytsar@bionet.nsc.ru (M.V.Z.); maslova@bionet.nsc.ru (E.A.M.)
2. Novosibirsk State University, 630090 Novosibirsk, Russia; Mor@niboch.nsc.ru
3. Perinatal Center of the Republic of Tyva, 667000 Kyzyl, Russia; marita.badyhoo@mail.ru
4. Yakut Scientific Centre of Complex Medical Problems, 677019 Yakutsk, Russia; barashkov2004@mail.ru
5. M.K. Ammosov North-Eastern Federal University, 677027 Yakutsk, Russia
6. Institute of Chemical Biology and Fundamental Medicine, Siberian Branch of the Russian Academy of Sciences, 630090 Novosibirsk, Russia; alex.bondar@mail.ru
* Correspondence: posukh@bionet.nsc.ru

Citation: Danilchenko, V.Y.; Zytsar, M.V.; Maslova, E.A.; Bady-Khoo, M.S.; Barashkov, N.A.; Morozov, I.V.; Bondar, A.A.; Posukh, O.L. Different Rates of the *SLC26A4*-Related Hearing Loss in Two Indigenous Peoples of Southern Siberia (Russia). *Diagnostics* **2021**, *11*, 2378. https://doi.org/10.3390/diagnostics11122378

Academic Editor: José M. Millán

Received: 16 November 2021
Accepted: 13 December 2021
Published: 17 December 2021

Publisher's Note: MDPI stays neutral with regard to jurisdictional claims in published maps and institutional affiliations.

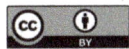

Copyright: © 2021 by the authors. Licensee MDPI, Basel, Switzerland. This article is an open access article distributed under the terms and conditions of the Creative Commons Attribution (CC BY) license (https://creativecommons.org/licenses/by/4.0/).

Abstract: Hereditary hearing loss (HL) is known to be highly locus/allelic heterogeneous, and the prevalence of different HL forms significantly varies among populations worldwide. Investigation of region-specific landscapes of hereditary HL is important for local healthcare and medical genetic services. Mutations in the *SLC26A4* gene leading to nonsyndromic recessive deafness (DFNB4) and Pendred syndrome are common genetic causes of hereditary HL, at least in some Asian populations. We present for the first time the results of a thorough analysis of the *SLC26A4* gene by Sanger sequencing in the large cohorts of patients with HL of unknown etiology belonging to two neighboring indigenous Turkic-speaking Siberian peoples (Tuvinians and Altaians). A definite genetic diagnosis based on the presence of biallelic *SLC26A4* mutations was established for 28.2% (62/220) of all enrolled Tuvinian patients vs. 4.3% (4/93) of Altaian patients. The rate of the *SLC26A4*-related HL in Tuvinian patients appeared to be one of the highest among populations worldwide. The *SLC26A4* mutational spectrum was characterized by the presence of Asian-specific mutations c.919-2A>G and c.2027T>A (p.Leu676Gln), predominantly found in Tuvinian patients, and c.2168A>G (p.His723Arg), which was only detected in Altaian patients. In addition, a novel pathogenic variant c.1545T>G (p.Phe515Leu) was found with high frequency in Tuvinian patients. Overall, based on the findings of this study and our previous research, we were able to uncover the genetic causes of HL in 50.5% of Tuvinian patients and 34.5% of Altaian patients.

Keywords: hearing loss; genetic diagnosis; *SLC26A4*; DFNB4; Tuvinians; Altaians; Southern Siberia; Russia

1. Introduction

Hearing loss (HL) is one of the most common sensory disorders affecting over 5% of the world's population [1]. Approximately half of all HL cases are attributed to genetic causes [2]. Hereditary HL includes many different syndromes with HL as one of the clinical symptoms and more common nonsyndromic forms. Over 160 nuclear genes are causally implicated in nonsyndromic HL with different types of inheritance: autosomal dominant—DFNA, autosomal recessive—DFNB, or X-linked—DFNX [3]. In addition, some mutations in mitochondrial DNA are also associated with HL [4]. Mutations in the *GJB2* gene (13q12.11, OMIM 121011) encoding transmembrane protein connexin 26 result in the nonsyndromic autosomal recessive deafness 1A (DFNB1A, OMIM 220290), which is one of the most common forms of HL in many populations, at least of Caucasian descent [5]. Testing of *GJB2* mutations is efficient for establishing a genetic diagnosis in many HL cases. However, the causes of HL in a large number of patients often remain unknown because of high locus/allelic heterogeneity and varying prevalence of hereditary HL in different populations.

Mutations in the *SLC26A4* gene (Solute carrier family 26, member 4/pendrin, 7q22.3, OMIM 605646) are considered to be the second commonest cause of hereditary HL in most world populations, at least in East Asia (Japan, Korea, China) and Mongolia [6–13]. The *SLC26A4* gene encodes pendrin, a protein belonging to the SLC26 anion transporter family, which is mostly expressed in tissues of the inner ear, thyroid, and kidneys and is involved in the transport of various anions [14,15]. In the inner ear, pendrin maintains anionic composition of endolymph by mediating Cl^-/HCO_3-exchange [16]. Mutations in the *SLC26A4* gene cause non-syndromic recessive deafness (DFNB4, OMIM 600791) and Pendred syndrome (PDS, OMIM 274600), which combines sensorineural HL and goiter. A prominent clinical characteristic of inner ear in the *SLC26A4*-related HL is the enlarged vestibular aqueduct (EVA) and other malformations of inner ear structures detected by computed tomography (CT) or magnetic resonance imaging (MRI) [17]. Two radiologic criteria are used to establish EVA: a historically earliest and most commonly used "Valvassori criteria" (a midpoint diameter of the vestibular aqueduct >1.5 mm) [18] and relatively recent "Cincinnati criteria" (a midpoint diameter ≥ 1.0 mm or an operculum diameter ≥ 2.0 mm) [19,20]. Murine model studies revealed pendrin to be responsible for maintenance of endocochlear potential and fluid homeostasis in the cochlea. The deficiency or dysfunction of pendrin causes endolymphatic hydrops with enlargement of the vestibular aqueduct and endolymphatic sac, as well as other abnormalities of the inner ear structures, being presumably a consequence of defects in anion and fluid transport [21]. However, the pathogenesis of EVA may also be attributed to other mechanisms since not all patients with detected EVA have the *SLC26A4*-related HL [22].

To date, more than 500 variants in the *SLC26A4* gene associated with a wide range of HL phenotypes have been reported (Human Gene Mutation Database: http://www.hgmd.cf.ac.uk/ac/index.php (accessed on 1 November 2021) [23]. Screening for *SLC26A4* mutations has become an important part of molecular genetic testing for HL, especially for patients with detected EVA. Nevertheless, despite numerous studies, the pathogenic contribution of *SLC26A4* to HL in different populations remains to be accurately estimated. First, this is due to the heterogeneity of the examined cohorts of patients in different studies, which varied in size and phenotypic characteristics of enrolled patients (pediatric or adult samples, cochlear implantees, patients with nonsyndromic sensorineural HL (NSHL), patients with diagnosed EVA or Pendred syndrome). Second, methods for the *SLC26A4* analysis varied from a target screening of only the most prevalent *SLC26A4* mutations to a thorough study of the *SLC26A4* coding and adjoined regions or the whole *SLC26A4* sequence by Sanger sequencing or NGS technology.

Different proportions of patients having biallelic *SLC26A4* mutations were revealed in a relatively limited number of large NSHL studies performed without preselection of patients with EVA or Pendred syndrome: 3.5% of sib pairs from the UK Caucasian child population [24], 0.9% of Czech patients [25], 2.9% of Brazilian patients [26], 6.3% (0–8.3%) of patients from different regions of Iran [27], 7.2% of patients from Pakistan [28], 3.5% of patients from southern India [29], 1.1% of Korean patients [6], 4.6% of the Vietnamese pediatric population [30], 1–1.5% of Mongolian patients [6,12], up to 15.3% of patients from different regions of mainland China [31–34], and 5.8% of Taiwanese patients [13]. A significantly higher proportion of biallelic *SLC26A4* mutations was found in the studies on cohorts of patients who were pre-screened for EVA, reaching 65–95% in Asian cohorts and approximately one-fourth of patients with nonsyndromic EVA in Caucasian cohorts, which is probably influenced by the different ethnicities of patients and an increased sensitivity of sequencing techniques [7,10,22,35–37].

In numerous studies, the *SLC26A4* mutation spectrum and prevalence were found to be very diverse around the world and were considered to be ethnic-specific since some ethnic groups appeared to have different mutational hotspots, although, so far, there are significantly fewer supporting data in comparison with the *GJB2* gene [6,11,38,39]. Meta-analysis performed by Lu et al. (2015) revealed 26 out of 272 different *SLC26A4* mutations that were in the top 10% of mutation rates in patients with HL worldwide. Among them, c.919-2A>G was the highest frequency *SLC26A4* mutation (62.4%) followed by c.2168A>G (p.His723Arg) (26.1%). Various sets of the *SLC26A4* mutations with frequencies of more than 5% were found only either in Asia or in Europe [39]. It is now evident that the *SLC26A4* mutation spectrum found in Asian populations is quite different from that in populations of Caucasian ancestry [11].

The concentration of the *SLC26A4*-related HL in a particular population or region is probably influenced by a certain population genetic structure and factors of population dynamics as were shown for some other forms of hereditary HL. Investigation of region-specific landscapes of the *SLC26A4*-related HL is important for local healthcare and medical genetic services.

Siberia, a large (over 13.1 million square kilometers) geographical region of the Russian Federation with a population of approximately 36 million in total, is a multiethnic region where, along with numerous Russians, live various indigenous Siberian peoples. Tuvinians (Tuvans) and Altaians, representing two indigenous Turkic-speaking peoples, live in the Republic of Tyva and the Republic of Altai, respectively, bordering each other in Southern Siberia. Both republics also border Mongolia in the south, and the Altai Republic borders China (in the south) and Kazakhstan (in the southwest). Tuvinians, about 250,000 people in total, according to the Russian Census of 2010, live mainly in the Tyva Republic. Besides the Tyva Republic, relatively small groups of Tuvinians also live in the northern part of Mongolia and in the Xinjiang Uygur Autonomous Region of China [40,41]. Tuvinians are one of the most ancient Turkic-speaking peoples inhabiting Central Asia and the Sayan-Altai region. Prolonged relations with residents of neighboring regions (Turkic-, Mongolic-, Ket-, and Samoyedic-speaking tribes) had a significant impact on the formation of the Tuvinian population [42,43]. The Altaians, about 70,000 people in total, according to the Russian Census of 2010, originated from several ancient Turkic-speaking tribes [44]. The archaeological, linguistic, anthropological, and historical evidence indicates similarities in the ethnogenesis of both Turkic-speaking Tuvinians and Altaians.

During our previous molecular genetic studies of the hereditary HL in Tuvinian and Altaian deaf patients, a genetic diagnosis based on the thorough testing for the *GJB2* gene and the target screening of several mutations in other HL-associated genes, was established in many HL cases [45–51]. Nevertheless, the causes of HL in a significant number of patients remained unknown.

Pathogenic variants in the *SLC26A4* gene are considered as a common cause of HL among many Asian populations; thus, the involvement of *SLC26A4* in the etiology of HL in Tuvinian and Altaian patients living in Southern Siberia (Russia) seems to be quite expected. In this regard, the aim of this work was to evaluate for the first time the *SLC26A4* pathogenic contribution to HL in Tuvinian and Altaian patients.

2. Materials and Methods

2.1. Study Subjects

2.1.1. Patients

The ethnically matched cohort of patients with HL of unknown etiology from Southern Siberia (Russia) included 170 Tuvinians (the Tyva Republic) and 62 Altaians (the Altai Republic). Analysis of pedigrees and family histories revealed that the group of examined Tuvinian patients consisted of 57 familial (two or more affected family members) and 111 single/sporadic (the only affected individual in family) HL cases while the group of Altaian patients included 36 familial and 26 single/sporadic HL cases. These patients were selected from the main groups of Tuvinian ($n = 220$) and Altaian ($n = 93$) patients and represent individuals in whom the causes of HL remained unknown after the thorough testing for the *GJB2* gene [45,48,49,51] and the target screening of several mutations in other genes (*MT-RNR1, MT-TS1, OTOF, RAI1*) [46,47,50]. Genomic DNA samples of Tuvinian patients were collected from 2010 to 2018, and DNA samples of Altaian patients were collected from 2001 to 2003 with the subsequent addition of samples in 2012.

The hearing status of patients was evaluated by otoscopic and pure-tone audiometry examinations at different times in the specialized audiological services located in the town of Kyzyl (the Tyva Republic) and the town of Gorno-Altaiisk (the Altai Republic). The severity of HL was defined as mild (25–40 dB), moderate (41–70 dB), severe (71–90 dB), or profound (above 90 dB). The majority of examined Tuvinian patients (164 individuals) had congenital or early onset severe-to-profound HL and six patients had moderate HL. Among Altaian patients, 30 individuals had severe-to-profound HL, 18 individuals had moderate HL, and for 14 Altaian patients the severity of HL was not determined. Other concomitant information was collected from local unspecialized medical services and by direct interview with the patients and their relatives. The CT scan of temporal bones in Tuvinian patients with biallelic *SLC26A4* mutations was performed in the Department of Diagnostic Radiology of the Republican Hospital No. 1 (Kyzyl, the Tyva Republic, Russia). Unfortunately, the examination of patients for thyroid dysfunction and/or a goiter using a perchlorate discharge test and a thyroid ultrasound was not available.

2.1.2. Control Samples

The control samples were represented by 157 unrelated Tuvinians and 141 unrelated Altaians from different regions of the Tyva Republic and the Altai Republic, respectively. None of them were registered by audiological services and had complained of hearing impairment.

2.1.3. Ethics Statement

Written informed consent was obtained from all individuals or their legal guardians before they participated in the study. The study was conducted in accordance with the Declaration of Helsinki, and the protocol was approved by the Bioethics Commission at the Institute of Cytology and Genetics SB RAS, Novosibirsk, Russia (Protocol No. 9, 24 April 2012).

2.2. Molecular Analysis

Genomic DNA was isolated from the buffy coat fraction of blood by a standard phenol-chloroform extraction method.

2.2.1. Mutation Analysis of the *SLC26A4* Gene

The *SLC26A4* gene sequence encompassing all 21 exons with flanking regions was analyzed by Sanger sequencing. Primer pairs designed to amplify corresponding PCR products and also used for Sanger sequencing are summarized in Supplementary Table S1. The PCR products were purified by sorption on Agencourt Ampure XP (Beckman Coulter, Indianapolis, IN, USA) and subjected to Sanger sequencing using a BigDye Terminator V.3.1 Cycle Sequencing Kit (Applied Biosystems, Waltham, MA, USA) with subsequent unincorporated dye removal by gel filtration on the Sephadex G-50 (GE Healthcare, Chicago, IL, USA). Sanger products were analyzed on an ABI 3130XL Genetic Analyzer (Applied Biosystems/Life Technologies, USA) in the SB RAS Genomics Core Facility (Institute of Chemical Biology and Fundamental Medicine SB RAS, Novosibirsk, Russia). DNA sequence variations were identified by comparison with the *SLC26A4* gene reference sequences: NC_000007.13 (https://www.ncbi.nlm.nih.gov/nuccore/NC_000007.13/ (accessed on 1 November 2021) and NC_000007.14 (https://www.ncbi.nlm.nih.gov/nuccore/NC_000007.14/ (accessed on 1 November 2021).

2.2.2. Screening of Pathogenic *SLC26A4* Variants in Control Samples

Screening of variants c.170C>A (exon 3), c.919-2A>G (intronic region between exons 7 and 8), c.1545T>G (exon 14), and c.2168A>G (exon 19) in control samples was performed by PCR-RFLP assays using primer pairs designed to amplify corresponding PCR products and restriction enzymes *Tru9 I, Hpa II, Pce I, Rsr2 I*, respectively (Supplementary Table S1).

Screening of variants c.2027T>A (exon 17) and c.2034+1G>A (intronic region between exons 17 and 18) in control samples was performed by Sanger sequencing.

2.3. Bioinformatics Tools

2.3.1. Bioinformatics Prediction Tools

Functional effect of c.1545T>G (p.Phe515Leu) variant was predicted using PolyPhen-2 (http://genetics.bwh.harvard.edu/pph2), PROVEAN (http://provean.jcvi.org), MutationTaster (http://www.mutationtaster.org/), FATHMM (http://fathmm.biocompute.org.uk/), MutationAssessor (http://mutationassessor.org/), Align-GVGD (http://agvgd.hci.utah.edu/), MutPred2 (http://mutpred.mutdb.org/), Condel (https://bbglab.irbbarcelona.org/fannsdb/), SNPs & GO (https://snps-and-go.biocomp.unibo.it/snps-and-go/), CADD (https://cadd.gs.washington.edu/), SIFT (https://sift.bii.a-star.edu.sg/) (Supplementary Table S2).

2.3.2. 3D Modeling of Pendrin Molecule Structure

The three-dimensional (3D) molecule structure of the wild-type and mutant p.Phe515Leu type of pendrin protein was predicted by the I-Tasser program (https://zhanglab.ccmb.med.umich.edu/I-TASSER/) [52–54] and was visualized by Swiss-PdbViewer v.4.1.0 (http://www.expasy.org/spdbv/) [55].

2.4. Statistical Methods

Two-tailed Fisher's exact test with a significance level of $p < 0.05$ was applied to compare allele frequencies between patients and controls.

3. Results

3.1. SLC26A4 Genotypes of Patients

Analysis of the *SLC26A4* gene was performed in ethnically matched cohorts of patients (170 Tuvinians and 62 Altaians) with HL of unknown etiology. Sequential analysis of the *SLC26A4* gene fragments by Sanger sequencing in a particular patient was continued until two recessive pathogenic *SLC26A4* variants were detected and, therefore, diagnosis could be made. The *SLC26A4* genotypes of patients are presented in Table 1. Thirteen different *SLC26A4* genotypes including recessive pathogenic *SLC26A4* variants were found in patients: four genotypes with homozygous variants, five genotypes with compound heterozygous variants, and four genotypes with single variants (Table 1).

In total, six different pathogenic or likely pathogenic *SLC26A4* variants were found in both cohorts of patients (Table 2). Among them, the variants c.170C>A (p.Ser57Ter), c.919-2A>G, c.2027T>A (p.Leu676Gln), c.2034+1G>A, and c.2168A>G (p.His723Arg) were previously found in patients with HL in different regions of the world while c.1545T>G (p.Phe515Leu) was a novel *SLC26A4* variant.

For patients who were homozygous or compound heterozygous for pathogenic *SLC26A4* variants ($n = 66$, comprising 62 Tuvinians and 4 Altaians), the genetic diagnosis "Hearing loss due to the presence of two recessive mutations in the *SLC26A4* gene" could be established. Thus, the pathogenic contribution of the *SLC26A4* gene to HL of patients, defined as the proportion of patients with biallelic recessive pathogenic *SLC26A4* variants among all enrolled Tuvinian and Altaian patients, could be estimated as 28.2% (62/220) and 4.3% (4/93), respectively. Only one recessive pathogenic *SLC26A4* allele was identified in 14 patients (13 Tuvinians and 1 Altaian) (Table 1).

Table 1. The *SLC26A4* genotypes in Tuvinian and Altaian patients.

	SLC26A4 Genotypes		Tuvinian Patents (n = 220)	Altaian Patents (n = 93)
	Homozygotes			
1	c.[919-2A>G];[919-2A>G] p.[splice acceptor variant];[splice acceptor variant]	intronic region between exons 7 and 8	30	-
2	c.[2027T>A];[2027T>A] p.[Leu676Gln];[Leu676Gln]	exon 17	4	-
3	c.[2168A>G];[2168A>G] p.[His723Arg];[His723Arg]	exon 19	-	2
4	c.[170C>A];[170C>A] p.[Ser57Ter];[Ser57Ter]	exon 3	1	-
	Total		35	2
	Compound heterozygotes			
5	c.[919-2A>G];[2027T>A] p.[splice acceptor variant];[Leu676Gln]	intronic region between exons 7 and 8/exon 17	14	2
6	c.[919-2A>G];[1545T>G] * p.[splice acceptor variant];[Phe515Leu] *	intronic region between exons 7 and 8/exon 14	8	-
7	c.[170C>A];[919-2A>G] p.[Ser57Ter];[splice acceptor variant]	exon 3/intronic region between exons 7 and 8	3	-
8	c.[919-2A>G];[2034+1G>A] p.[splice acceptor variant];[splice donor variant]	intronic region between exons 7 and 8/intronic region between exons 17 and 18	1	-
9	c.[1545T>G] *;[2027T>A] p.[Phe515Leu] *;[Leu676Gln]	exons 14/17	1	-
	Total		27	2
	Biallelic *SLC26A4* mutations in total		62 (28.2%)	4 (4.3%)
	Single heterozygotes			
10	c.[919-2A>G];[?] p.[splice acceptor variant];[?]	intronic region between exons 7 and 8	9	-
11	c.[1545T>G] *;[?] p.[Phe515Leu] *;[?]	exon 14	2	-
12	c.[170C>A];[?] p.[Ser57Ter];[?]	exon 3	1	-
13	c.[2027T>A];[?] p.[Leu676Gln];[?]	exon 17	1	1
	Total		13 (5.9%)	1 (1.1%)

The *SLC26A4* variations are designated at the nucleotide level (NC_000007.14, https://www.ncbi.nlm.nih.gov/nuccore/NC_000007.14/ (accessed on 1 November 2021) and amino acid level (NP_000432.1, https://www.ncbi.nlm.nih.gov/protein/NP_000432.1/ (accessed on 1 November 2021) at the top and bottom of each line, respectively. *—novel variant in the *SLC26A4* gene.

Table 2. Pathogenic variants in the *SLC26A4* gene found in Tuvinian and Altaian patients.

	SLC26A4 Variants		Location	Molecular Consequence	dbSNP ID	ClinVar (2021)
	Nucleotide	Amino Acid				
1	c.170C>A	p.Ser57Ter	exon 3	nonsense variant	rs111033200	pathogenic
2	c.919-2A>G	splice acceptor variant	intronic region between exons 7 and 8	splice acceptor	rs111033313	pathogenic
3	c.1545T>G *	p.Phe515Leu	exon 14	missense variant	not presented	not presented
4	c.2027T>A	p.Leu676Gln	exon 17	missense variant	rs111033318	pathogenic/likely pathogenic
5	c.2034+1G>A	splice donor variant	intronic region between exons 17 and 18	splice donor	rs759683649	likely pathogenic
6	c.2168A>G	p.His723Arg	exon 19	missense variant	rs121908362	pathogenic/likely pathogenic

*—novel variant in the *SLC26A4* gene.

Variant c.919-2A>G was the most frequent of all pathogenic *SLC26A4* variants detected in Tuvinian patients (95/137, 69.3%), followed by c.2027T>A (p.Leu676Gln) (24/137, 17.5%), c.1545T>G (p.Phe515Leu) (11/137, 8.0%), c.170C>A (p.Ser57Ter) (6/137, 4.4%), and c.2034+1G>A (1/137, 0.7%). Variant c.2168A>G (p.His723Arg) was prevalent in Altaian patients (4/9, 44.5%) followed by c.2027T>A (p.Leu676Gln) (3/9, 33.3%), and c.919-2A>G (2/9, 22.2%) (Figure 1).

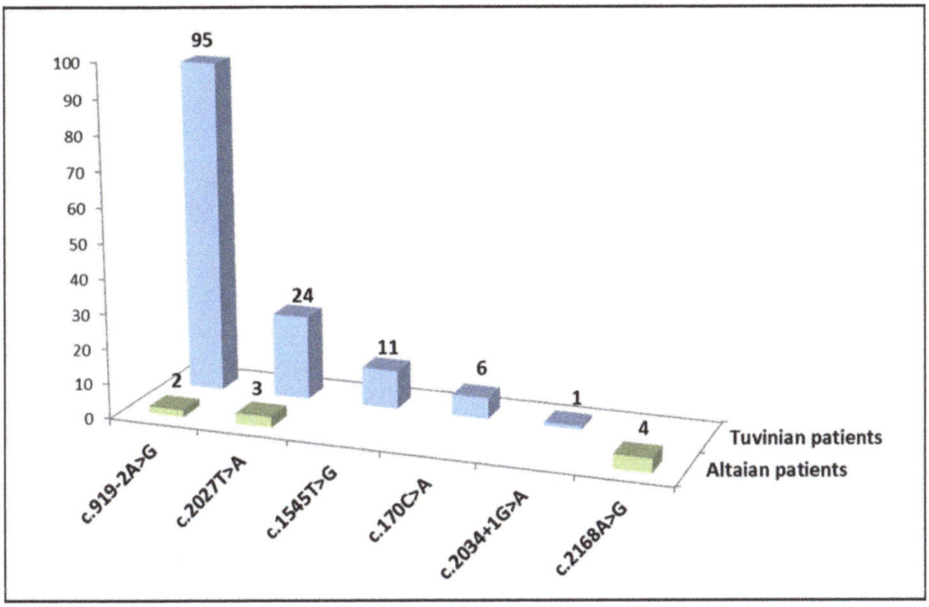

Figure 1. Distribution of pathogenic variants among all mutated *SLC26A4* alleles in Tuvinian and Altaian patients.

3.2. Novel SLC26A4 Variant c.1545T>G (p.Phe515Leu)

The c.1545T>G is a novel, previously undescribed, missense variant in exon 14 of *SLC26A4* leading to substitution of phenylalanine by leucine at amino acid position 515 (p.Phe515Leu) of the pendrin protein (Figure 2). This variant was found in 11 Tuvinian patients from 8 unrelated families: in 9 patients in a compound with already known *SLC26A4* mutations (c.919-2A>G or c.2027T>A) and in 2 patients in a heterozygous state (Table 1).

The analysis of available family members in one Tuvinian family where the c.1545T>G (p.Phe515Leu) variant was found revealed the segregation of c.1545T>G (p.Phe515Leu) with HL (Figure 2). Unfortunately, the testing of the relatives of other patients with this variant was not available to support strong segregation of c.1545T>G (p.Phe515Leu) with HL. In addition, the allelic frequency of c.1545T>G was estimated in the group of Tuvinian patients tested for c.1545T>G (137 individuals) and in the Tuvinian control sample. To exclude possible bias in the estimation of c.1545T>G frequency in a group of patients owing to the presence of a certain number of related individuals, we used a sample of unrelated patients formed by analysis of their pedigrees (121 individuals, 242 alleles) for a comparative analysis. The frequency of c.1545T>G in this sample of Tuvinian patients (3.7%, 9/242) was significantly higher than in the Tuvinian control sample (1.0%, 3/296) ($p = 0.03391$). We also evaluated a potential functional significance of this novel variant using 11 bioinformatics predictive software tools. Most of them predicted a potentially deleterious effect ("damaging"/"disease causing"/"possibly damaging") of this missense variant (Supplementary Table S2).

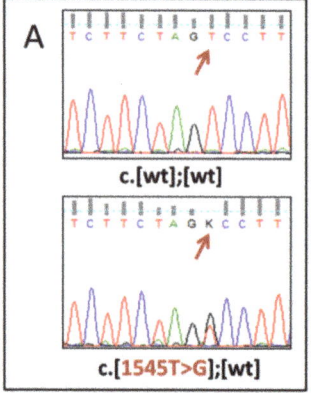
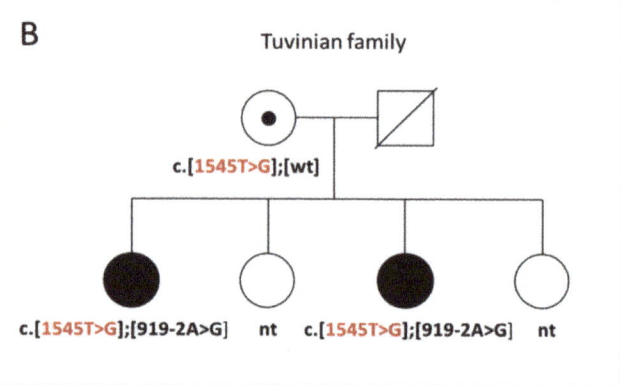
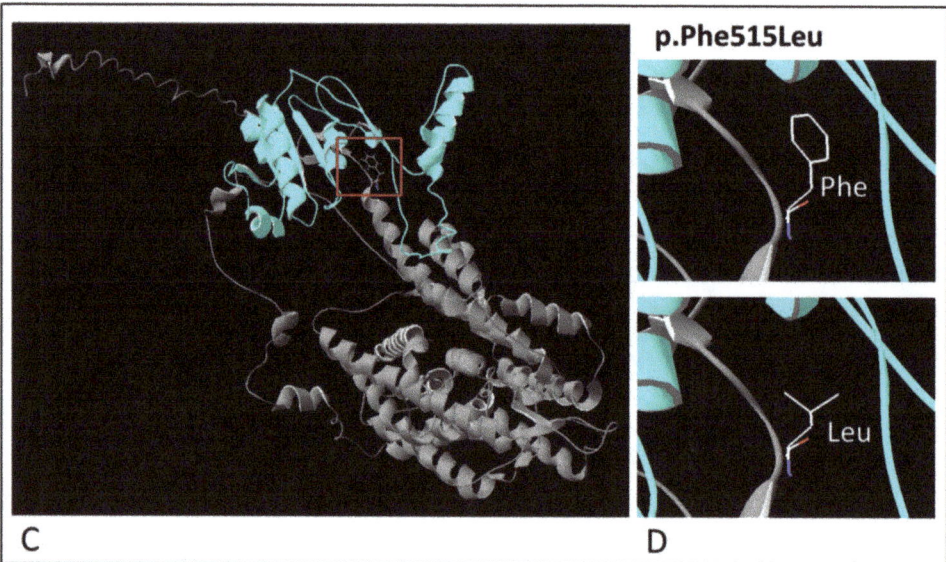

Figure 2. (**A**) Identification of variant c.1545T>G (p.Phe515Leu) by Sanger sequencing; (**B**) The pedigree of the Tuvinian family demonstrating the segregation of variant c.1545T>G (p.Phe515Leu) in compound with recessive mutation c.919-2A>G with HL. Deaf individuals are shown by black symbols; the variant c.1545T>G (p.Phe515Leu) is shown by red; nt—not tested; wt—wild-type; (**C**) The 3D structure of the pendrin protein with localization of variant p.Phe515Leu; (**D**) Close-up views of wild (Phe515) and mutant (Leu515) types of pendrin.

3.3. Carrier Frequency of Pathogenic SLC26A4 Variants in Tuvinian and Altaian Control Samples

Based on the prevalence of pathogenic *SLC26A4* variants in both groups of patients (Tuvinians and Altaians), we screened the most frequent pathogenic *SLC26A4* variants in appropriate ethnically matched control samples. Two pathogenic variants, c.919-2A>G and c.1545T>G, were found with frequencies of 5.1% (8/157) and 2.0% (3/148), respectively, among unrelated healthy Tuvinians, while none of the pathogenic *SLC26A4* variants were detected in the Altaian control sample (Table 3).

Table 3. The carrier frequency of pathogenic SLC26A4 variants in Tuvinian and Altaian control samples.

Pathogenic SLC26A4 Variants	Tuvinian Control Sample	Altaian Control Sample
c.919-2A>G	5.1% (8/157)	nt
c.1545T>G	2.0% (3/148)	nt
c.170C>A	0% (0/100)	nt
c.2027T>A	0% (0/157)	0% (0/123)
c.2034+1G>A	0% (0/157)	0% (0/123)
c.2168A>G	nt	0% (0/141)

nt—not tested.

The allelic frequency of each pathogenic SLC26A4 variant (except for the very rare c.2034+1G>A found in one Tuvinian patient) in both groups of patients (Tuvinians and Altaians) was significantly higher ($p < 0.05$) than in the corresponding ethnic controls. For a correct comparative analysis, the samples of unrelated patients were used.

3.4. Computed Tomography (CT) of the Temporal Bones in Tuvinian Patients

To elucidate the prevalence of the enlarged vestibular aqueduct (EVA) in Tuvinian patients homozygous or compound heterozygous for the SLC26A4 mutations, the temporal bone computed tomography (CT) was performed. Unfortunately, the CT examination was available only for 27 out of 62 Tuvinian patients with biallelic SLC26A4 mutations. These patients (15 females and 12 males, aged from 11 to 57 years old) belonged to 19 unrelated families. Clinical descriptions and CT medical reports of patients are presented in Supplementary Table S3. Among 27 patients who passed the CT examination, the genotype c.[919-2A>G];[919-2A>G] was prevalent (15 patients) followed by the genotype c.[919-2A>G];[2027T>A] (7 patients), and one of the other five genotypes (c.[919-2A>G];[1545T>G], c.[2027T>A];[2027T>A], c.[919-2A>G];[2034+1G>A], c.[170C>A];[170C>A] or c.[170C>A];[919-2A>G]) was found in single patients. The CT scans were interpreted by the specialists from the Department of Diagnostic Radiology of the Republican Hospital No. 1 (Kyzyl, the Tyva Republic, Russia) according to the most accepted "Valvassori" criterion for the definition of EVA [18]: a vestibular aqueduct was considered to be enlarged if its diameter was >1.5 mm at the midpoint between the common crus and the external aperture of the vestibular aqueduct on CT images. A total of 24 out of 27 examined patients had bilateral EVA varying from 1.5 to 5.1 mm; the vestibular aqueduct up to 1.5 mm in both ears was found in one patient; unilateral EVA was observed in two patients. The results showed that the degree of EVA in examined patients can differ in both ears of the same patient and is characterized by intrafamilial and interfamilial variability (Supplementary Table S3).

4. Discussion

4.1. The SLC26A4-Related HL in Tuvinian and Altaian Patients

In this study, we investigated the prevalence of the SLC26A4 pathogenic variants in Tuvinian and Altaian patients where the causes of HL remained unknown after thorough testing for the GJB2 gene [45,48,49,51] and target screening for several mutations in other genes (MT-RNR1, MT-TS1, OTOF, RAI1) [46,47,50]. Unlike most studies, in which the SLC26A4 gene was generally tested in the cohorts of patients with already diagnosed EVA, the patients in our study were not preselected by the presence of EVA. This approach allowed us to estimate the overall pathogenic contribution of SLC26A4 mutations in HL in total groups of Tuvinian ($n = 220$) and Altaian patients ($n = 93$). The presence of biallelic recessive pathogenic SLC26A4 variants explained the etiology of HL (DFNB4) in 28.2% (62/220) of Tuvinian patients and in 4.3% (4/93) of Altaian patients (Table 1). To our knowledge, the rate of the SLC26A4-related HL in Tuvinian patients (28.2%) is one of the highest among populations worldwide. In addition, the significant difference in the prevalence of SLC26A4-caused HL (28.2% in Tuvinians vs. 4.3% in Altaians) among two neighboring indigenous Turkic-speaking Siberian peoples with a common ethnic background is an unexpected and interesting observation.

The enlarged vestibular aqueduct (EVA) detected by CT or MRI scanning is a specific feature of DFNB4 in the majority of patients with *SLC26A4* mutations. The EVA syndrome was first described in the study by Valvassori and Clemis (1978) where the vestibular aqueduct was considered as enlarged if its anteroposterior diameter was more than 1.5 mm in the midpoint of the post isthmic segment or halfway between the external aperture and the common crus [18]. Subsequently, these criteria were generally considered to be the defining characteristics of EVA in patients with HL. Based on a review of a pediatric HL database and the radiographic comparisons to a group of normal hearing children, Boston et al. (2007) and Vijayasekaran et al. (2007) proposed to define EVA as one that is 2 mm at the operculum and/or 1 mm at the midpoint [19,20]. Dewan et al. (2009) reported that the use of these criteria (referred to as "Cincinnati criteria") allowed identification of a large percentage (significantly greater than would have been identified by the Valvassori criterion) of pediatric cochlear implant patients with EVA who might otherwise have no known etiology for their deafness [56]. Currently, there are no uniform and standardized criteria for the diagnosis of EVA, and both criteria (the Valvassori criteria or the Cincinnati criteria) are used in different studies.

In our study, the temporal bone computed tomography (CT) was performed only in a limited number of Tuvinian patients (27 out of 62 patients homozygous or compound heterozygous for the *SLC26A4* mutations) because of the unavailability of CT examination for patients living in small remote villages in various administrative districts of the Tyva Republic. According to the conventional Valvassori criterion, bilateral EVA (a midpoint diameter from 1.5 to 5.1 mm) was observed in the majority (24 out of 27) of examined patients with different *SLC26A4* genotypes. The EVA degree differed in both ears of the same patient and was characterized by intrafamilial and interfamilial variability (Supplementary Table S3). When these results were reviewed using the Cincinnati criteria, all patients appeared to have bilateral EVA, except one with unilateral EVA (patient #17, male, 18 years old, genotype c.[919-2A>G];[919-2A>G]) (Supplementary Table S3). These results were consistent with the abundant data confirming EVA in the vast majority of patients with biallelic *SLC26A4* mutations. Unfortunately, the limited number of CT-examined patients did not allow us to identify any correlations of the EVA degree with a certain *SLC26A4* genotype.

4.2. Pathogenic SLC26A4 Variants in Tuvinians and Altaians

A total of six different pathogenic *SLC26A4* variants were identified in patients in our study (Table 2). Two of them, c.919-2A>G and c.2168A>G (p.His723Arg), were the most frequent among Tuvinian and Altaian patients, respectively (Figure 1).

The proportions of c.919-2A>G among all mutant *SLC26A4* alleles identified were 69.9% in Tuvinian patients and 22.2% in Altaian patients. The c.919-2A>G mutation (previously named IVS7-2A>G, rs111033313) is located at the splice site in the intron region between exons 7 and 8 and leads to a skipping of exon 8, with the formation of a stop codon at amino acid position 311 and finally a truncated form of pendrin molecule. This mutation was firstly identified in an extended inbred Turkish family [57]. In numerous subsequent studies, c.919-2A>G was often detected in deaf subjects from Asian countries (mainland China, Taiwan, Mongolia, Korea, and Japan) and observed with the highest frequency in China [6,8,12,13,39,58].

The c.2168A>G (p.His723Arg, rs121908362) mutation, detected only in Altaian patients, was one of the first *SLC26A4* mutations identified in patients with Pendred syndrome and EVA [59,60]. Subsequently, c.2168A>G (p.His723Arg) was found to be the predominant *SLC26A4* mutation in patients from Japan and Korea [6,10,61].

Thus, c.919-2A>G and c.2168A>G (p.His723Arg) are thought to be the most common *SLC26A4* mutations in Asian populations. High frequencies of c.2168A>G (p.His723Arg) in Japanese and Koreans, and c.919-2A>G in Han Chinese (Taiwanese) are probably the result of the founder effect [6,62].

Variant c.2027T>A (rs111033318) in exon 17 of the *SLC26A4* gene results in substitution of leucine by glutamine at position 676 (p.Leu676Gln) in the pendrin amino acid sequence. This variant was predicted to disrupt an α-helical domain of pendrin leading to altered trafficking of pendrin and its intracellular retention [63,64]. Variant c.2027T>A (p.Leu676Gln) appears to be specific for Asian populations, since it was previously detected, although relatively rare, in patients from China, Mongolia, and Korea [6,8,12,31,32,65,66]. In our study, unlike the studies in China, Mongolia, and Korea, variant c.2027T>A (p.Leu676Gln) was found in a significant number of patients (19 Tuvinians and 2 Altaians) and was the second most frequent pathogenic *SLC26A4* variant in both cohorts of examined patients.

The variant c.170C>A (rs111033200) in exon 3 of the *SLC26A4* gene was detected in our study only in five Tuvinian patients. This mutation leads to the formation of a stop codon at amino acid position 57 (p.Ser57Ter) at the NH_2-terminus of the pendrin molecule, and the protein is predicted to lack most of the important domains [67]. The c.170C>A (p.Ser57Ter) mutation was previously found in several deaf patients from India, China, Pakistan, Mexico, and Turkey [6,28,66–68].

Variant c.2034+1G>A was found in one Tuvinian patient in a compound heterozygous state with mutation c.919-2A>G. This mutation affects a donor splice site in intron 17 of the *SLC26A4* gene and has been classified as "likely pathogenic", since it is expected to disrupt RNA splicing and likely to result in the disrupted protein product. This variant has not been reported in the literature in individuals with *SLC26A4*-related conditions and currently presents only in population databases (rs759683649, ExAC: 0.009%). Detection of c.2034+1G>A in a deaf patient in our study supported the pathogenicity of this variant but additional data are required to prove that conclusively.

The missense variant c.1545T>G (NC_000007.13:g.107338487 T>G, p.Phe515Leu) (Figure 2) in exon 14 of *SLC26A4* was found for the first time in Tuvinian patients and the Tuvinian control sample. Several lines of evidence (segregation of c.1545T>G with HL in affected subjects from several unrelated families; significantly higher frequency of this variant in patients compared with ethnically matched controls; multiple computational predictions of its deleterious effect; current absence in the world human genome databases) support the presumed pathogenicity of this variant. It is worth noting that two other rare *SLC26A4* variants, c.1544T>C (NC_000007.13:g.107336484T>C, rs138132962) and c.1544T>G (NC_000007.13:g.107336484T>G), leading to amino acid substitutions at the same position 515 (NP_000432.1:p.Phe515Ser and NP_000432.1:p.Phe515Cys, respectively), were characterized as "pathogenic" (DEAFNESS VARIATION DATABASE https://deafnessvariationdatabase.org/ (accessed on 1 November 2021). Both c.1544T>C and c.1544T>G in compound with other *SLC26A4* mutations were previously found in Chinese or Turkish patients, respectively [66,69].

In total, we revealed a relatively narrow spectrum of *SLC26A4* mutations in Tuvinian and Altaian patients, which was characterized by the presence of Asian-specific variants—c.919-2A>G (predominant in Tuvinians), c.2168A>G (p.His723Arg) (found only in Altaians), and also c.2027T>A (p.Leu676Gln), whose frequency in Tuvinians was significantly higher than in other populations worldwide. In addition, a high frequency of a novel, likely pathogenic, variant c.1545T>G (p.Phe515Leu) was observed in Tuvinian patients.

4.3. Comparative Analysis of Genetic Causes of HL in Tuvinian and Altaian Patients

We compared the ascertained genetic causes of HL in Tuvinian and Altaian patients by combining the results of the *SLC26A4* analysis performed in this study with the data from our previous studies aimed at elucidating the genetic components of HL in these indigenous peoples of Southern Siberia [45–51]. In total, we revealed the genetic causes of HL in 50.5% of Tuvinian patients and in 34.5% of Altaian patients (Figure 3).

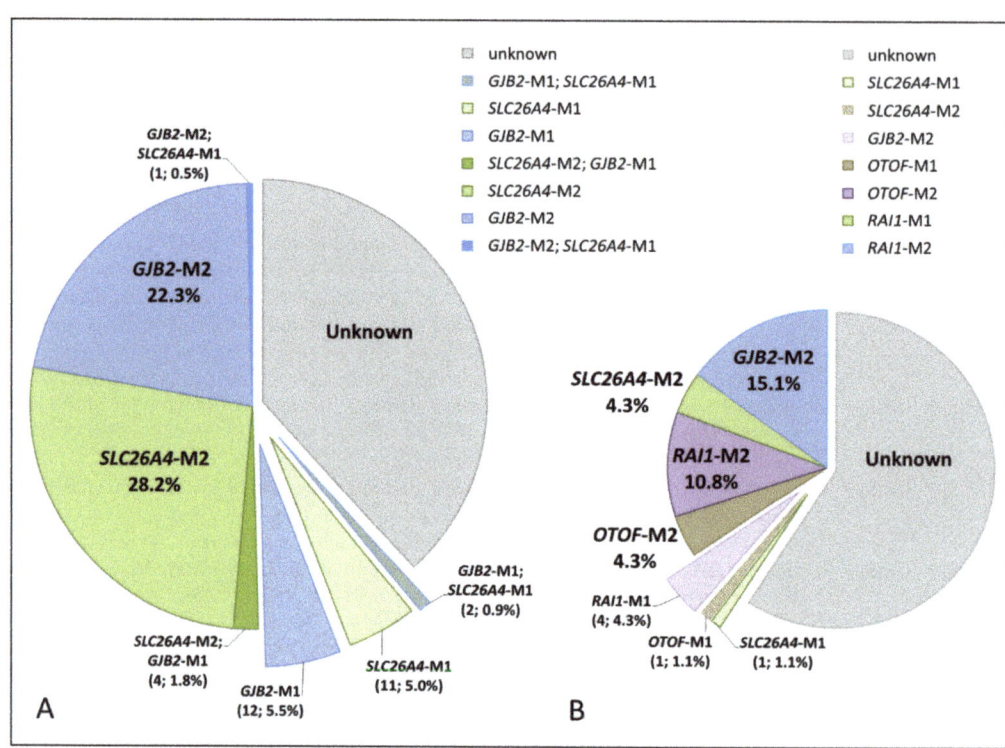

Figure 3. The genetic causes of HL in Tuvinian (**A**) and Altaian (**B**) patients. *SLC26A4*-M2 and *SLC26A4*-M1—biallelic and monoallelic *SLC26A4* mutations, respectively; *GJB2*-M2 and *GJB2*-M1—biallelic and monoallelic *GJB2* mutations, respectively; *RAI1*-M2 and *RAI1*-M1—biallelic and monoallelic mutation c.5254G>A (p.Gly1752Arg) in the *RAI1* gene, respectively; *OTOF*-M2 and *OTOF*-M1—biallelic and monoallelic mutation c.1111C>G (p.Gly371Arg) in the *OTOF* gene, respectively; unknown—no pathogenic variants were found in the studied genes. The pie chart area is proportional to the size of each examined group.

Along with 66 patients with biallelic *SLC26A4* genotypes, 14 patients (13 Tuvinians and 1 Altaian) were the carriers of a single recessive *SLC26A4* pathogenic variant (Table 1). Most of them had severe-to-profound HL. Our previous *GJB2* gene testing revealed biallelic *GJB2* mutations in 49 out of 220 Tuvinian patients (22.3%) while 18 (8.2%) Tuvinian patients appeared to be the coincidental carriers of one pathogenic *GJB2* allele [48]. When we compared the results of the *SLC26A4* testing in Tuvinian patients with their *GJB2* genotypes, four patients with the *SLC26A4*-related HL were also the carriers of one pathogenic *GJB2* allele and two patients were coincidently *GJB2*- and *SLC26A4*-heterozygotes. Moreover, additional *SLC26A4* testing revealed heterozygous *SLC26A4* variant c.1545T>G (p.Phe515Leu) in one Tuvinian patient with biallelic *GJB2* mutations (Figure 3).

A relatively large proportion of deaf individuals carrying only one recessive *SLC26A4* pathogenic variant has been reported in many studies [35,70–72], and diagnostic interpretation in such cases remains problematical. Several assumptions have been made to resolve this issue: HL in these patients could be caused by an uncertain impact of the *SLC26A4* gene (the presence of yet undetected regulatory or deep-intronic variants and intragenic exon deletions); HL could be the result of digenic inheritance; these patients could be only the coincidental carriers of one pathogenic *SLC26A4* variant and, consequently, other factors (other genes or environmental impacts) caused their HL.

A thorough analysis of all 21 exons and adjacent regions in *SLC26A4* did not reveal any other pathogenic variants in our *SLC26A4* monoallelic patients. There were no statistically significant differences in the frequency of monoallelic *SLC26A4* mutations among Tuvinian patients in whom two pathogenic *SLC26A4* mutations were not identified, compared to the Tuvinian control sample (data not shown). Thus, although we cannot completely rule out any unrecognized *SLC26A4* variants in other regions of the *SLC26A4* sequence or large deletions, the *SLC26A4* monoallelic patients in our samples were more likely to be coincidental carriers of a single *SLC26A4* pathogenic variant, and other factors (other genes or environmental impacts) could have caused their HL.

5. Conclusions

In conclusion, thorough testing of the *SLC26A4* gene is essential for establishing a genetic diagnosis of HL in the indigenous populations of Southern Siberia. The data obtained in this study provide important targeted information for genetic counseling of affected Tuvinian and Altaian families and enrich the current information on the *SLC26A4* gene variability worldwide.

Supplementary Materials: The following are available online at https://www.mdpi.com/article/10.3390/diagnostics11122378/s1, Table S1: Primers for PCR/Sanger sequencing and PCR-RFLP assays. Table S2: Bioinformatic predictions of the functional significance of a novel missense variant c.1545T>G (p.Phe515Leu) in the *SLC26A4* gene. Table S3: Clinical descriptions of Tuvinian patients with biallelic *SLC26A4* mutations.

Author Contributions: Conceptualization, O.L.P.; Methodology, V.Y.D., O.L.P., A.A.B. and I.V.M.; Formal analysis, V.Y.D., M.V.Z., A.A.B. and I.V.M.; Investigation, V.Y.D., M.V.Z., E.A.M., M.S.B.-K., A.A.B. and I.V.M.; Resources, O.L.P., V.Y.D. and M.V.Z.; Data curation, O.L.P., V.Y.D. and M.S.B.-K.; Writing—original draft preparation, O.L.P., V.Y.D.; Writing—review and editing, O.L.P., V.Y.D., M.V.Z., E.A.M., N.A.B., A.A.B. and I.V.M.; Supervision, O.L.P. All authors have read and agreed to the published version of the manuscript.

Funding: This work was supported by the Ministry of Education and Science of the Russian Federation (grant #2019-0546/FSUS-2020-0040 to O.L.P, V.Y.D., E.A.M., and grant #FSRG-2020-0016 to N.A.B.), by the Budget Projects of the Institute of Cytology and Genetics SB RAS (#AAAA-A19-119100990053-4 to V.Y.D., M.V.Z., and #0259-2021-0014 to O.L.P.), and by the RFBR grants (#17-29-06016_ofi_m and #20-015-00328_A to O.L.P.).

Institutional Review Board Statement: The study was conducted in accordance with the Declaration of Helsinki, and the protocol was approved by the Bioethics Commission at the Institute of Cytology and Genetics SB RAS, Novosibirsk, Russia (Protocol No. 9, 24 April 2012).

Informed Consent Statement: Written informed consent was obtained from all individuals or their legal guardians before they participated in the study.

Data Availability Statement: The data presented in this study are available in this article and Supplementary Materials.

Acknowledgments: The authors are sincerely grateful to all participants of the study. We also wish to acknowledge physicians Mongush B.B. and Shavyraa B.N. (the Department of Diagnostic Radiology of the Republican Hospital No. 1, Kyzyl, the Tyva Republic, Russia) for carrying out the temporal CT scanning and analysis of CT scans.

Conflicts of Interest: The authors declare no conflict of interest.

References

1. World Health Organization. Available online: https://www.who.int/en/news-room/fact-sheets/detail/deafness-and-hearing-loss (accessed on 1 April 2021).
2. Morton, C.C.; Nance, W.E. Newborn Hearing Screening—A Silent Revolution. *N. Engl. J. Med.* **2006**, *354*, 2151–2164. [CrossRef]
3. Van Camp, G.; Smith, R.J.H. Hereditary Hearing Loss Homepage. Available online: https://hereditaryhearingloss.org (accessed on 4 October 2021).
4. MITOMAP: A Human Mitochondrial Genome Database. 2019. Available online: http://www.mitomap.org (accessed on 1 November 2021).
5. Del Castillo, F.J.; del Castillo, I. DFNB1 Non-syndromic Hearing Impairment: Diversity of Mutations and Associated Phenotypes. *Front. Mol. Neurosci.* **2017**, *10*, 428. [CrossRef] [PubMed]

6. Park, H.J.; Shaukat, S.; Liu, X.Z.; Hahn, S.H.; Naz, S.; Ghosh, M.; Kim, H.N.; Moon, S.K.; Abe, S.; Tukamoto, K.; et al. Origins and frequencies of *SLC26A4* (*PDS*) mutations in east and south Asians: Global implications for the epidemiology of deafness. *J. Med. Genet.* **2003**, *40*, 242–248. [CrossRef] [PubMed]
7. Albert, S.; Blons, H.; Jonard, L.; Feldmann, D.; Chauvin, P.; Loundon, N.; Sergent-Allaoui, A.; Houang, M.; Joannard, A.; Schmerber, S.; et al. *SLC26A4* gene is frequently involved in nonsyndromic hearing impairment with enlarged vestibular aqueduct in Caucasian populations. *Eur. J. Hum. Genet.* **2006**, *14*, 773–779. [CrossRef] [PubMed]
8. Wang, Q.J.; Zhao, Y.L.; Rao, S.Q.; Guo, Y.F.; Yuan, H.; Zong, L.; Guan, J.; Xu, B.C.; Wang, D.Y.; Han, M.K.; et al. A distinct spectrum of *SLC26A4* mutations in patients with enlarged vestibular aqueduct in China. *Clin. Genet.* **2007**, *72*, 245–254. [CrossRef] [PubMed]
9. Hilgert, N.; Smith, R.J.; Van Camp, G. Forty-six genes causing nonsyndromic hearing impairment: Which ones should be analyzed in DNA diagnostics? *Mutat. Res.* **2009**, *681*, 189–196. [CrossRef] [PubMed]
10. Miyagawa, M.; Nishio, S.Y.; Usami, S. Deafness Gene Study Consortium. Mutation spectrum and genotype-phenotype correlation of hearing loss patients caused by *SLC26A4* mutations in the Japanese: A large cohort study. *J. Hum. Genet.* **2014**, *59*, 262–268. [CrossRef]
11. Tsukada, K.; Nishio, S.Y.; Hattori, M.; Usami, S. Ethnic-specific spectrum of *GJB2* and *SLC26A4* mutations: Their origin and a literature review. *Ann. Otol. Rhinol. Laryngol.* **2015**, *124* (Suppl. S1), 61S–76S. [CrossRef]
12. Erdenechuluun, J.; Lin, Y.-H.; Ganbat, K.; Bataakhuu, D.; Makhbal, Z.; Tsai, C.-Y.; Lin, Y.-H.; Chan, Y.-H.; Hsu, C.-J.; Hsu, W.-C.; et al. Unique spectra of deafness-associated mutations in Mongolians provide insights into the genetic relationships among Eurasian populations. *PLoS ONE* **2018**, *13*, e0209797. [CrossRef]
13. Wu, C.C.; Tsai, C.Y.; Lin, Y.H.; Chen, P.Y.; Lin, P.H.; Cheng, Y.F.; Wu, C.M.; Lin, Y.H.; Lee, C.Y.; Erdenechuluun, J.; et al. Genetic Epidemiology and Clinical Features of Hereditary Hearing Impairment in the Taiwanese Population. *Genes* **2019**, *10*, 772. [CrossRef] [PubMed]
14. Everett, L.A.; Glaser, B.; Beck, J.C.; Idol, J.R.; Buchs, A.; Heyman, M.; Adawi, F.; Hazani, E.; Nassir, E.; Baxevanis, A.D.; et al. Pendred syndrome is caused by mutations in a putative sulphate transporter gene (PDS). *Nat. Genet.* **1997**, *17*, 411–422. [CrossRef] [PubMed]
15. Everett, L.A.; Morsli, H.; Wu, D.K.; Green, E.D. Expression pattern of the mouse ortholog of the Pendred's syndrome gene (Pds) suggests a key role for pendrin in the inner ear. *Proc. Natl. Acad. Sci. USA* **1999**, *96*, 9727–9732. [CrossRef] [PubMed]
16. Mount, D.B.; Romero, M.F. The SLC26 gene family of multifunctional anion exchangers. *Pflug. Arch.* **2004**, *447*, 710–721. [CrossRef] [PubMed]
17. Honda, K.; Griffith, A.J. Genetic architecture and phenotypic landscape of *SLC26A4*-related hearing loss. *Hum. Genet.* **2021**. [CrossRef]
18. Valvassori, G.E.; Clemis, J.D. The large vestibular aqueduct syndrome. *Laryngoscope* **1978**, *88*, 723–728. [CrossRef] [PubMed]
19. Boston, M.; Halsted, M.; Meinzen-Derr, J.; Bean, J.; Vijayasekaran, S.; Arjmand, E.; Choo, D.; Benton, C.; Greinwald, J. The large vestibular aqueduct: A new definition based on audiologic and computed tomography correlation. *Otolaryngol. Head Neck Surg.* **2007**, *136*, 972–977. [CrossRef] [PubMed]
20. Vijayasekaran, S.; Halsted, M.J.; Boston, M.; Meinzen-Derr, J.; Bardo, D.M.; Greinwald, J.; Benton, C. When is the vestibular aqueduct enlarged? A statistical analysis of the normative distribution of vestibular aqueduct size. *AJNR Am. J. Neuroradiol.* **2007**, *28*, 1133–1138. [CrossRef]
21. Dror, A.A.; Brownstein, Z.; Avraham, K.B. Integration of human and mouse genetics reveals pendrin function in hearing and deafness. *Cell Physiol. Biochem.* **2011**, *28*, 535–544. [CrossRef] [PubMed]
22. Roesch, S.; Rasp, G.; Sarikas, A.; Dossena, S. Genetic Determinants of Non-Syndromic Enlarged Vestibular Aqueduct: A Review. *Audiol. Res.* **2021**, *11*, 40. [CrossRef] [PubMed]
23. Stenson, P.D.; Mort, M.; Ball, E.V.; Chapman, R.; Evans, K.; Azevedo, L.; Hayden, M.; Heywood, S.; Millar, D.S.; Phillips, A.D.; et al. The Human Gene Mutation Database (HGMD®): Optimizing its use in a clinical diagnostic or research setting. *Hum. Genet.* **2020**, *139*, 1197–1207. [CrossRef]
24. Hutchin, T.; Coy, N.N.; Conlon, H.; Telford, E.; Bromelow, K.; Blaydon, D.; Taylor, G.; Coghill, E.; Brown, S.; Trembath, R.; et al. Assessment of the genetic causes of recessive childhood non-syndromic deafness in the UK—Implications for genetic testing. *Clin. Genet.* **2005**, *68*, 506–512. [CrossRef] [PubMed]
25. Pourová, R.; Janousek, P.; Jurovcík, M.; Dvoráková, M.; Malíková, M.; Rasková, D.; Bendová, O.; Leonardi, E.; Murgia, A.; Kabelka, Z.; et al. Spectrum and frequency of *SLC26A4* mutations among Czech patients with early hearing loss with and without Enlarged Vestibular Aqueduct (EVA). *Ann. Hum. Genet.* **2010**, *74*, 299–307. [CrossRef] [PubMed]
26. Nonose, R.W.; Lezirovitz, K.; de Mello Auricchio, M.T.B.; Batissoco, A.C.; Yamamoto, G.L.; Mingroni-Netto, R.C. Mutation analysis of *SLC26A4* (Pendrin) gene in a Brazilian sample of hearing-impaired subjects. *BMC Med. Genet.* **2018**, *19*, 73. [CrossRef] [PubMed]
27. Koohiyan, M. A systematic review of *SLC26A4* mutations causing hearing loss in the Iranian population. *Int. J. Pediatr. Otorhinolaryngol.* **2019**, *125*, 1–5. [CrossRef]
28. Anwar, S.; Riazuddin, S.; Ahmed, Z.M.; Tasneem, S.; Ateeq-ul-Jaleel; Khan, S.Y.; Griffith, A.J.; Friedman, T.B.; Riazuddin, S. SLC26A4 mutation spectrum associated with DFNB4 deafness and Pendred's syndrome in Pakistanis. *J. Hum. Genet.* **2009**, *54*, 266–270. [CrossRef]
29. Chandru, J.; Jeffrey, J.M.; Pavithra, A.; Vanniya, S.P.; Devi, G.N.; Mahalingam, S.; Karthikeyen, N.P.; Srisailapathy, C.R.S. Genetic analysis of *SLC26A4* gene (pendrin) related deafness among a cohort of assortative mating families from southern India. *Eur. Arch. Otorhinolaryngol.* **2020**, *277*, 3021–3035. [CrossRef]

30. Han, J.J.; Nguyen, P.D.; Oh, D.Y.; Han, J.H.; Kim, A.R.; Kim, M.Y.; Park, H.R.; Tran, L.H.; Dung, N.H.; Koo, J.W.; et al. Elucidation of the unique mutation spectrum of severe hearing loss in a Vietnamese pediatric population. *Sci. Rep.* **2019**, *9*, 1604. [CrossRef]
31. Guo, Y.F.; Liu, X.W.; Guan, J.; Han, M.K.; Wang, D.Y.; Zhao, Y.L.; Rao, S.Q.; Wang, Q.J. *GJB2*, *SLC26A4* and mitochondrial DNA A1555G mutations in prelingual deafness in Northern Chinese subjects. *Acta Otolaryngol.* **2008**, *128*, 297–303. [CrossRef] [PubMed]
32. Chai, Y.; Huang, Z.; Tao, Z.; Li, X.; Li, L.; Li, Y.; Wu, H.; Yang, T. Molecular etiology of hearing impairment associated with nonsyndromic enlarged vestibular aqueduct in East China. *Am. J. Med. Genet. A* **2013**, *161A*, 2226–2233. [CrossRef] [PubMed]
33. Xiang, Y.B.; Tang, S.H.; Li, H.Z.; Xu, C.Y.; Chen, C.; Xu, Y.Z.; Ding, L.R.; Xu, X.Q. Mutation analysis of common deafness-causing genes among 506 patients with nonsyndromic hearing loss from Wenzhou city, China. *Int. J. Pediatr. Otorhinolaryngol.* **2019**, *122*, 185–190. [CrossRef] [PubMed]
34. Zhang, M.; Han, Y.; Zhang, F.; Bai, X.; Wang, H. Mutation spectrum and hotspots of the common deafness genes in 314 patients with nonsyndromic hearing loss in Heze area, China. *Acta Otolaryngol.* **2019**, *139*, 612–617. [CrossRef] [PubMed]
35. Pang, X.; Chai, Y.; Chen, P.; He, L.; Wang, X.; Wu, H.; Yang, T. Mono-allelic mutations of *SLC26A4* is over-presented in deaf patients with non-syndromic enlarged vestibular aqueduct. *Int. J. Pediatr. Otorhinolaryngol.* **2015**, *79*, 1351–1353. [CrossRef]
36. Rah, Y.C.; Kim, A.R.; Koo, J.W.; Lee, J.H.; Oh, S.H.; Choi, B.Y. Audiologic presentation of enlargement of the vestibular aqueduct according to the *SLC26A4* genotypes. *Laryngoscope* **2015**, *125*, E216–E222. [CrossRef] [PubMed]
37. Tian, Y.; Xu, H.; Liu, D.; Zhang, J.; Yang, Z.; Zhang, S.; Liu, H.; Li, R.; Tian, Y.; Zeng, B.; et al. Increased diagnosis of enlarged vestibular aqueduct by multiplex PCR enrichment and next-generation sequencing of the *SLC26A4* gene. *Mol. Genet. Genom. Med.* **2021**, *9*, e1734. [CrossRef] [PubMed]
38. Du, W.; Guo, Y.; Wang, C.; Wang, Y.; Liu, X. A systematic review and meta-analysis of common mutations of *SLC26A4* gene in Asian populations. *Int. J. Pediatr. Otorhinolaryngol.* **2013**, *77*, 1670–1676. [CrossRef] [PubMed]
39. Lu, Y.J.; Yao, J.; Wei, Q.J.; Xing, G.Q.; Cao, X. Diagnostic Value of *SLC26A4* Mutation Status in Hereditary Hearing Loss With EVA: A PRISMA-Compliant Meta-Analysis. *Medicine* **2015**, *94*, e2248. [CrossRef]
40. Mongush, M.V. Tuvans of Mongolia and China. *Int. J. Cent. Asian Stud.* **1996**, *1*, 225–243.
41. Chen, Z.; Zhang, Y.; Fan, A.; Zhang, Y.; Wu, Y.; Zhao, Q.; Zhou, Y.; Zhou, C.; Bawudong, M.; Mao, X.; et al. Brief communication: Y-chromosome haplogroup analysis indicates that Chinese Tuvans share distinctive affinity with Siberian Tuvans. *Am. J. Phys. Anthropol.* **2011**, *144*, 492–497. [CrossRef]
42. Vainshtein, S.I.; Mannay-Ool, M.H. *History of Tyva*, 2nd ed.; Science: Novosibirsk, Russia, 2001. (In Russian)
43. Mannai-ool, M.K. *Tuvan People. The Origin and Formation of the Ethnos*; Nauka Publ.: Novosibirsk, Russia, 2004; pp. 99–166. (In Russian)
44. Potapov, L.P. *Ethnical Structure and Origin of Altaians*; Nauka: Leningrad, Russia, 1969. (In Russian)
45. Posukh, O.; Pallares-Ruiz, N.; Tadinova, V.; Osipova, L.; Claustres, M.; Roux, A.-F. First molecular screening of deafness in the Altai Republic population. *BMC Med. Genet.* **2005**, *6*, 12. [CrossRef] [PubMed]
46. Dzhemileva, L.U.; Posukh, O.L.; Tazetdinov, A.M.; Barashkov, N.A.; Zhuravskiĭ, S.G.; Ponidelko, S.N.; Markova, T.G.; Tadinova, V.N.; Fedorova, S.A.; Maksimova, N.R.; et al. Analysis of mitochondrial 12S rRNA and tRNA(Ser(UCN)) genes in patients with nonsyndromic sensorineural hearing loss from various regions of Russia. *Genetika* **2009**, *45*, 982–991. (In Russian) [CrossRef]
47. Churbanov, A.Y.; Karafet, T.M.; Morozov, I.V.; Mikhalskaia, V.Y.; Zytsar, M.V.; Bondar, A.A.; Posukh, O.L. Whole Exome Sequencing Reveals Homozygous Mutations in *RAI1*, *OTOF*, and *SLC26A4* Genes Associated with Nonsyndromic Hearing Loss in Altaian Families (South Siberia). *PLoS ONE* **2016**, *11*, e0153841. [CrossRef]
48. Posukh, O.L.; Zytsar, M.V.; Bady-Khoo, M.S.; Danilchenko, V.Y.; Maslova, E.A.; Barashkov, N.A.; Bondar, A.A.; Morozov, I.V.; Maximov, V.N.; Voevoda, M.I. Unique mutational spectrum of the *GJB2* Gene and its pathogenic contribution to deafness in Tuvinians (Southern Siberia, Russia): A high prevalence of rare variant c.516G>C (p.Trp172Cys). *Genes* **2019**, *10*, 429. [CrossRef]
49. Posukh, O.L.; (Institute of Cytology and Genetics, Novosibirsk, Russia). Personal communication, 2019.
50. Danilchenko, V.Y.; (Institute of Cytology and Genetics, Novosibirsk, Russia). Personal communication, 2020.
51. Zytsar, M.V.; Bady-Khoo, M.S.; Danilchenko, V.Y.; Maslova, E.A.; Barashkov, N.A.; Morozov, I.V.; Bondar, A.A.; Posukh, O.L. High Rates of Three Common *GJB2* Mutations c.516G>C, c.-23+1G>A, c.235delC in Deaf Patients from Southern Siberia Are Due to the Founder Effect. *Genes* **2020**, *11*, 833. [CrossRef] [PubMed]
52. Zhang, Y. I-TASSER server for protein 3D structure prediction. *BMC Bioinform.* **2008**, *9*, 40. [CrossRef] [PubMed]
53. Roy, A.; Kucukural, A.; Zhang, Y. I-TASSER: A unified platform for automated protein structure and function prediction. *Nat. Protoc.* **2010**, *5*, 725–738. [CrossRef] [PubMed]
54. Yang, J.; Yan, R.; Roy, A.; Xu, D.; Poisson, J.; Zhang, Y. The I-TASSER Suite: Protein structure and function prediction. *Nat. Methods* **2015**, *12*, 7–8. [CrossRef] [PubMed]
55. Guex, N.; Peitsch, M.C. SWISS-MODEL and the Swiss-PdbViewer: An environment for comparative protein modeling. *Electrophoresis* **1997**, *18*, 2714–2723. [CrossRef]
56. Dewan, K.; Wippold, F.J., 2nd; Lieu, J.E. Enlarged vestibular aqueduct in pediatric sensorineural hearing loss. *Otolaryngol. Head Neck Surg.* **2009**, *140*, 552–558. [CrossRef] [PubMed]
57. Coucke, P.J.; van Hauwe, P.; Everett, L.A.; Demirhan, O.; Kabakkaya, Y.; Dietrich, N.L.; Smith, R.J.; Coyle, E.; Reardon, W.; Trembath, R.; et al. Identification of two different mutations in the *PDS* gene in an inbred family with Pendred syndrome. *J. Med. Genet.* **1999**, *36*, 475–477.

58. Dai, P.; Li, Q.; Huang, D.; Yuan, Y.; Kang, D.; Miller, D.T.; Shao, H.; Zhu, Q.; He, J.; Yu, F.; et al. *SLC26A4* c.919-2A>G varies among Chinese ethnic groups as a cause of hearing loss. *Genet. Med.* **2008**, *10*, 586–592. [CrossRef] [PubMed]
59. Van Hauwe, P.; Everett, L.A.; Coucke, P.; Scott, D.A.; Kraft, M.L.; Ris-Stalpers, C.; Bolder, C.; Otten, B.; de Vijlder, J.J.; Dietrich, N.L.; et al. Two frequent missense mutations in Pendred syndrome. *Hum. Mol. Genet.* **1998**, *7*, 1099–1104. [CrossRef]
60. Usami, S.; Abe, S.; Weston, M.D.; Shinkawa, H.; van Camp, G.; Kimberling, W.J. Non-syndromic hearing loss associated with enlarged vestibular aqueduct is caused by *PDS* mutations. *Hum. Genet.* **1999**, *104*, 188–192. [CrossRef] [PubMed]
61. Shin, J.W.; Lee, S.C.; Lee, H.K.; Park, H.J. Genetic screening of *GJB2* and *SLC26A4* in Korean cochlear implantees: Experience of Soree ear clinic. *Clin. Exp. Otorhinolaryngol.* **2012**, *5* (Suppl. S1), S10–S13. [CrossRef] [PubMed]
62. Wu, C.C.; Yeh, T.H.; Chen, P.J.; Hsu, C.J. Prevalent *SLC26A4* mutations in patients with enlarged vestibular aqueduct and/or Mondini dysplasia: A unique spectrum of mutations in Taiwan, including a frequent founder mutation. *Laryngoscope* **2005**, *115*, 1060–1064. [CrossRef] [PubMed]
63. Gillam, M.P.; Sidhaye, A.R.; Lee, E.J.; Rutishauser, J.; Stephan, C.W.; Kopp, P. Functional characterization of pendrin in a polarized cell system. Evidence for pendrin-mediated apical iodide efflux. *J. Biol. Chem.* **2004**, *279*, 13004–13010. [CrossRef] [PubMed]
64. Yoon, J.S.; Park, H.J.; Yoo, S.Y.; Namkung, W.; Jo, M.J.; Koo, S.K.; Park, H.Y.; Lee, W.S.; Kim, K.H.; Lee, M.G. Heterogeneity in the processing defect of *SLC26A4* mutants. *J. Med. Genet.* **2008**, *45*, 411–419. [CrossRef]
65. Lee, H.J.; Jung, J.; Shin, J.W.; Song, M.H.; Kim, S.H.; Lee, J.H.; Lee, K.A.; Shin, S.; Kim, U.K.; Bok, J.; et al. Correlation between genotype and phenotype in patients with bi-allelic *SLC26A4* mutations. *Clin. Genet.* **2014**, *86*, 270–275. [CrossRef]
66. Zhao, J.; Yuan, Y.; Huang, S.; Huang, B.; Cheng, J.; Kang, D.; Wang, G.; Han, D.; Dai, P. KCNJ10 may not be a contributor to nonsyndromic enlargement of vestibular aqueduct (NSEVA) in Chinese subjects. *PLoS ONE* **2014**, *9*, e108134. [CrossRef]
67. Khan, M.R.; Bashir, R.; Naz, S. *SLC26A4* mutations in patients with moderate to severe hearing loss. *Biochem. Genet.* **2013**, *51*, 514–523. [CrossRef] [PubMed]
68. Cengiz, F.B.; Yilmazer, R.; Olgun, L.; Sennaroglu, L.; Kirazli, T.; Alper, H.; Olgun, Y.; Incesulu, A.; Atik, T.; Huesca-Hernandez, F.; et al. Novel pathogenic variants underlie *SLC26A4*-related hearing loss in a multiethnic cohort. *Int. J. Pediatr. Otorhinolaryngol.* **2017**, *101*, 167–171. [CrossRef]
69. Uzumcu, A.; Uyguner, O.; Ulubil-Emiroglu, M.; Hafiz, G.; Baserer, N.; Eris, H.; Basaran, S.; Wollnik, B. Compound heterozygosity for novel and known mutations in *SLC26A4* cause large vestibular aqueduct. *Balkan J. Med. Genet.* **2006**, *9*, 105.
70. Pryor, S.P.; Madeo, A.C.; Reynolds, J.C.; Sarlis, N.J.; Arnos, K.S.; Nance, W.E.; Yang, Y.; Zalewski, C.K.; Brewer, C.C.; Butman, J.A.; et al. *SLC26A4/PDS* genotype-phenotype correlation in hearing loss with enlargement of the vestibular aqueduct (EVA): Evidence that Pendred syndrome and non-syndromic EVA are distinct clinical and genetic entities. *J. Med. Genet.* **2005**, *42*, 159–165. [CrossRef] [PubMed]
71. Pique, L.M.; Brennan, M.L.; Davidson, C.J.; Schaefer, F.; Greinwald, J., Jr.; Schrijver, I. Mutation analysis of the *SLC26A4*, *FOXI1* and *KCNJ10* genes in individuals with congenital hearing loss. *PeerJ* **2014**, *2*, e384. [CrossRef] [PubMed]
72. Smits, J.J.; de Bruijn, S.E.; Lanting, C.P.; Oostrik, J.; O'Gorman, L.; Mantere, T.; DOOFNL Consortium; Cremers, F.P.M.; Roosing, S.; Yntema, H.G.; et al. Exploring the missing heritability in subjects with hearing loss, enlarged vestibular aqueducts, and a single or no pathogenic *SLC26A4* variant. *Hum. Genet.* **2021**. [CrossRef]

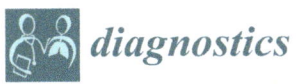

Case Report

When Familial Hearing Loss Means Genetic Heterogeneity: A Model Case Report

Camille Cenni [1,2], Luke Mansard [2], Catherine Blanchet [3,4], David Baux [2,5], Christel Vaché [2,5], Corinne Baudoin [2], Mélodie Moclyn [2], Valérie Faugère [2], Michel Mondain [3], Eric Jeziorski [6], Anne-Françoise Roux [2,5,†] and Marjolaine Willems [1,*,†]

1. Département de Génétique Médicale, Maladies Rares et Médecine Personnalisée, CHU Montpellier, Université de Montpellier, 34090 Montpellier, France; camille.cenni@chu-montpellier.fr
2. Laboratoire de Génétique Moléculaire, CHU Montpellier, Université de Montpellier, 34090 Monpellier, France; l-mansard@chu-montpellier.fr (L.M.); david.baux@inserm.fr (D.B.); christel.vache@inserm.fr (C.V.); corinne.baudoin@inserm.fr (C.B.); melodie.moclyn@inserm.fr (M.M.); valerie.faugere@inserm.fr (V.F.); anne-francoise.roux@inserm.fr (A.-F.R.)
3. Service ORL, CHU Montpellier, Université de Montpellier, 34090 Montpellier, France; c-blanchet@chu-montpellier.fr (C.B.); m.mondain@chu-montpellier.fr (M.M)
4. Centre National de Référence Maladies Rares "Affections Sensorielles Génétiques", CHU Montpellier, Université de Montpellier, 34090 Montpellier, France
5. INM, Université de Montpellier, INSERM U1298, 34090 Montpellier, France
6. Service de Pédiatrie Générale, Infectiologie et Immunologie Clinique, CHU Montpellier, Université de Montpellier, 34090 Montpellier, France; e-jeziorski@chu-montpellier.fr
* Correspondence: m-willems@chu-montpellier.fr
† These authors contributed equally to this work.

Abstract: We describe a family with both hearing loss (HL) and thrombocytopenia, caused by pathogenic variants in three genes. The proband was a child with neonatal thrombocytopenia, childhood-onset HL, hyper-laxity and severe myopia. The child's mother (and some of her relatives) presented with moderate thrombocytopenia and adulthood-onset HL. The child's father (and some of his relatives) presented with adult-onset HL. An HL panel analysis, completed by whole exome sequencing, was performed in this complex family. We identified three pathogenic variants in three different genes: *MYH9*, *MYO7A* and *ACTG1*. The thrombocytopenia in the child and her mother is explained by the *MYH9* variant. The post-lingual HL in the paternal branch is explained by the *MYO7A* variant, absent in the proband, while the congenital HL of the child is explained by a de novo *ACTG1* variant. This family, in which HL segregates, illustrates that multiple genetic conditions coexist in individuals and make patient care more complex than expected.

Keywords: familial hearing loss; multiple diagnoses; non-syndromic hearing loss; *ACTG1*; *MYH9*

1. Introduction

Hereditary hearing loss (HL) is the most common sensory-neural deficit and is characterized by a high degree of genetic and phenotypic heterogeneity. More than 70% of genetic HL is non-syndromic (non-syndromic hearing loss, NSHL) and can follow a pattern of autosomal recessive (AR) inheritance in 75–80% of cases, autosomal dominant (AD) inheritance in 20–25% of cases and X-linked inheritance in 1–1.5% of cases [1]. More than 120 responsible genes have been identified to date (https://hereditaryhearingloss.org/, last reviewed in 17 December 2020), of which there are at least 45 genes in patients with ADNSHL. Some of them are also involved in syndromic entities.

The development of massively parallel sequencing (MPS), which allows the study of thousands of genes simultaneously, whole exome and whole genome, has allowed one to highlight the concept of "atypical phenotype" as instances of dual or more molecular diagnoses [2]. The occurrence of multiple molecular diagnoses in a single individual has been reported in 2–7.2% of cases [2,3].

In this article, we describe a family with both HL and thrombocytopenia caused by pathogenic variants in *MYO7A*, *ACTG1* and *MYH9* genes.

2. Materials and Methods

2.1. Clinical Report

The proband was 3 years old when referred, issued from unrelated Caucasian parents (Figure 1A). She was born at term after a normal pregnancy, without cytomegalovirus infection. All birth parameters were normal (50th centile), and otoacoustic emissions were present at birth. She presented neonatal thrombopenia (between 1000 and 3000 platelets/mm^3) with subependymal and retinal hemorrhages without clinical severity, treated by two platelet transfusions and one immunoglobulin infusion. At 6 months, she had a normal platelet count (160,000/mm^3). She was able to walk at 18 months and had normal development. An absence of language at 18 months led to the diagnosis of evolutive moderate-to-severe sensorineural HL (Figure 1B). A subsequent analysis at 2 and 2.5 years confirmed an asymptomatic and chronic thrombocytopenia. At 7 years and 9 months of age, she weighed 24.5 kg (70th centile), measured 126 cm (75th centile) and her head circumference was 52.5 cm (30th centile). She presented some ecchymoses but no severe hemorrhages, a ligamental hyper-laxity and advanced myopia (-7 diopters in the right eye and -10.5 diopters in the left eye) associated with large optic discs.

In the paternal branch, at least five men over two generations presented with evolutive, sensorineural HL, with an onset in the third decade (Figure 1A,B), suggesting an AD sensorineural HL inheritance. Four women, from three generations, in the maternal branch, presented with non-severe thrombopenia, between 20,000 and 100,000 platelets/mm^3, associated with a sensorineural HL, with an onset of around 40 years of age (Figure 1A,B). The proband's mother developed mild deafness at 40 years old.

2.2. Molecular Analysis

Informed consent for genetic analysis was obtained from the family in compliance with national ethics regulations. DNA from all affected members was isolated from peripheral blood samples by standard procedures.

2.2.1. NSHL Gene Panel Sequencing

Both proband and father underwent MPS gene panel testing. In total, 74 NSHL genes were screened using the NimbleGen SeqCap EZ Choice technology [4]. Each exon (coding and non-coding) and its surrounding 50 bp intronic sequences, referenced in RefSeq or Ensembl, was targeted. Sequencing was performed on an Illumina MiSeq instrument (version 2 chemistry), and we used the MiSeqReporter software (v2.5) for the secondary analysis of the generated data. Variant calling files (VCFs) were automatically included in our in-house database system (USHVaM2), which also handled variant annotation. Lastly, variants of interest were confirmed by Sanger sequencing, and segregation analysis was performed on available members of the family.

2.2.2. Whole Exome Sequencing (WES)

Genomic DNA was obtained from blood samples belonging to the proband and her parents. Library preparation was performed with the Nimbelgen SeqCap EZ MedExome kit (Roche Technology) according to the manufacturer's instructions. Exome-enriched libraries were sequenced using the Illumina NextSeq system (Illumina, San Diego, CA, USA). Bioinformatic analysis of sequencing data was based on an in-house pipeline (https://github.com/beboche/nenufaar, accessed on 17 December 2019) generate a merged BAM and VCF file for the family. Quality data revealed more than 91% of the target nucleotides covered at 30X for individuals with an average coverage of 120X. Tertiary analysis involved the MobiDL captainAchab workflow (https://github.com/mobidic/MobiDL, accessed on 17 December 2019), based on ANNOVAR [5], MPA [6] and Captain-ACHAB (https://github.com/mobidic/Captain-ACHAB, accessed on 17 December 2019).

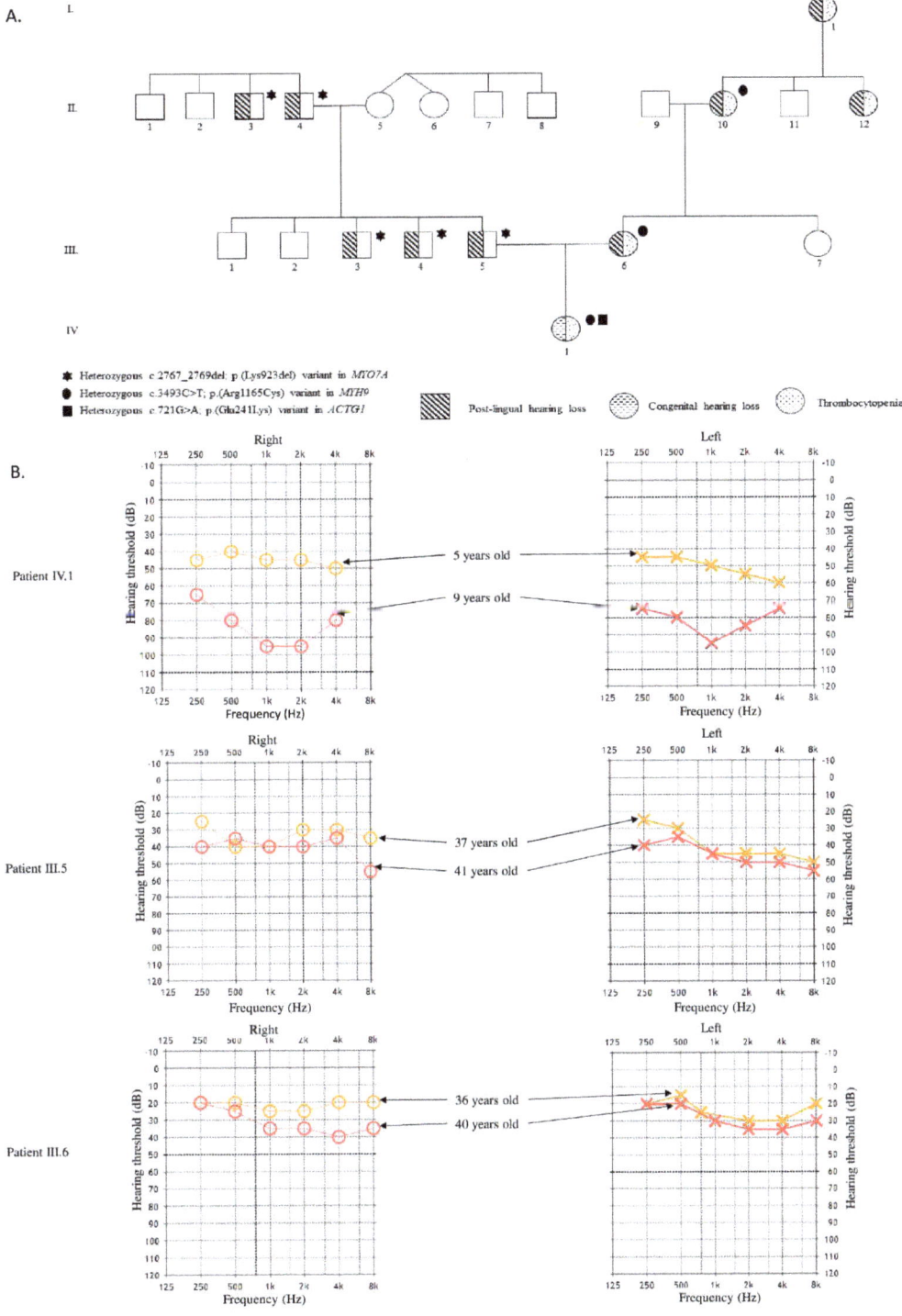

Figure 1. (**A**): Pedigree of the family. (**B**): Audiograms of proband and her parents.

3. Results

The gene panel study identified two heterozygous variants in *MYH9* and in *ACTG1* in the proband (Figure 1A).

The c.3493C>T; p.(Arg1165Cys) variation in *MYH9* (NM_002473.5) has already been reported to be implicated in *MYH9* syndromic disease [7]. The mother and maternal grandmother were also heterozygous for this variant. The c.721G>A; p.(Glu241Lys) variant in the *ACTG1* gene (NM_001614.4) has already previously been detected in a family with ADNSHL [8]. This variant was absent in the parents, supporting a de novo occurrence, although a germline mosaicism could not be excluded. Gene panel testing was then performed for the father to elucidate the origin of his HL, and the c.2767_2769del; p.(Lys923del) variation in the *MYO7A* gene (NM_000260.3) was identified. It was absent from the control population databases (GnomAD, dbSNP). Sanger analysis confirmed the segregation of the variant in all the hearing-impaired members of the paternal branch. It is classified as likely pathogenic according to ACMG criteria [9]. We submitted this variant to the ClinVar database in NCBI (www.ncbi.nlm.nih.gov/clinvar/, accession number: VCV000930183.1, accessed on 19 June 2020).

WES was performed on the trio to explain the hyper-laxity and the myopia diagnosed in the proband, but no additional variants of interest could be identified.

4. Discussion

In conclusion, alterations in three different genes are responsible for the symptoms present in this family. The thrombocytopenia and the HL segregating in the maternal branch are explained by the *MYH9* variant. The child's HL is explained by the de novo *ACTG1* variant, and the HL on her father's side is explained by the *MYO7A* variant.

We report a new variant in the *MYO7A* gene, p.(Lys923del), resulting in an in-frame loss of a conserved lysine residue at codon 923, which segregates with the disease in this family, compatible with AD transmission. The *MYO7A* (*276903) encodes an unconventional myosin and is expressed in the pigment epithelium, the photoreceptor cells of the retina and the human embryonic cochlear and vestibular neuroepithelia [10]. Pathogenic alterations have been reported to cause syndromic HL (Usher syndrome type 1B, #276900) [10] or NSHL (DFNB2, #600060 and DFNA11, #601317) [10,11]. DFNA11 is characterized by a symmetric and progressive neurosensory HL with post-lingual onset. However, the degree of HL can be significantly different within the same family or among patients in the same age group [11]. Liu et al. had previously reported a family with DFNA11 and an in-frame 9-bp deletion leading to the loss of three residues, including two lysines at codons 887 and 888 [11]. Both this mutation and our variant are located in the same single alpha-helix (SAH) region. The SAH regions are rich in charged residues, which are predicted to stabilize the alpha-helical structure by ionic bonds and are constant force springs in proteins [12]. We concluded that p.(Leu923del) is a new dominant pathogenic variant.

The *ACTG1* gene (*102560) encodes actin gamma 1, a member of a highly conserved cytoskeletal protein family that plays fundamental roles in nearly all aspects of eukaryotic cell biology. This protein is particularly abundant in the specialized hair cells of the inner ear. *ACTG1* was identified as a causative gene for ADNSHL (DFNA20/26, #604717) [13]. Patients present with progressive post-lingual HL, and the age of onset ranges between the first and the fourth decades. Very early-onset or pre-lingual-onset HL has already been described [13]. *ACTG1* is also implicated in Baraitser–Winter syndrome type 2 (BWS2, #614583), which is a rare developmental syndrome characterized by dysmorphism traits, intellectual disability and congenital anomalies [14]. However, no genotype–phenotype correlation has been made to explain both syndromic and non-syndromic diseases linked to *ACTG1* [13]. We reviewed the *ACTG1* variants to compare the position in the gene and in the protein domains, the difference between the wild-type and the mutated residues, the impact on the conformation and the protein interactions. Any of the variants implicated in one or the other diseases are heterozygous missense. We compared 35 different variants: 11 implicated in the BWS2 (31%) and 24 in the DFNA20/26 (69%). Variants are distributed over the entire gene without regional clusters (Figure 2). No variant is involved in both BWS2 and DFNA20/26. Interestingly, two different variants alter the same residue: p.(Glu334Gln) involved in BWS2 and p.(Glu334Asp) in DFNA20/26. We evaluated the possible alteration of the conformation and the interactions with other molecules through the Hope3D website (https://www3.cmbi.umcn.nl/hope/input/, accessed on 19 June 2020) [15]. We found that more 8/11 BWS2 variants (73%) than 9/24 DFNA20/26 variants (37.5%) could alter the conformation of the gamma-actin based on the residues' size or polarity difference. We also found that only 1/11 BWS2 variants (9%) whereas 9/24 DFNA20/26 variants (37.5%) could alter the "predicted" interaction between the protein and its ligands. However, the functional consequences of *ACTG1* heterozygous missense in BWS2 and DFNA20/26 still remain unclear. Rivière et al. suggested that BWS2 represents the severe end of a spectrum of cytoplasmic actin-associated phenotypes that begins with DFNA20/26 and extends to BWS2 [16].

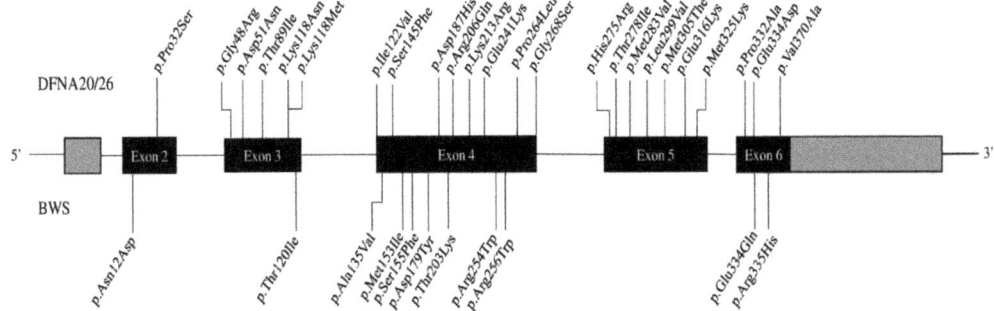

Figure 2. *ACTG1* variants. Schematic representation of the full-length *ACTG1* gene showing the different exons and locations of the reported variants. Variants associated with DFNA20/26 are indicated above the gene and those associated with BWS2 are below the gene.

We found no explanation for the severe myopia and hyper-laxity. BWS2 is associated with ocular features, including microphthalmia or coloboma [17], and articular features with progressive joint stiffness, which are not similar to those observed in our patient. Therefore, we cannot conclude whether the hyper-laxity and myopia observed in our patient are related to the extra-auditory features from the *ACTG1*-related disorder.

5. Conclusions

Prior to molecular investigations, we postulated that the proband had inherited two AD adulthood-onset HL defects, explaining a more severe and childhood-onset phenotype. However, we were surprised to find a de novo *ACTG1* variant as the cause of her HL.

In this study, we show that it is necessary to perform systematic and unbiased molecular studies in several individuals within a family when phenotypes resemble one another but are not the same. This is especially true in pathologies such as HL, which is frequent and genetically heterogeneous.

Author Contributions: Investigation, C.C., L.M., C.B. (Catherine Blanchet), M.M. (Michel Mondain), E.J. and M.W.; Data curation, C.V.; Writing—original draft preparation, C.C.; Writing—review and editing, L.M., D.B., C.B. (Catherine Blanchet), C.V., M.M. (Mélodie Moclyn), C.B. (Corinne Baudoin) and V.F.; Supervision, A.-F.R. and M.W. All authors have read and agreed to the published version of the manuscript.

Funding: This research received no external funding.

Institutional Review Board Statement: Institutional Review Board (IRB) of CHU de Montpellier: 2018_IRB-MTP_05-05 obtained on the 15 June 2018.

Informed Consent Statement: Informed consent was obtained from all subjects involved in the study.

Data Availability Statement: Not applicable.

Conflicts of Interest: The authors declare no conflict of interest.

References

1. Smith, R.J.H.; Hildebrand, M.S.; Shearer, A.E.; Adam, M.P.; Ardinger, H.H.; Pagon, R.A.; Wallace, S.E.; Bean, L.J.H.; Mirzaa, G.; Amemiya, A. Deafness and hereditary hearing loss overview. In *GeneReviews*; University of Washington: Seattle, WA, USA, 1999.
2. Posey, J.E.; Harel, T.; Liu, P.; Rosenfeld, J.A.; James, R.A.; Coban Akdemir, Z.H.; Walkiewicz, M.; Bi, W.; Xiao, R.; Ding, Y.; et al. Resolution of disease phenotypes resulting from multilocus genomic variation. *N. Engl. J. Med.* **2017**, *376*, 21–31. [CrossRef] [PubMed]
3. Smith, E.D.; Blanco, K.; Sajan, S.A.; Hunter, J.M.; Shinde, D.N.; Wayburn, B.; Rossi, M.; Huang, J.; Stevens, C.A.; Muss, C.; et al. A retrospective review of multiple findings in diagnostic exome sequencing: Half are distinct and half are overlapping diagnoses. *Genet. Med.* **2019**, *21*, 2199–2207. [CrossRef] [PubMed]
4. Baux, D.; Vaché, C.; Blanchet, C.; Willems, M.; Baudoin, C.; Moclyn, M.; Faugère, V.; Touraine, R.; Isidor, B.; Dupin-Deguine, D.; et al. Combined genetic approaches yield a 48% diagnostic rate in a large cohort of French hearing-impaired patients. *Sci. Rep.* **2017**, *7*, 16783. [CrossRef] [PubMed]
5. Wang, K.; Li, M.; Hakonarson, H. ANNOVAR: Functional annotation of genetic variants from high-throughput sequencing data. *Nucleic Acids Res.* **2010**, *38*, e164. [CrossRef] [PubMed]
6. Yauy, K.; Baux, D.; Pegeot, H.; Van Goethem, C.; Mathieu, C.; Guignard, T.; Morales, R.J.; Lacourt, D.; Krahn, M.; Lehtokari, V.L.; et al. MoBiDiC prioritization algorithm, a free, accessible, and efficient pipeline for single-nucleotide variant annotation and prioritization for next-generation sequencing routine molecular diagnosis. *J. Mol. Diagn.* **2018**, *20*, 465–473. [CrossRef] [PubMed]
7. Kunishima, S.; Matsushita, T.; Kojima, T.; Amemiya, N.; Choi, Y.M.; Hosaka, N.; Inoue, M.; Jung, Y.; Mamiya, S.; Matsumoto, K.; et al. Identification of six novel *MYH9* mutations and genotype-phenotype relationships in autosomal dominant macrothrombocytopenia with leukocyte inclusions. *J. Hum. Genet.* **2001**, *46*, 722–729. [CrossRef]
8. Morín, M.; Bryan, K.E.; Mayo-Merino, F.; Goodyear, R.; Mencía, Á.; Modamio-Høybjør, S.; del Castillo, I.; Cabalka, J.M.; Richardson, G.; Moreno, F.; et al. In vivo and in vitro effects of two novel gamma-actin (*ACTG1*) mutations that cause DFNA20/26 hearing impairment. *Hum. Mol. Genet.* **2009**, *18*, 3075–3089. [CrossRef] [PubMed]
9. Richards, S.; Aziz, N.; Bale, S.; Bick, D.; Das, S.; Gastier-Foster, J.; Grody, W.W.; Hegde, M.; Lyon, E.; Spector, E.; et al. Standards and guidelines for the interpretation of sequence variants: A joint consensus recommendation of the American College of Medical Genetics and Genomics and the Association for Molecular Pathology. *Genet. Med.* **2015**, *17*, 405–424. [CrossRef] [PubMed]
10. Friedman, T.B.; Sellers, J.R.; Avraham, K.B. Unconventional myosins and the genetics of hearing loss. *Am. J. Med. Genet.* **1999**, *89*, 147–157. [CrossRef]
11. Liu, X.Z.; Walsh, J.; Tamagawa, Y.; Kitamura, K.; Nishizawa, M.; Steel, K.P.; Brown, S.D. Autosomal dominant non-syndromic deafness caused by a mutation in the myosin VIIA gene. *Nat. Genet.* **1997**, *17*, 268–269. [CrossRef] [PubMed]
12. Wolny, M.; Batchelor, M.; Knight, P.J.; Paci, E.; Dougan, L.; Peckham, M. Stable single alpha-helices are constant force springs in proteins. *J. Biol. Chem.* **2014**, *289*, 27825–27835. [CrossRef] [PubMed]
13. Lee, C.G.; Jang, J.; Jin, H.S. A novel missense mutation in the *ACTG1* gene in a family with congenital autosomal dominant deafness: A case report. *Mol. Med. Rep.* **2018**, *17*, 7611–7617. [CrossRef] [PubMed]
14. Di Donato, N.; Rump, A.; Koenig, R.; Der Kaloustian, V.M.; Halal, F.; Sonntag, K.; Krause, C.; Hackmann, K.; Hahn, G.; Schrock, E.; et al. Severe forms of Baraitser-Winter syndrome are caused by *ACTB* mutations rather than *ACTG1* mutations. *Eur. J. Hum. Genet.* **2014**, *22*, 179–183. [CrossRef] [PubMed]
15. Venselaar, H.; Te Beek, T.; Kuipers, R.; Hekkelman, M.; Vriend, G. Protein structure analysis of mutations causing inheritable diseases. An e-science approach with life scientist friendly interfaces. *BMC Bioinform.* **2010**, *11*, 548. [CrossRef] [PubMed]
16. Rivière, J.B.; Van Bon, B.W.; Hoischen, A.; Kholmanskikh, S.S.; O'Roak, B.J.; Gilissen, C.; Gijsen, S.; Sullivan, C.T.; Christian, S.L.; Abdul-Rahman, O.A.; et al. De novo mutations in the actin genes *ACTB* and *ACTG1* cause Baraitser-Winter syndrome. *Nat. Genet.* **2012**, *44*, 440–444. [CrossRef] [PubMed]
17. Rainger, J.; Williamson, K.A.; Soares, D.C.; Truch, J.; Kurian, D.; Gillessen-Kaesbach, G.; Seawright, A.; Prendergast, J.; Halachev, M.; Wheeler, A.; et al. A recurrent de novo mutation in *ACTG1* causes isolated ocular coloboma. *Hum. Mutat.* **2017**, *38*, 942–946. [CrossRef] [PubMed]

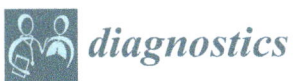

Case Report

An Atypical Case of Head Tremor and Extensive White Matter in an Adult Female Caused by 3-Hydroxy-3-methylglutaryl-CoA Lyase Deficiency

Nassim Boutouchent [1], Julie Bourilhon [2,3], Bénédicte Sudrié-Arnaud [1], Antoine Bonnevalle [2], Lucie Guyant-Maréchal [3], Cécile Acquaviva [4], Loréna Dujardin-Ippolito [1], Soumeya Bekri [1], Ivana Dabaj [5] and Abdellah Tebani [1,*]

1. Normandie University, UNIROUEN, INSERM U1245, CHU Rouen, Department of Metabolic Biochemistry, 76000 Rouen, France; Nassim.Boutouchent@chu-rouen.fr (N.B.); b.sudrie-Arnaud@chu-rouen.fr (B.S.-A.); L.Dujardin-Ippolito@chu-rouen.fr (L.D.-I.); soumeya.bekri@chu-rouen.fr (S.B.)
2. Rouen University Hospital, CHU de Rouen, Department of Neurology, 76000 Rouen, France; Julie.Bourilhon@chu-rouen.fr (J.B.); Antoine.Bonnevalle@chu-rouen.fr (A.B)
3. Department of Neurophysiology, Rouen University Hospital, 76000 Rouen, France; Lucie.Guyant@chu-rouen.fr
4. Department of Biochemistry and Molecular Biology, Inborn Errors of Metabolism, Center of Biology and Pathology Est, CHU Lyon, 69310 Bron, France; cecile.acquaviva-bourdain@chu-lyon.fr
5. Normandie University, UNIROUEN, INSERM U1245, CHU Rouen, Department of Neonatal Pediatrics, Intensive Care and Neuropediatrics, 76000 Rouen, France; ivana.dabaj@chu-rouen.fr
* Correspondence: abdellah.tebani@chu-rouen.fr

Abstract: 3-Hydroxy-3-methylglutaryl-CoA (HMG-CoA) Lyase deficiency (HMGLD) (OMIM 246450) is an autosomal recessive genetic disorder caused by homozygous or compound heterozygous variants in the *HMGCL* gene located on 1p36.11. Clinically, this disorder is characterized by a life-threatening metabolic intoxication with a presentation including severe hypoglycemia without ketosis, metabolic acidosis, hyper-ammoniemia, hepatomegaly and a coma. HMGLD clinical onset is within the first few months of life after a symptomatic free period. In nonacute periods, the treatment is based on a protein- and fat-restricted diet. L-carnitine supplementation is recommended. A late onset presentation has been described in very few cases, and only two adult cases have been reported. The present work aims to describe an incidental discovery of an HMGLD case in a 54-year-old patient and reports a comprehensive review of clinical and biological features in adult patients to raise awareness about the late-onset presentation of this disease.

Keywords: HMGLD; *HMGCL*; HMG-CoA lyase deficiency; NGS; inherited metabolic diseases

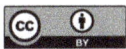

1. Introduction

The 3-Hydroxy-3-methylglutaryl-CoA Lyase (HMG-CoA Lyase) enzyme is involved in both L-Leucine catabolism and ketone bodies anabolism (Figure 1). HMG-CoA Lyase deficiency (HMGLD) (OMIM 246450) is an autosomal recessive genetic disorder caused by homozygous or compound heterozygous pathogenic variants in the *HMGCL* gene located on 1p36.11. Clinically, this disorder is characterized by a life-threatening metabolic intoxication with a presentation including severe hypoglycemia without ketosis, metabolic acidosis, hyperammonemia, hepatomegaly and, invariably, a coma state triggered by an energy crisis such as an infection, vaccination or low dietary intake [1,2]. HMGLD clinical onset is within the first few months of life after a symptomatic free period. Indeed, the metabolic crisis occurs in ~70% of cases before the age of 1 year [1]. In addition, several neurological manifestations such as epilepsy, lethargy and irritability as well as non-neurological manifestations including hepatomegaly, anaemia and eating difficulties have been reported in older children [2]. The diagnosis is based on (i) a urine organic acids analysis with a typical profile including high levels of 3-Hydroxy-3-MethylGlutaric, 3-MethylGlutaric, 3-MethylGlutaconic and 3-HydroxyIsovaleric acids [3], and (ii) an acylcarnitine profile revealing a high level of 3-hydroxy-isovalerylcarnitine with a decreased free carnitine concentration [3] (Figure 1). The molecular study of the *HMGCL* gene enables one to confirm the diagnosis. Fifty-one pathogenic variants have been reported in the Public Human Gene Database (HGMD—http://www.hgmd.cf.ac.uk/ac/index.php—1 May 2021).

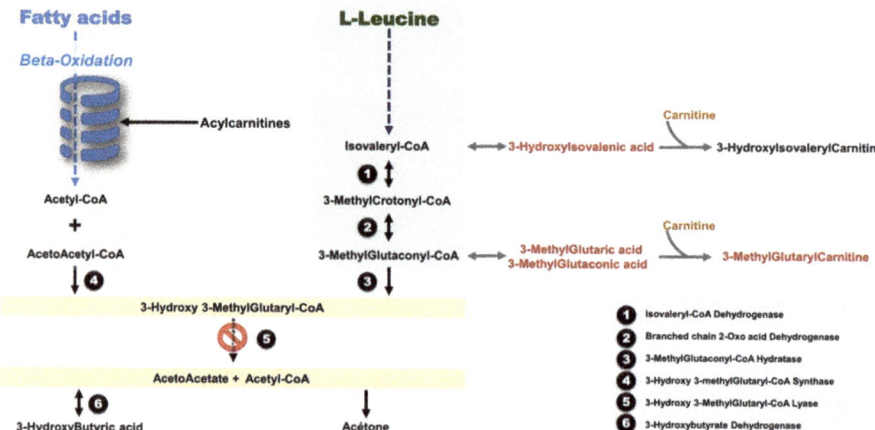

Figure 1. Overview of the involved metabolic pathways in the 3-Hydroxy-3-methylglutaryl-CoA Lyase (HMG-CoA Lyase) metabolism.

Hypoglycemia and ketone bodies shortage may underlie the pathophysiological mechanisms of this disease since acetoacetate and 3-hydroxybutyrate, named ketone bodies, are used as primary substrates for energy supply by several organs such as the central nervous system and the cardiac and skeletal muscles. Moreover, a redox balance disruption through the accumulation of toxic metabolites and a decreased carnitine level may contribute to the metabolic crisis [4,5]. This hypothesis is supported by an in vivo animal study suggesting that the long-term accumulation of key metabolites in HMGCLD induces an increase in the level of oxidative stress correlated with brain toxicity. These data could possibly account for the neurological presentation of this disease [6].

In nonacute periods, the treatment is based on a protein- and fat-restricted diet, and L-carnitine supplementation is recommended. The latter has a major role in organic acids' removal and their urinary elimination, and thus it acts as an antioxidant agent by reducing metabolites' accumulation [2,7]. Besides, a recent report highlights the efficacy of sodium DL-3-hydroxybutyrate as an adjuvant treatment for HMG-CoA lyase [8].

A late-onset presentation has been described in very few cases. Some cases have been reported in infancy and late childhood [9,10], while, to our knowledge, only two adult cases have been described [11,12]. The present work aims to describe an incidental discovery of an HMGLD case in a 54-year-old patient and reports a comprehensive review of clinical and biological features in adult patients in order to get more insight into the late-onset presentation of this disease.

2. Patient and Methods

2.1. Case Description

A fifty-four year old female patient presented with cervical dystonia and head tremor with lateral movement (no-no) from age 48. The past medical history includes an unexplained coma for three days at the age of three years, followed by childhood epilepsy. Seizures were controlled by phenobarbital given until the age of 14 years. She also suffered from substituted hypothyroidism, hypercholesterolemia and hypertension (regulated by appropriate therapy). She does not have any learning difficulties or developmental delay. She was born from non-consanguineous parents. The family history reveals that her older sister had epilepsy and severe mental retardation. The clinical examination confirmed a right laterocollis associated with a no-no head tremor. No cerebellar syndrome has been noticed. In addition, routine biological tests have shown a moderate hyperammonaemia of 69 µmol/L (normal range: 11–35 µmol/L), absence of acid-base disorders and a normal glycemia of 5.1 mmol/L (reference range: 4–6 mmol/L). Of note, the analysis of cerebrospinal fluid showed a moderate hyperproteinorachia (0.62 g/L; N < 0.4).

2.2. Brain Magnetic Resonance Imaging (MRI)

A cerebral MRI was performed using T2 weighting Fluid Attenuated Inversion Recovery (FLAIR) sequences associated with a long echo time (TE) [13]. This technique makes the CSF signal null and improves the detection of brain parenchyma lesions [14], making it very useful for cerebral imaging.

2.3. Biochemical Investigations

For urinary organic acids, urines samples were subjected to derivatization with N,O-bis(trimethylsilyl)trifluroacetamide and trimethylchlorosilane. Derivatized samples were injected into a Shimadzu QP-2010 Plus GC-MS operating in split mode. The metabolites were analyzed as trimethylsilyl compounds. Heptadecanoic acid was used as an internal standard. A Blood Acylcarnitine Profile on a dried blood spot was generated using butylation derivatization (ChromSystems®, Munich, Germany) and measured by MS/MS on a 4000 QTRAP (Sciex®, Concord, ON, Canada). The acylcarnitine butylated esters were acquired by precursor ion scanning of 85 m/z in positive ion mode.

2.4. Molecular Analysis

Genomic DNAs were tested by next-generation sequencing (NGS) using a custom design based on a SeqCap EZ Solution-Based Enrichment strategy (Roche NimbleGen, Madison, WI, USA). Targeted sequencing capture probes were custom designed by Roche NimbleGen. Targeted regions include exons and exon-intron boundaries (exon ± 25 nt), 5′- and 3′-UTR regions of genes involved in inborn metabolic diseases, including HMGCL gene. Sequencing was performed on a NextSeq500 sequencer using the NextSeq500 Mid Output Kit v2 (300 cycles) chemistry (Illumina, San Diego, CA, USA). Bioinformatic analyses were performed using a homemade pipeline according to the GATK Best Practices recommendations (PMID: 25431634). Putative identified pathogenic variants were verified by conventional dideoxy sequencing using the BigDye Terminator v.3.1 Cycle Sequencing Kit (Life Technologies, Carlsbad, CA, USA). Variants were named according to HGVS recommendations, using the NM_000191 sequence. Analyses of the variants were performed with Alamut v2.11 software (Interactive Biosoftware, Rouen, France), and scoring of 5′ and 3′ splice sites was performed using Neural Network Splice Prediction (NNSplice), MaxEntScan, Splice site Finder Like, GeneSplicer, Human Splicing Finder (HSF).

3. Results

3.1. Brain MRI

The brain MRI revealed severe symmetrical supratentorial with confluent periventricular and subcortical white matter hyperintensities on T2-FLAIR (Figure 2A–C) weighted images without abnormal contrast enhancement. Interestingly, the temporal lobes and u-fibers are minimally involved (Figure 2D–F). The basal ganglia, brainstem and cerebellum are spared (Figure 2).

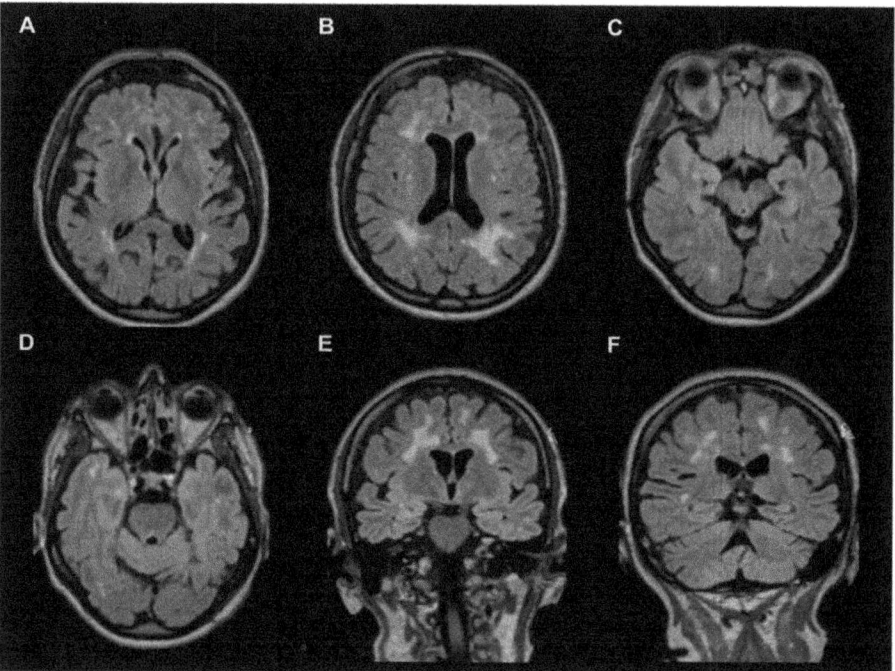

Figure 2. (**A–C**) Axial T2-weighted magnetic resonance images show a high signal intensity in patchy, confluent periventricular and subcortical areas of the white matter with a clear predominance in supratentorial areas. The basal ganglia and brainstem did not show any abnormalities. (**D**) Axial T2-weighted magnetic resonance images and (**E**) coronal T2-weighted magnetic resonance images show a slight temporal lobe involvement. (**F**) Coronal T2-weighted magnetic resonance images show no cerebellar abnormalities.

3.2. Biochemical Investigations

HMGLD diagnosis has been achieved by the detection of an elevated urinary concentration of 3-Hydroxy-3-MethylGlutaric, 3-MethylGlutaric, 3-MethylGlutaconic and 3-HydroxyIsovaleric acids. The analysis of acylcarnitines revealed an increased level of 3-HydroxyIsovalerylcarnitine, which supports the diagnosis (Table 1). Interestingly, a normal range of carnitine concentration has been retrieved without any therapeutic supplementation.

Table 1. Overview of the biochemical investigation results.

Investigation	Metabolite	Concentration	Reference Range
Urinary Organic Acids (mmol/mol of Creatinine)	3-Hydroxy-3-MethylGlutaric acid	304	<200
	3-hydroxyIsovaleric acid	143	<50
	3-methylGlutaric acid	54	<5
	3-methylGlutaconic acid	399	<25
Blood Carnitines (µmol/L)	Carnitine	20	15–35
	3-hydroxyIsovalerylcarnitine	3.73	<0.38

3.3. Molecular Analysis

HMGCL gene sequencing enabled the characterization of two pathogenic variants: NM_000191.2:c.144G>C-p.Lys48Asn, a variant previously described [15], and c.60+1G>C-p ? The latter has never been described and is predicted to abolish the splicing donor site and to cause exon 1 skipping. The allelic segregation was not performed as the DNA samples from the parents were not available for us.

4. Discussion

HMGCLD is a rare inborn error of ketone bodies synthesis and leucine degradation. It has a typical onset in the first few months of life with an initial presentation mimicking Reye syndrome, including recurrent vomiting, seizures and impaired vigilance [1]. The long-term outcome in older children is characterized by neurological complications such as epileptic seizures, muscular hypotonia and tremor associated with marked white matter lesions in the brain MRI [2]. The clinical expression of inborn errors of metabolism (IEM) is now viewed as a severity continuum with a wide clinical spectrum spanning from a severe presentation in the prenatal or neonatal period to moderate or even asymptomatic adult forms. The adult presentation of this IEM is underdiagnosed, and therefore the awareness of adult physicians is still to be improved. Here, we report an adult presentation of HMGCLD aiming to widen the clinical knowledge of this rare disease and raise awareness among the different stakeholders involved in the management of IEM.

To the best of our knowledge, only two adult presentations have been reported so far (Supplementary Table S1). Reimão et al. described a 29-year-old man with no prior medical history who presented with a sudden-onset coma, profound hypoglycemia, hyperammonaemia and metabolic acidosis without ketosis. The patient died with multi-organic failure within five days [12]. Bischof et al. reported the case of a 36-year-old woman with an acute episode of hypoglycaemia, hyperproteinorachia (0.73 g/L) and generalized seizures [11]. Her medical history is marked by recurrent episodes of somnolence and hypoglycemia starting from the neonatal period. During childhood, she presented seizures and developmental delay. This patient had carnitine supplementation, and some clinical features improved markedly [11]. In contrast, our patient's adult onset was not revealed by a metabolic decompensation, and the neurological impairment was in the forefront of the clinical picture. It is worth noting that our patient presented with cervical dystonia and head tremor. Regarding the head tremor, this feature has been observed in 9% of the reported cases [2], while the cervical dystonia has not been reported yet in HMGCLD and could thus be incidental. Indeed, considering the age of our patient, idiopathic dystonia cannot be excluded.

Biochemical investigations retrieved typical urine organic acids and blood acylcarnitine profiles. Molecular analysis confirmed the diagnosis by the identification of two heterozygous pathogenic variants (NM_000191.2:c.144G>C-p.Lys48Asn and c.60+1G>C-p ?).

The MRI findings in our case are very close to those described by Bischof et al. [11] with a supratentorial confluent leukoencephalopathy sparing basal ganglia. The U-fibers are slightly involved in our patient, while they were spared in the patient described by Bischof et al. [11]. The patient described by Reimão et al. [12] presented with a prominent clinical expression and a more severe leukoencephalopathy and U-fibers' involvement. Interestingly, the brainstem and cerebellum were normal too. Temporal involvement was not reported in either of the reported cases. It is interesting to note the absence of the brainstem involvement and the basal ganglia, which are usually affected in hypertensive leukoencephalopathy. Likewise, the predominance of the lesions in supratentorial areas with a relative sparing of the temporal lobes is not in favor of CADASIL disease [16].

5. Conclusions

Although HMGLD is quite a rare condition, it should be considered in cases with extensive white matter lesions with relatively spared brainstem and temporal lobes. The integrative interpretation of imaging, biochemical and molecular findings enable one to reach the diagnosis of this treatable condition.

Supplementary Materials: The following are available online at https://www.mdpi.com/article/10.3390/diagnostics11091561/s1, Table S1: Clinical data overview.

Author Contributions: Conceptualization, A.T. and S.B.; data curation, N.B., B.S.-A., J.B., L.D.-I., A.B., L.G.-M., C.A. and I.D.; writing—original draft preparation, N.B., J.B. and S.B.; writing—review and editing, A.T.; supervision, S.B. All authors have read and agreed to the published version of the manuscript.

Funding: This research received no external funding.

Institutional Review Board Statement: The study was conducted according to the guidelines of the Declaration of Helsinki, and approved by the Rouen University Hospital Review Board (E2021-59).

Informed Consent Statement: Informed consent was obtained from the patient.

Data Availability Statement: All data that support the findings are included in the manuscript and in the supplemental data.

Conflicts of Interest: The authors declare no conflict of interest.

References

1. Gibson, K.M.; Breuer, J.; Nyhan, W.L. 3-hydroxy-3-methylglutaryl-coenzyme a lyase deficiency: Review of 18 reported patients. *Eur. J. Pediatr.* **1988**, *148*, 180–186. [CrossRef] [PubMed]
2. Grünert, S.C.; Schlatter, S.M.; Schmitt, R.N.; Gemperle-Britschgi, C.; Mrázová, L.; Balcı, M.C.; Bischof, F.; Çoker, M.; Das, A.M.; Demirkol, M.; et al. 3-hydroxy-3-methylglutaryl-coenzyme a lyase deficiency: Clinical presentation and outcome in a series of 37 patients. *Mol. Genet. Metab.* **2017**, *121*, 206–215. [CrossRef] [PubMed]
3. Duran, M.; Ketting, D.; Wadman, S.K.; Jakobs, C.; Schutgens, R.B.; Veder, H.A. Organic acid excretion in a patient with 3-hydroxy-3-methylglutaryl-coa lyase deficiency: Facts and artefacts. *Clin. Chim. Acta Int. J. Clin. Chem.* **1978**, *90*, 187–193. [CrossRef]
4. Dos Santos Mello, M.; Ribas, G.S.; Wayhs, C.A.; Hammerschmidt, T.; Guerreiro, G.B.; Favenzani, J.L.; Sitta, Â.; de Moura Coelho, D.; Wajner, M.; Vargas, C.R. Increased oxidative stress in patients with 3-hydroxy-3-methylglutaric aciduria. *Mol. Cell Biochem.* **2015**, *402*, 149–155. [CrossRef] [PubMed]
5. Leipnitz, G.; Vargas, C.R.; Wajner, M. Disturbance of redox homeostasis as a contributing underlying pathomechanism of brain and liver alterations in 3-hydroxy-3-methylglutaryl-coa lyase deficiency. *J. Inherit. Metab. Dis.* **2015**, *38*, 1021–1028. [CrossRef] [PubMed]
6. Leipnitz, G.; Seminotti, B.; Haubrich, J.; Dalcin, M.B.; Dalcin, K.B.; Solano, A.; de Bortoli, G.; Rosa, R.B.; Amaral, A.U.; Dutra-Filho, C.S.; et al. Evidence that 3-hydroxy-3-methylglutaric acid promotes lipid and protein oxidative damage and reduces the nonenzymatic antioxidant defenses in rat cerebral cortex. *J. Neurosci. Res.* **2008**, *86*, 683–693. [CrossRef] [PubMed]
7. Delgado, C.A.; Balbueno Guerreiro, G.B.; Diaz Jacques, C.E.; de Moura Coelho, D.; Sitta, A.; Manfredini, V.; Wajner, M.; Vargas, C.R. Prevention by l-carnitine of DNA damage induced by 3-hydroxy-3-methylglutaric and 3-methylglutaric acids and experimental evidence of lipid and DNA damage in patients with 3-hydroxy-3-methylglutaric aciduria. *Arch. Biochem. Biophys.* **2019**, *668*, 16–22. [CrossRef] [PubMed]
8. Bhattacharya, K.; Matar, W.; Tolun, A.A.; Devanapalli, B.; Thompson, S.; Dalkeith, T.; Lichkus, K.; Tchan, M. The use of sodium dl-3-hydroxybutyrate in severe acute neuro-metabolic compromise in patients with inherited ketone body synthetic disorders. *Orphanet. J. Rare Dis.* **2020**, *15*, 53. [CrossRef] [PubMed]
9. Pierron, S.; Giudicelli, H.; Moreigne, M.; Khalfi, A.; Touati, G.; Caruba, C.; Rolland, M.O.; Acquaviva, C. Late onset 3-hmg-coa lyase deficiency: A rare but treatable disorder. *Arch. Pediatr.* **2010**, *17*, 10–13. [CrossRef] [PubMed]
10. Yilmaz, O.; Kitchen, S.; Pinto, A.; Daly, A.; Gerrard, A.; Hoban, R.; Santra, S.; Sreekantam, S.; Frost, K.; Pigott, A.; et al. 3-hydroxy-3-methylglutaryl-coa lyase deficiency: A case report and literature review. *Nutr. Hosp.* **2018**, *35*, 237–244. [PubMed]
11. Bischof, F.; Nägele, T.; Wanders, R.J.; Trefz, F.K.; Melms, A. 3-hydroxy-3-methylglutaryl-coa lyase deficiency in an adult with leukoencephalopathy. *Ann. Neurol.* **2004**, *56*, 727–730. [CrossRef] [PubMed]
12. Reimão, S.; Morgado, C.; Almeida, I.T.; Silva, M.; Corte Real, H.; Campos, J. 3-hydroxy-3-methylglutaryl-coenzyme a lyase deficiency: Initial presentation in a young adult. *J. Inherit. Metab. Dis.* **2009**, *32*, S49–S52. [CrossRef] [PubMed]
13. Hajnal, J.V.; Bryant, D.J.; Kasuboski, L.; Pattany, P.M.; De Coene, B.; Lewis, P.D.; Pennock, J.M.; Oatridge, A.; Young, I.R.; Bydder, G.M. Use of fluid attenuated inversion recovery (flair) pulse sequences in mri of the brain. *J. Comput. Assist Tomogr.* **1992**, *16*, 841–844. [CrossRef] [PubMed]
14. Stuckey, S.L.; Goh, T.D.; Heffernan, T.; Rowan, D. Hyperintensity in the subarachnoid space on flair mri. *AJR Am. J. Roentgenol.* **2007**, *189*, 913–921. [CrossRef] [PubMed]
15. Carrasco, P.; Menao, S.; López-Viñas, E.; Santpere, G.; Clotet, J.; Sierra, A.Y.; Gratacós, E.; Puisac, B.; Gómez-Puertas, P.; Hegardt, F.G.; et al. C-terminal end and aminoacid lys48 in hmg-coa lyase are involved in substrate binding and enzyme activity. *Mol. Genet. Metab.* **2007**, *91*, 120–127. [CrossRef] [PubMed]
16. Stojanov, D.; Vojinovic, S.; Aracki-Trenkic, A.; Tasic, A.; Benedeto-Stojanov, D.; Ljubisavljevic, S.; Vujnovic, S. Imaging characteristics of cerebral autosomal dominant arteriopathy with subcortical infarcts and leucoencephalopathy (cadasil). *Bosn. J. Basic Med. Sci.* **2015**, *15*, 1–8. [CrossRef] [PubMed]

Correlation of Genotype and Perinatal Period, Time of Diagnosis and Anthropometric Data before Commencement of Recombinant Human Growth Hormone Treatment in Polish Patients with Prader–Willi Syndrome

Agnieszka Lecka-Ambroziak [1,*], Marta Wysocka-Mincewicz [1], Katarzyna Doleżal-Ołtarzewska [2], Agata Zygmunt-Górska [2], Teresa Żak [3], Anna Noczyńska [3], Dorota Birkholz-Walerzak [4], Renata Stawerska [5], Maciej Hilczer [5], Monika Obara-Moszyńska [6], Barbara Rabska-Pietrzak [6], Elżbieta Gołębiowska [7], Adam Dudek [7], Elżbieta Petriczko [8], Mieczysław Szalecki [1,9] and on behalf of the Polish Coordination Group for rhGH Treatment [†]

[1] Department of Endocrinology and Diabetology, The Children's Memorial Health Institute, 04-730 Warsaw, Poland; m.wysocka@ipczd.pl (M.W.-M.); m.szalecki@ipczd.pl (M.S.)
[2] Department of Paediatric and Adolescent Endocrinology, University Children's Hospital, 30-663 Cracow, Poland; drkate@tlen.pl (K.D.-O.); endodim@cm-uj.krakow.pl (A.Z.-G.)
[3] Department of Endocrinology and Diabetology of Children and Adolescents, Wroclaw Medical University, 50-368 Wroclaw, Poland; kep@usk.wroc.pl (T.Ż.); anna.noczynska@umed.wroc.pl (A.N.)
[4] Department of Paediatrics, Diabetology and Endocrinology, Medical University of Gdansk, 80-952 Gdansk, Poland; debirkhol@wp.pl
[5] Department of Endocrinology and Metabolic Diseases, Polish Mother's Memorial Hospital—Research Institute, 93-338 Lodz, Poland; renata.stawerska@umed.lodz.pl (R.S.); maciej.hilczer@umed.lodz.pl (M.H.)
[6] Department of Paediatric Endocrinology and Rheumatology, Institute of Paediatrics, Poznan University of Medical Sciences, 60-572 Poznan, Poland; m.moszynska@ump.edu.pl (M.O.-M.); b.rabska@ump.edu.pl (B.R.-P.)
[7] II Clinic of Paediatrics, Endocrinology and Paediatric Diabetology, Clinical Regional Hospital No 2, 35-301 Rzeszow, Poland; sekretariat@szpital2.rzeszow.pl (E.G.); dudek.ad@wp.pl (A.D.)
[8] Department of Paediatrics, Endocrinology, Diabetology, Metabolic Disorders and Cardiology of Developmental Age, Pomeranian Medical University, 71-242 Szczecin, Poland; elzbieta.petriczko@pum.edu.pl
[9] Collegium Medicum, Jan Kochanowski University, 25-317 Kielce, Poland
* Correspondence: aleckaambroziak@gmail.com
[†] The Polish Coordination Group for rhGH Treatment members that participated in the study are listed in the Acknowledgments.

Abstract: Genotype–phenotype correlation in patients with Prader–Willi syndrome (PWS) has still not been fully described. We retrospectively analysed data of 147 patients and compared groups according to genetic diagnosis: paternal deletion of chromosome 15q11-q13 (DEL 15, $n = 81$), maternal uniparental disomy (UPD 15, $n = 10$), excluded DEL 15 (UPD 15 or imprinting centre defect, UPD/ID, $n = 30$). Group DEL 15 had an earlier genetic diagnosis and recombinant human growth hormone (rhGH) start ($p = 0.00$), with a higher insulin-like growth factor 1 (IGF1) level compared to group UPD/ID ($p = 0.04$). Among perinatal characteristics, there was only a tendency towards lower birth weight SDS in group UPD 15 ($p = 0.06$). We also compared data at rhGH start in relation to genetic diagnosis age—group 1: age ≤ 9 months, group 2: >9 months ≤ 2 years, group 3: > 2 years. Group 1 had the earliest rhGH start ($p = 0.00$), with lower body mass index (BMI) SDS ($p = 0.00$) and a tendency towards a higher IGF1 level compared to group 3 ($p = 0.05$). Genetic background in children with PWS is related to time of diagnosis and rhGH start, with a difference in IGF1 level before the therapy, but it seems to have little impact on perinatal data. Early genetic diagnosis leads to early rhGH treatment with favourable lower BMI SDS.

Keywords: Prader–Willi syndrome; imprinting disorder; recombinant human growth hormone; insulin-like growth factor 1

1. Introduction

Prader–Willi syndrome (PWS) is a rare disease with an estimated prevalence of 1 in 15,000 to 1 in 30,000. It had been previously recognised on the basis of clinical diagnostic criteria, but nowadays it should be confirmed by molecular genetic testing. PWS is a first recognised human genetic imprinting disorder and results from a lack of paternally inherited genes on chromosome 15q11-q13, which can be caused by paternal deletion (DEL 15, 65–75%), maternal uniparental disomy (UPD 15, 20–30%) or an imprinting centre defect (ID, estimated for 1–3%).

Among the imprinted genes are: *SNURF-SNRPN* (*SNRPN* upstream reading frame-small nuclear ribonucleoprotein polypeptide N), *MKRN3* (makorin RING-finger protein 3), *MAGEL2* (MAGE Family Member L2), *NDN* (Necdin protein), *C15orf2* (chromosome 15 open reading frame 2) and more than 70 C/D box snoRNA genes (*SNORDs*). The exact contribution of these genes to PWS is still not fully understood [1–4].

The main clinical features of PWS are mostly age-dependent and consist, in the first months of life, of marked hypotonia, global psychomotor delay, and moderate to severe difficulties in feeding with failure to thrive. This period is usually followed by a lack of satiety and obesity developing from early childhood that lead, if untreated, to morbid obesity. Other typical features in patients with PWS are hypogonadotropic hypogonadism, with almost universal cryptorchidism in male newborns, short stature, and cognitive and behaviour dysfunction [4–9]. However, the latest studies show a more complex phenotype in patients with PWS than had been established before. We are now more aware of heterogeneity of gonadal dysfunction, both hypogonadotropic and primary gonadal [10–13]. There are also studies confirming frequent premature adrenarche which does not influence the central puberty course or recombinant human growth hormone (rhGH) effectiveness [14]. The recent studies showed very importantly that we can also distinguish more age-specific nutritional phases in most patients with PWS [15–20]. According to Miller et al., in childhood we can describe the following phases (median age): 1a, until 9 months of life, characterised by feeding difficulties and decreased appetite; 1b, until 25 months, with improved feeding and appetite; 2a, until 4.5 years, when weight increases without increased appetite; 2b, until 8 years, with increased appetite and calorie intake. In a further phase, 3, that lasts until adulthood, patients are hyperphagic and show insatiable appetite [19]. The rhGH treatment together with multidisciplinary care has been a well-established approach to patients with PWS and it seems to positively influence not only the natural history of body composition and psychomotor development but also the above-described natural phases of PWS nutritional phenotype [21–27].

Although PWS is a rare disease, it can serve as a model of hypothalamic function disruption and, therefore, understanding PWS can help both scientists and clinicians better understand and maintain other diseases with a similar background, such as hypothalamic tumours before and after neurosurgery interventions. Moreover, we still lack full recognition of the influence of specific missing genes on hypothalamus dysfunction and its impact on PWS phenotype [2–4,28]. Studies regarding the relationship between the genotype and newborn phenotype have been conducted, but the results are not explicit [29–33]. There is also little data for anthropometric characteristics before rhGH treatment in relation to the molecular type of diagnosis. The latest research does not give concordant results regarding overall anthropometric differences between the genetic subtypes [34–37]. In the study by Butler et al. in 2019, regarding both paediatric and adult patients, with only part of them treated with rhGH, there was no difference in body mass index (BMI) identified, based on the genetic subtype [34]. In the recently published paper by Shepherd et al. in 2020, describing paediatric population, detailed information regarding rhGH treatment was not reported and no difference in height was found for males in both PWS subtypes (DEL 15 vs. non-DEL 15), with decreased height in females with non-DEL 15 for older ages. Weight and BMI were higher in the DEL 15 group, which suggests that these patients are more prone to obesity [35]. These results correspond with the findings by Mahmoud and Leonenko et al. in a multicentre study of a large cohort of 355 patients, published this year [36]. However, the authors of the above studies did not analyse the characteristics of patients with PWS with a different molecular diagnosis at the start of rhGH therapy.

We conducted our research to try to answer the question of whether the type of molecular diagnosis significantly influences the perinatal characteristics of newborns with PWS, the time of genetic diagnosis and the age of rhGH commencement as well as anthropometric parameters and insulin-like growth factor 1 (IGF1) level before the therapy. Furthermore, we investigated the patients' anthropometric and IGF1 values at the time of rhGH start in relation to the age of genetic diagnosis.

2. Material and Methods

We retrospectively analysed data (medical records and questionnaires filled in by clinicians) regarding time and type of molecular diagnosis, perinatal characteristics, and anthropometric and biochemical data before commencement of rhGH treatment in 147 patients, 69 girls (46.94%) and 78 boys (53.06%), from 12 paediatric endocrine centres in Poland, in the years 2002–2016. The rhGH treatment was accepted by the Polish Coordination Group for rhGH Treatment.

We have grouped the patients according to the subtype of genetic diagnosis: group DEL 15, $n = 81$ (55.1%), group UPD 15, $n = 10$ (6.80%). In 20 patients, the DEL 15 has been excluded and the diagnosis can be either UPD 15 or ID, and in 7 of them (4.76% of the whole cohort) DEL15 was excluded but further molecular studies have not been documented. Therefore, we created a third group of patients, with excluded DEL 15 diagnosis, group UPD/ID, $n = 30$ (20.41%). In 36 patients (24.49%), the abnormality in methylation pattern of *SNRPN* was confirmed, but the exact type of genetic diagnosis has been pending—in 1 patient the genetic report was not included in the documentation. As the exact molecular diagnosis in this group of patients had not been established, the group can be very heterogeneous and the patients may present with all possible molecular types of PWS diagnosis. Therefore, they were not analysed separately.

Subsequently, we analysed the data regarding the rhGH start according to the age of genetic diagnosis. We were directed by the age-depended nutritional phases, as described above. We divided our cohort into 3 groups: group 1: age ≤ 9 months, group 2: >9 months ≤ 2 years, group 3: > 2 years of life.

The height and BMI were assessed according to the Polish growth and BMI standards charts, and the BMI SDS was calculated using the LMS method (method to obtain SD, LMS parameters: Lambda for the skew, Mu for the median, and Sigma for the generalized coefficient of variation). IGF1 was evaluated with a radioimmunoassay technique.

The study was approved by the CMHI Bioethics Committee, 7/KBE/2019, 20 March 2019.

3. Data Analysis

Statistical analyses were performed using TIBCO Software Inc. (2017) Statistica version 13 StatSoft Company. Results are expressed as mean values and standard deviation scores (±SDS) and additionally as median (minimal-maximal value) for the age of diagnosis and therapy start. Data were checked for normality of distribution using the Shapiro–Wilk test, and data with skewness were log or square transformed to normal distribution if possible. Differences between the groups were tested by unpaired t-Student test or Mann–Whitney U test, as appropriate. Correlations between the assessed parameters were evaluated with Pearson correlation and Spearman rank correlation, dependent on distribution. Differences between the dependent variables were analysed by t-Student test for dependent variables or Wilcoxon test as appropriate. A p level <0.05 was recognized as statistically significant.

4. Results

The details regarding the perinatal period are presented in Table 1.

Table 1. Clinical characteristics at birth (the mean value ± standard deviation score, SDS).

PWS Group	All Patients	DEL 15	UPD 15	UPD/ID
Number of patients (%)	N = 147	N = 81 (55.10)	N = 10 (6.80)	N = 30 (20.41)
F/M (%)	69/78 (46.94/53.06)	43/38 (53.09/46.91)	1/9 (10/90)	11/19 (36.67/63.33)
Weeks of gestation	38.68 ± 2.65	38.76 ± 2.31	39.33 ± 2.29	38.50 ± 3.26
Apgar score 1st minute	7.36 ± 2.25	7.75 ± 1.94	7.70 ± 1.64	7.41 ± 1.82
Apgar score 10th minute	8.41 ± 1.20	8.41 ± 1.24	ND	8.27 ± 0.90
Weight [g]	2692.91 ± 534.95	2720.40 ± 527.70	2547.00 ± 471.03	2646 ± 558.21
Weight SDS	−1.88 ± 1.29	−1.85 ± 1.26	−2.69 ± 0.92 ($p = 0.06$) *	−1.91 ± 1.30
Length [cm]	52.13 ± 4.42	52.46 ± 4.16	51.20 ± 4.26	51.11 ± 5.83
Length SDS	1.20 ± 1.90	1.28 ± 1.99	0.27 ± 1.61	0.84 ± 2.15

PWS—Prader–Willi syndrome, DEL 15—deletion of chromosome 15q11-13, UPD 15—uniparental disomy, ID—imprinting defect, F/M—female/male, ND—not done. * group UPD 15 vs. DEL 15.

The mean values of week of gestation, Apgar score (AS) at the 1st and 10th minute of life and length SDS at gestation were within the normal range in the whole cohort ($n = 147$) and in the groups DEL 15, UPD 15 and UPD/ID. The mean birth weight was above −2 SDS, apart from the group UPD 15 (−2.69 ± 0.92). This difference was marked but did not reach statistical significance ($p = 0.06$). Below, we present the more detailed neonatal characteristics within the groups.

Group DEL 15—$n = 81$, 43 girls, 38 boys; 18 patients (22.22%) were born prematurely (31–37 weeks of pregnancy), most of the patients by caesarean section (49 patients, 60.49%). Thirty-six patients (44.44%) were born small for gestational age (SGA), according to the birth weight SDS, four patients according to both the birth weight and length. Thirty-two newborns (39.51%) had a lower AS of 1–7 points in the first minute of life. Six patients (28.40%) presented with serious complications within the neonatal period (mainly intrauterine infection, breathing difficulties and intraventricular haemorrhage (IVH), less often hypoglycaemia, seizures, gastrointestinal bleeding, thrombocytopenia, congenital heart defect). Cryptorchidism was present in 30 out of 38 boys (79%), and orchidopexy was performed in 23 boys, aged 2.95 ± 2.73 years.

Group UPD—$n = 10$, one girl, nine boys; two patients (20%) were born prematurely (35–36 weeks of pregnancy), most of the patients by caesarean section and as SGA (eight patients, 80%) with birth weight <2 SDS, one patient with both birth weight and length <2 SDS, and five (50%) with a lower AS of 5–7 points in the first minute of life. Three patients (30%) presented with serious neonatal complications (serious breathing difficulties, IVH, intrauterine infection). Cryptorchidism was present in all boys, and eight underwent orchidopexy at the age 7.15 ± 5.49 years.

Group UPD/ID—$n = 30$, 11 girls, 19 boys; eight patients (26.67%) were born prematurely (30–37 weeks of pregnancy), most of the patients by caesarean section (19 patients, 63.33%) and as SGA (16 patients, 53.33%) with birth weight <−2 SDS, two patients with both birth weight and length <−2 SDS, one patient with only birth length <−2 SDS, and half of the group with a lower AS of 1–7 points in the first minute of life. Six patients (20%) presented with serious neonatal complications (serious breathing difficulties, IVH, intrauterine infection, hepatitis). Cryptorchidism was present in almost all boys (18 boys, 94.74%), and 13 of them underwent orchidopexy at the age 5.82 ± 4.83 years.

There was a statistical significant difference in the age of genetic diagnosis between the group DEL 15 and group UPD 15 ($p = 0.003$), as well as group UPD/ID ($p = 0.00$) (Table 2).

Table 2. The age of PWS genetic diagnosis and the data at the start of rhGH treatment (the mean value ± standard deviation score, SDS; median (minimal-maximal value) for the age of diagnosis and rhGH start).

PWS Group	All Patients	DEL 15	UPD 15	UPD/ID
Number of patients (%)	N = 147	N = 81 (55.10)	N = 10 (6.80)	N = 30 (20.41)
F/M (%)	69/78 (46.94/53.06)	43/38 (53.09/46.91)	1/9 (10/90)	11/19 (36.67/63.33)
Age of diagnosis [years]	1.67 ± 2.39 0.53 (0.02–12.49)	1.38 ± 2.33 0.41 (0.02–12.49)	3.84 ± 2.86 4.1 (0.13–7.31) ($p = 0.003$) *	3.13 ± 2.72 2.55 (0.09–8.84) ($p = 0.00$) *
Age of rhGH start [years]	4.55 ± 3.74 3.03 (0.58–17.43)	4.24 ± 3.81 2.64 (0.58–16.75)	7.30 ± 3.03 8.31 (3.29–10.62) ($p = 0.003$) *	6.42 ± 3.74 5.62 (0.85–17.43) ($p = 0.00$)*
rhGH dose (IU/kg/week; mg/kg/day)	0.58 ± 0.16; 0.028 ± 0.008	0.57 ± 0.14; 0.027 ± 0.007	0.61 ± 0.13; 0.029 ± 0.006	0.60 ± 0.16; 0.029 ± 0.008
Height [cm]	96.62 ± 23.31	95.23 ± 24.18	111.78 ± 15.65	107.85 ± 20.34
Height SDS	−2.11 ± 1.50	−1.95 ± 1.53	−2.45 ± 1.07	−2.18 ± 1.57
BMI	18.05 ± 3.99	17.79 ± 3.78	20.55 ± 4.24	19.31 ± 3.40
BMI SDS	0.41 ± 1.55	0.39 ± 1.61	1.16 ± 0.91 ($p = 0.14$) *	0.86 ± 1.29 ($p = 0.15$) *
IGF1 [ng/mL]	70.31 ± 55.06	75.80 ± 64.56	84.11 ± 47.63	71.93 ± 38.79
IGF1 SDS	−0.89 ± 0.43	−0.83 ± 0.46	−1.03 ± 0.55	−1.03 ± 0.43 ($p = 0.04$) **

PWS—Prader–Willi syndrome, DEL 15—deletion of chromosome 15q11-13, UPD 15—uniparental disomy, ID—imprinting defect, F/M—female/male, rhGH—recombinant human growth hormone, BMI—body mass index, IGF1—insulin-like growth factor 1. * group UPD 15 vs. DEL 15, UPD/ID vs. DEL 15, ** group UPD/ID vs. DEL 15.

Children with DEL 15 were diagnosed much earlier, in the mean age within the 2nd year of life, whereas the groups UPD 15 and UPD/ID in the 4th year of life. The difference was even more evident when analysing the median values, with the age of diagnosis in the group DEL 15 of 5 months of age.

There was also a later start of rhGH treatment in the groups UPD 15 and UPD/ID compared to the group DEL 15 ($p = 0.003$, $p = 0.00$). The mean height SDS was below −2 SDS in the groups UPD 15 and UPD/ID, and −1.95 SDS in group DEL 15, with the mean BMI SDS within the normal range in the whole population of patients at the beginning of the therapy. We did not confirm any statistical difference in the height and BMI SDS at the start of the treatment within the groups. However, there was a tendency towards the higher BMI SDS in the groups UPD 15 and UPD/ID ($p = 0.14$, $p = 0.15$). We found a positive correlation between the age of genetic diagnosis and BMI SDS in the group DEL 15, as well as in the group UPD/ID ($r = 0.27$, $p = 0.014$ and $r = 0.38$, $p = 0.044$, respectively), but no correlation was found with the height SDS.

Interestingly, comparison of the results of birth length and height before the start of the treatment expressed in SDS showed a higher SDS for birth length in all the groups ($p = 0.00$).

The mean IGF1 level before rhGH therapy was close to −1 SDS in the patients from all the groups ($n = 142$), with a significantly lower IGF1 SDS value in the group UPD/ID vs. DEL 15 ($p = 0.04$). When we correlated the mean birth anthropometric parameter SDS with IGF1 SDS, we did not find the statistically significant correlations in the groups DEL 15 and UPD/ID. The details regarding the data before the rhGH start are presented in Table 2.

Furthermore, we analysed the patients' data according to the age of genetic diagnosis: group 1: age ≤9 months, group 2: >9 months ≤2 years, group 3: >2 years of life (Table 3).

Table 3. The age of PWS genetic diagnosis and the data at the start of rhGH treatment depending on the age of PWS molecular diagnosis (the mean value ± standard deviation score, SDS; median (minimal-maximal value) for the age of diagnosis and rhGH start).

PWS Group	Group 1	Group 2	Group 3
Number of patients (%)	n = 82 (55.8)	n = 25 (17)	n = 40 (27.2)
F/M (%)	39/43 (47.56/52.44)	13/12 (52/48)	17/23 (42.50/57.50)
Age of diagnosis [years]	0.25 ± 0.18 0.21 (0.02–0.71)	1.35 ± 0.36 1.22 (0.79–1.93) ($p = 0.00$) *	5.00 ± 2.56 4.33 (2.06–12.49) ($p = 0.00$) *
Age of rhGH start [years]	2.60 ± 2.28 1.97 (0.58–13.09)	4.86 ± 3.39 3.53 (1.59-12.56) ($p = 0.00$) *	8.44 ± 3.43 8.28 (2.91–17.43) ($p = 0.00$) *
rhGH dose (IU/kg/week; mg/kg/day)	0.57 ± 0.14; 0.027 ± 0.007	0.58 ± 0.15; 0.027 ± 0.007	0.60 ± 0.21; 0.029 ± 0.01
Height [cm]	84.57 ± 16.78	99.88 ± 21.04	119.81 ± 18.33
Height SDS	−2.13 ± 1.52	−2.02 ± 1.61	−2.10 ± 1.44
BMI	16.21 ± 2.60	18.79 ± 3.44	21.52 ± 4.35
BMI SDS	−0.21 ± 1.62	1.14 ± 1.26 ($p = 0.00$) **	1.24 ± 0.79 ($p = 0.00$) **
IGF1 [ng/mL]	52.46 ± 36.44	79.72 ± 64.76	101.87 ± 66.44
IGF1 SDS	−0.84 ± 0.27	−0.87 ± 0.43	−1.01 ± 0.64 ($p = 0.052$) ***

PWS—Prader–Willi syndrome, F/M—female/male, rhGH—recombinant human growth hormone, BMI—body mass index, IGF1—insulin-like growth factor 1, group 1: age ≤9 months, group 2: >9 months ≤2 years, group 3: >2 years of life, * group 2 vs. 1, group 3 vs. 1, group 3 vs. 2, ** group 2 vs. 1, group 3 vs. 1, *** group 3 vs. 1.

Group 1—n = 82, 39 girls, 43 boys; DEL 15 was diagnosed in 51 (62.2%), UPD 15 in 2 (2.44%), UPD/ID in 8 (9.76%), abnormality in methylation pattern of *SNRPN* in 23 (28.05%) patients. Group 2—n = 25, 13 girls, 12 boys; DEL 15 was diagnosed in 12 (48%), UPD 15 in 2 (8%), UPD/ID in 6 (24%), abnormality in methylation pattern of *SNRPN* in 7 (28%) patients. Group 3—n = 40, 17 girls, 23 boys; DEL 15 was diagnosed in 18 (45%), UPD 15 in 6 (15%), UPD/ID in 16 (40%), abnormality in methylation pattern of *SNRPN* in 6 (15%) patients.

The patients with early genetic diagnosis started rhGH treatment significantly earlier than children diagnosed >9 months of age, with a lower BMI SDS than in group 3 but similar height SDS to groups 2 and 3. BMI SDS was correlated with the age of diagnosis in the oldest group ($r = 0.41$, $p = 0.01$). The IGF 1 SDS was higher in the first group compared to group 3, but did not reach statistical significance ($p = 0.052$).

As we cover 15 years in our analysis, and in those years a number of advances in diagnosis and treatment occurred, we looked in more detail at the data of patients diagnosed in the years 2002–2009: n = 94 (63.95%), F/M (%) 38/56 (40.43/59.57), DEL15 n = 51 (54.26%), UPD 15 n = 9 (9.58%), UPD/ID n = 21 (22.34%), abnormality in methylation pattern of *SNRPN* n = 22 (23.40%); and in the years 2010–2016: n = 53 (36.05%), F/M (%) 31/22 (58.49/41.51), DEL15 n = 30 (56.60%), UPD 15 n = 1 (1.89%), UPD/ID n = 9 (16.98%), abnormality in methylation pattern of *SNRPN* n = 14 (26.42%). As expected, we found a significant difference in the age of diagnosis and the age of rhGH commencement between the groups, with the older age in the patients diagnosed in the years 2002–2009 vs. 2010–2016: 1.85 ± 2.08 years, med 1.01 (0.02–7.31) vs. 1.35 ± 2.84 years, med 0.26 (0.04–12.49), $p = 0.00$ and 5.67 ± 3.68 years, med 4.53 (0.93–17.43) vs. 2.57 ± 2.97 years, med 1.63 (0.58–14.55), $p = 0.00$, respectively. Analysis of the perinatal data showed only a tendency toward higher AS in the first minute of life in the patients diagnosed in the years 2010–2016: 7.80 ± 2.06 vs. 7.11 ± 2.32, $p = 0.08$.

Among the anthropometric characteristics before rhGH start, the patients diagnosed in the years 2002–2009 presented with higher BMI SDS: 0.71 ± 1.26 vs. −0.12 ± 1.85, $p = 0.002$.

Interestingly, height SDS as well as IGF1 SDS and rhGH dose were comparable between those groups of children.

5. Discussion

Compared to the recent literature, our findings show more frequent SGA characteristics among newborns with PWS. In our cohort of patients, both with DEL 15 and with UPD/ID, more than half of the patients were born by caesarean section, and half of the groups presented as SGA, mainly according to the birth weight, and with lower Apgar score. Close to 25% were born prematurely and with serious complications within the neonatal period. Among the perinatal anthropometric results, there was only a tendency towards the lower birth weight SDS in the group UPD 15. Singh et al., in their study in 2018, analysed data of 355 patients with PWS from the Rare Diseases Clinical Research Network (RDCRN) PWS registry and found that 54% were born by caesarean section, 26% were born prematurely and 34% were born with a low birth weight, and also no significant differences in the genetic subtypes were noted [29]. Bar et al., in a 2017 analysis of 61 newborns with PWS, reported 67% born by caesarean section, 20% prematurely and 30% newborns small for gestational age, and the data regarding the details within the genetic subtypes were not reported [30]. Salvatoni et al. in 2019 in a large cohort of 252 male and 244 female newborns with PWS confirmed only decreased birth length in females with DEL 15 vs. those with UPD 15 [31]. In a paper published in 2019, among 102 Chinese children with PWS, the authors observed a higher frequency of premature newborns in group UPD 15, the characteristic that was comparable in our groups of patients with DEL 15 and UPD 15 (22 and 20%). There was a difference in the frequency of cryptorchidism, with 57.3% in the group DEL 15 and 74.1% in the group UPD 15 [32]. In our cohort, cryptorchidism was present in 79% of boys in the group DEL 15, while it was almost a universal feature in the groups UPD and UPD/ID.

We presented new data regarding the age of diagnosis and the age of rhGH start in different PWS genetic subtypes. The patients in the group DEL 15 were diagnosed and started the treatment earlier in comparison to the groups UPD and UPD/ID. These data may suggest that the clinical manifestation of PWS in the case of patients with DEL 15 is more evident, even in view of the tendency to the lower mean weight SDS in the group UPD 15. However, we do not have the precise data regarding the incidence and severity of hypotonia or feeding difficulties in the neonatal period as well as dysmorphic features in all the patients. Therefore, we cannot formulate a definitive explanation for the difference in the time of diagnosis between children with different molecular diagnosis. Interestingly, the mean height and BMI SDS were closer to the normal mean values in the group DEL 15 at the start of the rhGH treatment, although these differences did not reach statistical significance. It may be explained by the earlier rhGH start, following the earlier diagnosis. It may be also speculated that the clinical, mainly dysmorphic features of PWS, other than short stature or higher BMI, are more relevant in the children with DEL 15. The DEL 15 phenotype has been described as a classic PWS phenotype that may therefore lead to the earlier diagnosis and start of the therapy [28,36]. The evident difference between the birth length SDS and height SDS before the start of the treatment in our research, independent of the genetic subtype, may indicate that there is a significant decrease in postnatal growth in children with PWS, regardless the specific molecular diagnosis. The mean IGF1 SDS values at the rhGH start were within the normal range for age and sex in all the genetic subtypes. There was a significantly lower IGF1 SDS in the group UPD/ID vs. DEL 15 that may again correspond to the later rhGH start in this group of patients. However, the height SDS did not differ between the groups.

Our research includes a new analysis of the time of diagnosis and start of the treatment within the different nutritional phases. The early genetic diagnosis (≤9 months of age) in the period of the phenotype of hypotonia and feeding difficulties with possible failure to thrive leads to the significantly earlier rhGH start. However, the mean beginning of the treatment was still in the 3rd year of life (median age close to the end of the 2nd year), when the weight tends to increase but still without increased appetite. Children diagnosed >9 months ≤2 years started the therapy in the 5th year of life (median 4th year), close to the period of increased appetite. The patients that were diagnosed at >4.5 years started the treatment even later, in the 9th year of life, when the individuals with PWS experience hyperphagia and insatiable appetite [19]. Moreover, early genetic diagnosis leads to the possible favourable lower BMI SDS and the tendency towards a higher IGF1 level at the rhGH treatment start. It may be probably explained by the younger age when the nutritional behaviour is more appropriate for healthy children and hypothetical growth hormone deficiency is less expressed. Interestingly, the height SDS still did not show any differences at the rhGH start. In the view of the positive effects of rhGH therapy in modifying not only the anthropometric characteristics but hypothetically also the satiety and appetite behaviour, it seems to be a crucial step to diagnose PWS in the first months of life and therefore start the treatment early [38,39]. Commencement of the rhGH therapy, which has a potential beneficial influence on metabolic state, as well as on psychomotor development, before the nutritional phase of increased appetite may modify the subsequent nutritional phenotype of patients with PWS. Moreover, early diagnosis has a potential influence on better multidisciplinary care with healthier nutritional habits, even before the rhGH therapy. However, analysing our cohort of patients, we have to take into consideration that some of them were born in the years before rhGH therapy was available in Poland cost-free for children with PWS (2006). Only a few of them were treated before with families' own resources. This may explain the discrepancy between the early diagnosis and relatively late start of the treatment in some of the patients. Although most of the patients were diagnosed in the years 2002–2009, they were significantly older at the time of genetic diagnosis as well as at the start of rhGH treatment, with a higher BMI SDS.

Finally, our research confirmed the need for specific molecular diagnosis in all patients with PWS, which is important not only for further genetic counselling but also for a better understanding of the possible future phenotype. In the analysed cohort, almost 25% of patients had the abnormality in the methylation pattern of *SNRPN*, but the exact type of genetic diagnosis has not yet been made and almost 5% of children had DEL15 excluded, but further molecular studies have not been documented. It may be partially explained by the early years of the genetic diagnostic process when not all of the molecular methods were widely available. However, the frequency of non-specific molecular diagnosis was close to 25% in the patients diagnosed in the years 2002–2009 as well as in the years 2010–2016. In a population-based observation of 160 Australian children with PWS in the years 1951–2012, published in 2015, there was a significant part of missing the exact molecular diagnosis: 58% in the years 1973–1981, with no UPD 15 diagnosis, and 17% in the years 2003–2012, with 45% of UPD 15. Similarly to our results, a quarter of the cohort was born prematurely and half of the analysed group as SGA [40]. In a lately published study showing outcomes of rhGH treatment in patients with PWS, there are also data with a high percentage of non-defined molecular diagnosis. In a large cohort of 522 prepubertal children and 173 adolescents with PWS treated with rhGH in the years 1987–2012 (Pfizer International Growth Database, KIGS), reported by Bakker et al. in 2017, the diagnosis of PWS was confirmed by genetic studies in 79% in both groups of patients, and in 14% and 20% of those, respectively, the exact genetic aberration was unknown. It seems that the remaining 21% of patients were still diagnosed on the basis of clinical criteria. The rhGH treatment was initiated at the mean age of 4.4 ± 2.9 and 8.2 ± 2.7 years, respectively [41]. Another large group of children treated with rhGH was analysed by Sävendahl et al. in 2019 and Angulo et al. in 2020 with the data from The American Norditropin Studies (ANSWER, years 2002–2016) and NordiNet International Outcome Study (NordiNet IOS, years 2006–2016, Europe) [42,43]. There were 234 and 132 paediatric patients with PWS, with the detailed analysis of 78 and 67 patients, respectively, but without reports regarding the genetic type and age of diagnosis. The mean age at baseline was 4.67 ± 5.00 and 4.91 ± 4.88 years [42]. There were no data on the anthropometric values at baseline in relation to the exact molecular diagnosis presented in the above studies regarding rhGH treatment. However, we can see that the later therapy start was more common in the previous years, similarly to our results. We acknowledge the limitations of our research. As this is a retrospective multicentre study, including the data from 15 years of patients' observation, not all the information may be fully precise. Questionnaires were filled in by clinicians from 12 endocrine centres; therefore, no strict standardization across all providers regarding documentation was present.

6. Conclusions

In our study, we presented new data regarding the influence of the genetic background in children with PWS on the time of diagnosis and rhGH start, with a significantly earlier genetic diagnosis and commencement of the therapy in children with DEL 15. This molecular type of diagnosis is also related to the possible favourable higher IGF1 level and the tendency towards lower BMI SDS before rhGH treatment. The type of genetic diagnosis seems to have little impact on perinatal data, with only the tendency towards lower birth weight SDS in the group UPD 15.

Additionally, we presented a new analysis of the time of diagnosis and start of the therapy in regard to the different nutritional phases in patients with PWS. Diagnosis in the nutritional phase 1a, before the 9th month of age, leads to earlier rhGH treatment, with the start early in the phase 2a when increased appetite is not yet observed and again with favourable lower BMI SDS and the tendency towards a higher IGF1 level.

In conclusion, we confirmed the importance of the early exact molecular type of diagnosis in patients with PWS and found differences in the circumstances of rhGH commencement between PWS genetic subtypes.

Author Contributions: Conceptualization, A.L.-A. and M.S.; Data curation, A.L.-A., K.D.-O., A.Z.-G., A.N., T.Ż., D.B.-W., R.S., M.H., M.O.-M., B.R.-P., E.G., A.D., E.P.; Formal analysis, A.L.-A. and M.W.-M.; Investigation, A.L.-A., K.D.-O., A.Z.-G., A.N., T.Ż., D.B.-W., R.S., M.H., M.O.-M., B.R.-P., E.G., A.D., E.P.; Methodology, A.L.-A., M.W.-M. and M.S.; Supervision, M.S.; Writing—original draft, A.L.-A.; Writing—review and editing, A.L.-A., M.W.-M. and M.S. All authors have read and agreed to the published version of the manuscript.

Funding: This research received no external funding.

Institutional Review Board Statement: The study was conducted according to the guidelines of the Declaration of Helsinki and approved by the Bioethics Committee of the Children's Memorial Health Institute (7/KBE/2019, 20 March 2019).

Informed Consent Statement: Written informed patient/parent consent was waived in this study due to the retrospective and anonymous character of the research, in accordance with the Bioethics Committee of the Children's Memorial Health Institute's decision.

Data Availability Statement: The data presented in this study are available on request from the corresponding author. The data are not publicly available due to ethical restrictions.

Acknowledgments: The Polish Coordination Group for rhGH Treatment members that participated in the study: Barbara Kalina-Faska, Ewa Małecka-Tendera, Department of Paediatrics, Endocrinology and Diabetes, Medical University of Silesia, Katowice, Poland; Anna Wędrychowicz, Jerzy Starzyk, Department of Paediatric and Adolescent Endocrinology, University Children's Hospital, Cracow, Poland; Marek Niedziela, Department of Paediatric Endocrinology and Rheumatology, Institute of Paediatrics, Poznan University of Medical Sciences, Poznan, Poland; Artur Mazur, II Clinic of Paediatrics, Endocrinology and Paediatric Diabetology, Clinical Regional Hospital No 2, Rzeszow, Poland; Mieczysław Walczak, Department of Paediatrics, Endocrinology, Diabetology, Metabolic Disorders and Cardiology of Developmental Age, Pomeranian Medical University, Szczecin, Poland; Andrzej Kędzia, Department of Clinical Auxology and Paediatric Nursing, Poznan University of Medical Sciences, Poznan, Poland; Jolanta Nawrotek, II Clinic of Paediatrics, Regional Specialist Children's Hospital, Kielce, Poland; Elżbieta Moszczyńska, Department of Endocrinology and Diabetology, The Children's Memorial Health Institute, Warsaw, Poland. The authors wish to acknowledge the contribution to the study of Agnieszka Bogusz-Wójcik, Kamila Marszałek-Dziuba, Department of Endocrinology and Diabetology, Agata Skórka, Department of Medical Genetics,

The Children's Memorial Health Institute, Warsaw, Poland; Katarzyna Majewska, Department of Clinical Auxology and Paediatric Nursing, Poznan University of Medical Sciences, Poznan, Poland. We would like to address special acknowledgments for the significant contribution to the research to our dear colleagues: Maria Kalina, Department of Paediatrics, Endocrinology and Diabetes, Medical University of Silesia, Katowice, Poland and Urszula Oczkowska, Endocrinology Outpatient Clinic, Institute of Mother and Child, Warsaw, Poland.

Conflicts of Interest: The authors declare no conflict of interest.

References

1. Goldstone, A.P.; Holland, A.J.; Hauffa, B.P.; Hokken-Koelega, A.C.; Tauber, M. On behalf of speakers and contributors at the Second Expert Meeting of the Comprehensive Care of Patients with PWS. Recommendations for the diagnosis and management of Prader-Willi syndrome. *J. Clin. Endocrinol. Metab.* **2008**, *93*, 4183–4197. [CrossRef]
2. Cassidy, S.B.; Schwartz, S.; Miller, J.L.; Driscoll, D.J. Prader-Willi syndrome. *Genet. Med.* **2012**, *14*, 10–26. [CrossRef]
3. Butler, M.G.; Duis, J. Chromosome 15 Imprinting Disorders: Genetic Laboratory Methodology and Approaches. *Front. Pediatr.* **2020**, *8*, 154. [CrossRef] [PubMed]
4. Kanber, D.; Giltay, J.; Wieczorek, D.; Zogel, C.; Hochstenbach, R.; Caliebe, A.; Kuechler, A.; Horsthemke, B.; Buiting, K. A paternal deletion of MKRN3, MAGEL2 and NDN does not result in Prader–Willi syndrome. *Eur. J. Hum. Genet.* **2009**, *17*, 582–590. [CrossRef] [PubMed]
5. Duis, J.; van Wattum, P.J.; Scheimann, A.; Salehi, P.; Brokamp, E.; Fairbrother, L.; Childers, A.; Shelton, A.R.; Bingham, N.C.; Shoemaker, A.H.; et al. A multidisciplinary approach to the clinical management of Prader–Willi syndrome. *Mol. Genet. Genom. Med.* **2019**, *7*, e514. [CrossRef] [PubMed]
6. Emerick, J.E.; Vogt, K.S. Endocrine manifestations and management of Prader-Willi syndrome. *Int. J. Pediatric Endocrinol.* **2013**, *2013*, 14. [CrossRef]
7. Miller, J.L. Approach to the child with Prader-Willi syndrome. *J. Clin. Endocrinol. Metab.* **2012**, *97*, 3837–3844. [CrossRef] [PubMed]
8. Alves, C.; Franco, R.R. Prader-Willi syndrome: Endocrine manifestations and management. *Arch. Endocrinol. Metab.* **2020**, *64*, 3. [CrossRef]
9. Mann, N.P.; Butler, G.E. Prader-Willi syndrome: Clinical features and management. *Paediatr. Child. Health* **2009**, *19*, 473–478. [CrossRef]
10. Goldstone, A.P. Prader-Willi syndrome: Advances in genetics, pathophysiology and treatment. *Trends Endocrinol. Metab.* **2004**, *15*, 12–20. [CrossRef]
11. Napolitano, L.; Barone, B.; Morra, S.; Celentano, G.; La Rocca, R.; Capece, M.; Morgera, V.; Turco, C.; Caputo, V.F.; Spena, G.; et al. Hypogonadism in Patients with Prader Willi Syndrome: A Narrative Review. *Int. J. Mol. Sci.* **2021**, *22*, 1993. [CrossRef]
12. Gross-Tsur, V.; Hirsch, H.J.; Benarroch, F.; Eldar-Geva, T. The FSH-inhibin axis in Prader-Willi syndrome: Heterogeneity of gonadal dysfunction. *Reprod. Biol. Endocrinol.* **2012**, *10*, 2–7. [CrossRef] [PubMed]
13. Hirsch, H.J.; Eldar-Geva, T.; Bennaroch, F.; Pollak, Y.; Gross-Tsur, V. Sexual dichotomy of gonadal function in Prader-Willi syndrome from early infancy through the fourth decade. *Hum. Reprod.* **2015**, *30*, 2587–2596. [CrossRef]
14. Lecka-Ambroziak, A.; Wysocka-Mincewicz, M.; Marszałek-Dziuba, K.; Rudzka-Kocjan, A.; Szalecki, M. Premature Adrenarche in Children with Prader-Willi Syndrome Treated with Recombinant Human Growth Hormone Seems to Not Influence the Course of Central Puberty and the Ecacy and Safety of the Therapy. *Life* **2020**, *10*, 237. [CrossRef] [PubMed]
15. Butler, M.G.; Kimonis, V.; Dykens, E.; Gold, J.A.; Miller, J.; Tamura, R.; Driscoll, D.J. Prader–Willi syndrome and early-onset morbid obesity NIH rare disease consortium: A review of natural history study. *Am. J. Med. Genet. A* **2018**, *176*, 368–375. [CrossRef] [PubMed]
16. Khan, M.J.; Gerasimidis, K.; Edwards, C.A.; Shaikh, M.G. Mechanisms of Obesity in Prader-Willi Syndrome. *J. Ped. Obes.* **2018**, *13*, 3–13. [CrossRef] [PubMed]
17. Crinò, A.; Fintini, D.; Bocchini, S.; Grugni, G. Obesity management in Prader–Willi syndrome: Current perspectives. *Diabetes, Metabolic Syndrome and Obesity. Targets Ther.* **2018**, *11*, 579–593.
18. Gantz, M.G.; Andrews, S.M.; Wheeler, A.C. Food and Non-Food-Related Behavior across Settings in Children with Prader–Willi Syndrome. *Genes* **2020**, *11*, 204. [CrossRef]
19. Miller, J.L.; Lynn, C.H.; Driscoll, D.C.; Goldstone, A.P.; Gold, J.A.; Kimonis, V.; Dykens, E.; Butler, M.G.; Shuster, J.J.; Driscoll, D.J. Nutritional phases in Prader-Willi syndrome. *Am. J. Med. Genet. Part A* **2011**, *155*, 1040–1049. [CrossRef]
20. Butler, J.V.; Whittington, J.E.; Holland, A.J.; McAllister, C.J.; Goldstone, A.P. The transition between the phenotypes of Prader-Willi syndrome during infancy and early childhood. *Dev. Med. Child. Neurol.* **2010**, *52*, e88–e93. [CrossRef]
21. Deal, C.L.; Tony, M.; Hoybye, C.; Allen, D.B.; Tauber, M.; Christiansen, J.S.; Growth Hormone in Prader-Willi Syndrome Clinical Care Guidelines Workshop Participants. Growth Hormone Research Society Workshop Summary. Consensus guidelines for recombinant human growth hormone therapy in Prader-Willi syndrome. *J. Clin. Endocrinol. Metab.* **2013**, *98*, E1072–E1087. [CrossRef]

22. De Lind van Wijngaarden, R.F.A.; Siemensma, E.P.C.; Festen, D.A.M.; Otten, B.J.; van Mil, E.G.; Rotteveel, J.; Odink, R.J.H.; Bindels-de Heus, G.C.B.K.; van Leeuwen, M.; Haring, D.A.J.P.; et al. Efficacy and safety of long-term continuous growth hormone treatment in children with Prader-Willi syndrome. *J. Clin. Endocrinol. Metab.* **2009**, *94*, 4205–4215. [CrossRef]
23. Carrel, A.L.; Myers, S.E.; Whitman, B.Y.; Eickhoff, J.; Allen, D.B. Long-term growth hormone therapy changes the natural history of body composition and motor function in children with Prader-Willi syndrome. *J. Clin. Endocrinol. Metab.* **2010**, *95*, 1131–1136. [CrossRef]
24. Bakker, N.E.; Kuppens, R.J.; Siemensma, E.P.C.; Tummers-de Lind van Wijngaarden, R.F.A.; Festen, D.A.M.; Bindels-de Heus, G.C.B.; Bocca, G.; Haring, D.A.J.P.; Hoorweg-Nijman, J.J.G.; Houdijk, E.C.A.M.; et al. Eight years of growth hormone treatment in children with Prader-Willi syndrome: Maintaining the positive effects. *J. Clin. Endocrinol. Metab.* **2013**, *98*, 4013–4022. [CrossRef]
25. Donze, S.H.; Damen, L.; Mahabier, E.F.; Hokken-Koelega, A.C.S. Improved Mental and Motor Development during 3 Years of GH Treatment in Very Young Children with Prader-Willi Syndrome. *J. Clin. Endocrinol. Metab.* **2018**, *103*, 3714–3719. [CrossRef]
26. Bakker, N.E.; Siemensma, E.P.C.; van Rijn, M.; Festen, D.; Hokken-Koelega, A.C.S. Beneficial Effect of Growth Hormone Treatment on Health-Related Quality of Life in Children with Prader-Willi Syndrome: A Randomized Controlled Trial and Longitudinal Study. *Horm. Res. Paediatr.* **2015**, *84*. [CrossRef]
27. Luo, Y.; Zheng, Z.; Yang, Y.; Bai, X.; Yang, H.; Zhu, H.; Pan, H.; Chen, S. Effects of growth hormone on cognitive, motor, and behavioral development in Prader-Willi syndrome children: A meta-analysis of randomized controlled trials. *Endocrine* **2021**, *71*, 321–330. [CrossRef]
28. Costa, R.A.; Ferreira, I.R.; Cintra, H.A.; Gomes, L.H.F. Guida LdC. Genotype-Phenotype Relationships and Endocrine Findings in Prader-Willi Syndrome. *Front. Endocrinol.* **2019**, *10*, 864. [CrossRef]
29. Singh, P.; Mahmoud, R.; Gold, J.A.; Miller, J.L.; Roof, E.; Tamura, R.; Dykens, E.; Butler, M.G.; Driscoll, D.J.; Kimonis, V. A multicenter study of maternal and neonatal outcomes in individuals with Prader-Willi syndrome. *J. Med. Genet.* **2018**, *55*, 594–598. [CrossRef]
30. Bar, C.; Diene, G.; Molinas, C.; Bieth, E.; Casper, C.; Tauber, M. Early diagnosis and care is achieved but should be improved in infants with Prader-Willi syndrome. *Orphanet J. Rare Dis.* **2017**, *12*, 118. [CrossRef]
31. Salvatoni, A.; Moretti, A.; Grugni, G.; Agosti, M.; Azzolini, S.; Bonaita, V.; Cianci, P.; Corica, D.; Crinò, A.; DelVecchio, M.; et al. Anthropometric characteristics of newborns with Prader-Willi syndrome. *Am. J. Med. Genet.* **2019**, *179*, 2067–2074. [CrossRef]
32. Ge, M.M.; Gao, Y.Y.; Wu, B.B.; Yan, K.; Qin, Q.; Wang, H.; Zhou, W.; Yang, L. Relationship between phenotype and genotype of 102 Chinese newborns with Prader–Willi syndrome. *Mol. Biol. Rep.* **2019**, *46*, 4717–4724. [CrossRef] [PubMed]
33. Bacheré, N.; Diene, G.; Delagnes, V.; Molinas, C.; Moulin, P.; Tauber, M. Early Diagnosis and Multidisciplinary Care Reduce the Hospitalization Time and Duration of Tube Feeding and Prevent Early Obesity in PWS Infants. *Horm. Res.* **2008**, *69*, 45–52. [CrossRef] [PubMed]
34. Butler, M.G.; Matthews, N.A.; Patel, N.; Surampalli, A.; Gold, J.A.; Khare, M.; Thompson, T.; Cassidy, S.B.; Kimonis, V.E. Impact of genetic subtypes of Prader–Willi syndrome with growth hormone therapy on intelligence and body mass index. *Am. J. Med. Genet. A* **2019**, *179*, 1826–1835. [CrossRef]
35. Shepherd, D.A.; Vos, N.; Reid, S.M.; Godler, D.E.; Guzys, A.; Moreno-Betancur, M.; Amor, D.J. Growth Trajectories in Genetic Subtypes of Prader–Willi Syndrome. *Genes* **2020**, *11*, 736. [CrossRef] [PubMed]
36. Mahmoud, R.; Leonenko, A.; Butler, M.G.; Flodman, P.; Gold, J.A.; Miller, J.L.; Roof, E.; Dykens, E.; Driscoll, D.J.; Kimonis, V. Influence of Molecular Classes and Growth Hormone Treatment on Growth and Dysmorphology in Prader-Willi Syndrome: A Multicenter Study. *Clin. Genet.* **2021**. [CrossRef] [PubMed]
37. Oldzej, J.; Manazir, J.; Gold, J.A.; Mahmoud, R.; Osann, K.; Flodman, P.; Cassidy, S.B.; Kimonis, V.E. Molecular subtype and growth hormone effects on dysmorphology in Prader–Willi syndrome. *Am. J. Med. Genet.* **2020**, *182A*, 169–175. [CrossRef] [PubMed]
38. Magill, L.; Laemmer, C.; Woelfle, J.; Fimmers, R.; Gohlke, B. Early start of growth hormone is associated with positive effects on auxology and metabolism in Prader-Willi-syndrome. *Orphanet J. Rare Dis.* **2020**, *15*, 283. [CrossRef] [PubMed]
39. Corripio, R.; Tubau, C.; Calvo, L.; Brun, C.; Capdevila, N.; Larramona, H.; Gabau, E. Safety and effectiveness of growth hormone therapy in infants with Prader-Willi syndrome younger than 2 years: A prospective study. *J. Pediatr. Endocrinol. Metab.* **2019**, *32*, 879–884. [CrossRef]
40. Lionti, T.; Reid, S.M.; White, S.M.; Rowell, M.M. A population-based profile of 160 Australians with Prader-Willi syndrome: Trends in diagnosis, birth prevalence and birth characteristics. *Am. J. Med. Genet. A* **2015**, *167A*, 371–378. [CrossRef]
41. Bakker, N.E.; Lindberg, A.; Heissler, J.; Wollmann, H.A.; Camacho-Hübner, C.; Hokken-Koelega, A.C.; on behalf of the KIGS Steering Committee. Growth Hormone Treatment in Children with Prader-Willi Syndrome: Three Years of Longitudinal Data in Prepubertal Children and Adult Height Data from the KIGS Database. *J. Clin. Endocrinol. Metab.* **2017**, *102*, 1702–1711. [CrossRef]
42. Sävendahl, L.; Polak, M.; Backeljauw, P.; Blair, J.; Miller, B.S.; Rohrer, T.R.; Pietropoli, A.; Ostrow, V.; Ross, J. Treatment of Children with GH in the United States and Europe: Long-Term Follow-Up from NordiNet® IOS and ANSWER Program. *J. Clin. Endocrinol. Metab.* **2019**, *104*, 4730–4742. [CrossRef] [PubMed]
43. Angulo, M.; Abuzzahab, M.J.; Pietropoli, A.; Ostrow, V.; Kelepouris, N.; Tauber, M. Outcomes in children treated with growth hormone for Prader-Willi syndrome: Data from the ANSWER Program® and NordiNet® International Outcome Study. *Int. J. Pediatr. Endocrinol.* **2020**, *2020*, 1–8. [CrossRef] [PubMed]

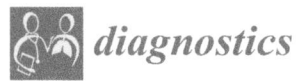

Review

Facilitations and Hurdles of Genetic Testing in Neuromuscular Disorders

Andrea Barp [1,*], Lorena Mosca [2] and Valeria Ada Sansone [1]

[1] The NEMO Clinical Center in Milan, Neurorehabilitation Unit, University of Milan, Piazza Ospedale Maggiore 3, 20162 Milano, Italy; valeria.sansone@centrocliniconemo.it
[2] Medical Genetics Unit, ASST Grande Ospedale Metropolitano Niguarda, Piazza Ospedale Maggiore 3, 20162 Milano, Italy; lorena.mosca@ospedaleniguarda.it
* Correspondence: andrea.barp@centrocliniconemo.it

Abstract: Neuromuscular disorders (NMDs) comprise a heterogeneous group of disorders that affect about one in every thousand individuals worldwide. The vast majority of NMDs has a genetic cause, with about 600 genes already identified. Application of genetic testing in NMDs can be useful for several reasons: correct diagnostic definition of a proband, extensive familial counselling to identify subjects at risk, and prenatal diagnosis to prevent the recurrence of the disease; furthermore, identification of specific genetic mutations still remains mandatory in some cases for clinical trial enrollment where new gene therapies are now approaching. Even though genetic analysis is catching on in the neuromuscular field, pitfalls and hurdles still remain and they should be taken into account by clinicians, as for example the use of next generation sequencing (NGS) where many single nucleotide variants of "unknown significance" can emerge, complicating the correct interpretation of genotype-phenotype relationship. Finally, when all efforts in terms of molecular analysis have been carried on, a portion of patients affected by NMDs still remain "not genetically defined". In the present review we analyze the evolution of genetic techniques, from Sanger sequencing to NGS, and we discuss "facilitations and hurdles" of genetic testing which must always be balanced by clinicians, in order to ensure a correct diagnostic definition, but taking always into account the benefit that the patient could obtain especially in terms of "therapeutic offer".

Keywords: neuromuscular disease; genetic testing; next generation sequencing; whole exome sequencing

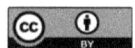

1. Introduction

Neuromuscular disorders (NMDs) comprise a clinically and genetically heterogeneous group of disorders that affect about one in every thousand individuals worldwide [1], representing a significant health burden to society. Skeletal muscle (muscular dystrophies, myotonic dystrophies type 1 and 2 (DM1 and DM2), congenital DM (CDM), congenital myopathies (CMs) and metabolic myopathies), skeletal muscle voltage-gated ion channels (periodic paralysis, congenital myotonia), neuromuscular junctions (myasthenic syndromes), nerves/motor neurons (Charcot–Marie–Tooth neuropathies (CMTs), amyotrophic lateral sclerosis (ALS), hereditary spastic paraplegias (HSPs) and spinal muscular atrophies (SMA)) can be primarily affected. Onset may occur at birth (SMA, CDM, CMDs, Pompe disease), during childhood (Duchenne muscular dystrophy (DMD), and many CMs, congenital muscular dystrophies (CMDs)), in adulthood (DM1/2, facioscapulohumeral dystrophy (FSHD). Some limb-girdle muscular dystrophies (LGMDs) and other muscular dystrophies) or have a predominant late-onset (ALS). Progression also varies amongst the different types, and amongst patients: it can be rapidly progressive since birth (e.g., SMA type 1) or even if onset is later in life (e.g., ALS with bulbar onset), or it may be slower over time (e.g., SMA type 3, LGMDs, FSHD, DM2, or hypokalemic periodic paralysis (HOP)) [2].

2. The Complexity of Diagnosing a Neuromuscular Disorder

Although NMDs are unique and the clinical presentation varies, they all share some common features: muscle weakness and wasting, often fasciculations, cramps, or muscle pain, and not uncommonly—symptoms of bulbar involvement like respiratory and swallowing problems and cranial nerve palsies [3]. There may be a significant phenotypic overlap amongst the different types of NMDs [4]. Moreover, this heterogeneous neuromuscular picture is often "complicated" by the fact that, in some patients disease penetrance is reduced, onset is variable just as is expressivity [5], and many patients may have predominantly extra-muscular symptoms as part of their disease. This in part accounts for the diagnostic delay, which is known to characterize many of these diseases. Several specialists and professionals may come into play at the time of the initial symptoms and there may be the need for many medical investigations, such as extensive biochemical blood tests, muscle magnetic resonance imaging (MRI) or other imaging techniques, neurophysiological assessments, muscle and/or nerve biopsies, lumbar puncture and other diagnostic tests [6,7]. Table 1 summarizes the multiple clinical presentations of the most frequent NMDs and the possible time-lag between initial symptoms and the clinical or genetic confirmation of disease.

Table 1. Main neuromuscular conditions and time lag between onset and diagnosis.

Neuromuscular Disease	Common Neuromuscular Presentation	Common Extramuscular Presentation	Time-Lag between Onset of Symptoms and Diagnosis
Duchenne muscular dystrophy (DMD)	Very high CK levels Proximal LL weakness Calves hypertrophy	Intellectual disability/autism	24 months [8]
Spinal muscular atrophy (SMA)	Hypotonia and respiratory failure (if birth onset) Proximal muscle weakness and absent DTRs (if adult onset)	–	4.7 ± 2.82 months (type 1) 15.6 ± 5.88 months (type 2) 4.34 ± 4.01 years (type 3) [9]
Congenital myotonic dystrophy (CDM)	Mixed hypotonia at birth	Intellectual disability Difficulty breathing Swallowing problems Talipes	Few days from birth [10]
Myotonic dystrophy type 1 (DM1)	Hand and foot dorsiflexor weakness Hand myotonia Bilteral ptosis Facial weakness	Early-onset cataracts Cardiac arrhythmias Syncope/cardiac arrest Gonadal failure Insulin resistance Excessive daytime sleepiness	7.3 ± 8.2 years [11]
Myotonic dystrophy type 2 (DM2)	High CK Difficulty climbing stairs Muscle pain	Early-onset cataracts Cardiac arrhythmias Insulin resistance Fatiguability	14.4 ± 12.8 years [11]
Facioscapulohumeral muscular dystrophy type 1 and 2 (FSHD1/2)	Proximal weakness in the UL Proximal and distal weakness in the LL Wing scapula Facial weakness	Retinal vasculopathy/Coat syndrome Right bundle branch block High frequency hearing loss Pectus excavatus	Variable, from few years to several years [12]
Amyotrophic lateral sclerosis (ALS)	Bulbar onset: dysarthria, dysphagia Spinal onset: weakness in the upper or lower limbs, usually distal	Loss of weight Fatigue Shortness of breath Cognitive impairment	12 months [13]

CK, creatin kinase; DTRs, deep tendon reflexes; LL, lower limb; UL, upper limb.

The vast majority of NMDs has a genetic cause, with about 600 genes already identified (see http://www.musclegenetable.fr/index.html, accessed date: 13 April 2021), and this number is still growing; pathogenic variants involved display autosomal recessive, autosomal dominant or X-linked inheritance [1] as well as mitochondrial inheritance. For different NMDs, many genes are involved (genetic heterogeneity) and a great variety of mutation types can be found in a single gene (allelic heterogeneity). The full mutational spectrum reported in NMDs includes single nucleotide variants, large deletions and duplications, small mutations, expansion repeats, epigenetic changes, dynamic mutations and atypical mutations or alterations occurring in regulatory regions as promoters, untranslated 5′/3′ regions, or intergenic segments [14]. While, on one hand, genetics facilitates the diagnostic process, it adds also complexity. Not infrequently, the family history is reported to be negative, or genetic testing in the family members or parents is inconclusive. In these cases, a de novo mutation should be considered, along with a somatic mosaicism in which a mutation may be present in some, but not all cells [15]. Moreover, despite the progress in genetics, there are still a number of patients with a probable NMD based on the clinical and laboratory data (e.g., neurophysiological studies and muscle biopsy results) in whom there is no genetic confirmation [16,17].

3. The Approach to Genetic Testing

Due to the significant costs of most molecular tests, in terms of both human resources and reagents, it is crucial to establish as precise a clinical diagnosis as possible. The most important step is to consider if the patient's symptoms may have a genetic origin. There are some features which can suggest a hereditary process: longstanding or slowly progressive deficits, clinical signs out of proportion to the patients' symptoms, early onset of them, similar symptoms reported in other family members, and the association with musculoskeletal abnormalities, such as pes cavus, scoliosis or contractures. Sometimes patients are unable to identify slowly progressive deficit or recognize similar symptoms in other family members, particularly if they have not received a confirmed diagnosis. Specific questions regarding early milestones, participation in sports, or other physically demanding activity is often necessary to reveal subtle deficits in neuromuscular function [15]. When clinicians have considered the possibility of a NMD, the second step is to localize the disease process (muscle, neuromuscular junction, peripheral nerve or motor neuron). In such a way, ancillary tests like neurophysiological testing, laboratory testing or muscle biopsy may be required to exclude other acquired disorders and narrow the differential diagnosis to allow for targeted molecular testing. Despite these measures, the diagnostic yield of neurogenetic testing can be low even if multiple tests are pursued. Table 2 describes some of the most common signs or symptoms, which may help clinicians to localize the site of lesion and better target the subsequent work up, including genetic testing.

Table 2. Main clinical findings and corresponding neuromuscular site of involvement, which can help to target the genetic analysis.

Main Neuromuscular Sign/Symptom	Possible/Probable Site of Lesion	Differential Diagnosis
Muscle weakness and stiffness, pseudobulbar signs, ↑↑ DTRs, Babinski and Hoffmann signs, clonus.	UMN	PLS ALS (UMN prevalent) HSP
Distal symmetric weakness, distal muscular atrophy, sensory and/or autonomic signs, ↓↓ DTRs, pes cavus, hammertoe deformities, leg atrophy. In general symptoms << signs.	Peripheral nerve	Genetic neuropathy (CMT)
Proximal muscle weakness and wasting, ↓↓ or absent DTRs, Gower's sign, no sensory symptoms.	Skeletal muscle, LMN	Muscular dystrophies SMA type 3
Young age, proximal muscle weakness, facial weakness, diffuse wasting, ↓↓ or absent DTRs, Gower's sign, bulbar signs, osteoskeletal deformities (pectus excavatus, scoliosis, tendon retractions, congenital hip dysplasia).	Skeletal muscle	CMs
Distal muscular weakness, grip myotonia, ↓↓ or absent DTRs, cataract, baldness, ptosis, bulbar signs.	Skeletal muscle	DM1
Proximal muscle weakness, normal or ↑↑ DTR, myotonia, myalgia, cataract	Skeletal muscle	DM2

Table 2. Cont.

Main Neuromuscular Sign/Symptom	Possible/Probable Site of Lesion	Differential Diagnosis
Limb fasciculations associated with muscle weakness and/or atrophy, ↓↓ or absent DTRs, no sensory symptoms	LMN Peripheral nerve	ALS (LMN prevalent) Kennedy disaease (note that a sensory neuropathy could be also present) Pure motor neuropahy
Limb fasciculations associated with muscle weakness and/or atrophy, ↓↓ or absent DTRs, no sensory symptoms, bulbar signs	LMN	ALS (LMN prevalent) Kennedy disaease
Mixed LMN and UMN signs in the same myotome (e.g., muscle wasting, ↑↑ DTRs, fasciculations, muscle stiffness), bulbar signs	LMN and UMN	Classic ALS
Episodic weakness and/or paralysis	Skeletal muscle (ion channel)	Channelopathies
Fluctuating weakness with fatiguability, no sensory symptoms	Neuromuscular junction	Myasthenia gravis
Isolated "foot drop"	Peripheral nerve LMN Skeletal muscle	Genetic or acquired neuropathy ALS DM1 FSHD Distal myopathy
Isolated "drop head"	LMN Neuromuscular junction Skeletal muscle	ALS Miasthenia gravis Muscular dystrophies Metabolic myopathies
Isolated "bulbar signs"	LMN Neuromuscular junction	ALS Myasthenia gravis
Hypotonia and/or respiratory failure at birth	LMN Neuromuscular junction Skeletal muscle	SMA type 1 Congenital myasthenia CDM CMDs CMs Congenital myopathies Metabolic myopathy (Pompe disease)

ALS, amyotrophic lateral sclerosis; CDM, congenital DM; CMs, congenital myopathies; CMDs, congenital muscular dystrophies; CMT, Charcot–Marie–Tooth; DM1/2, myotonic dystrophy type 1 and 2; DTRs, deep tendon reflexes; FSHD, facioscapulohumeral dystrophy; HSP, hereditary spastic paraparesis; LL, lower limb; LMN, lower motor neuron; PLS, primary lateral sclerosis; SMA, spinal muscular atrophy; UMN, upper motor neuron; ↑↑, increased; ↓↓, decreased; <<, less than.

4. The Evolution of Genetic Techniques and Their Application to NMDs

The scientific history of genetics began with the introduction of the fundamental laws of inheritance by Mendel in 1859, and was improved in 1910 by Morgan's experiments, which revealed that genes were responsible for the appearance of a specific phenotype located on chromosomes [18]. In 1953, Watson and Crick described the structure of DNA and showed that genetic information is represented by a sequence of nucleotides on its two strands [19]. The genetic code was finally uncovered in 1966, by defining that a sequence of adjacent three nucleotides (codon) codes for amino acids. All such findings brought a rapid improvement to the genetics field and to the development of new molecular technologies. The first genetic analysis was performed in the cytogenetics field, making possible the identification of a number of structure abnormalities of human chromosomes [18]. The detection of single nucleotides changes in DNA was instead rapidly developed after the setting-up of polymerase chain reaction (PCR) by Mullis and Smith in 1983, enabling the generation of thousands to millions of copies of a particular DNA sequence [20]. At first, PCR was applied to techniques widely used for known mutations screening. The need to detect every genetic variant was overcome by the introduction of chemical sequencing technology; in particular, the development in 1977 of the dideoxynucleotide chain termination sequencing by Sanger enabled DNA reading at base pair resolution. Quickly, thanks to the introduction of automated DNA sequencers, the manual method was improved and replaced by the automated one [18,21]. All such technological advances were useful in launching of the Human Genome Project in 1990; the draft of the human genome, first released in 2001, was then completed in 2003, leading to the release of the sequence of the entire human genome, the illustration of the vast genetic diversity in humans, and the identification of a large number of disease genes [6,22]. Such a project also contributed to the improvement of sequencing technology, up to the development in 2005 of next generation sequencing (NGS). In contrast to Sanger sequencing, which involves reading of contiguous piece of DNA 1 base at time, NGS utilizes massively parallel sequencing to generate millions of short reads (100–200 base pairs each) at once, which are then aligned to a reference sequence (Figure 1).

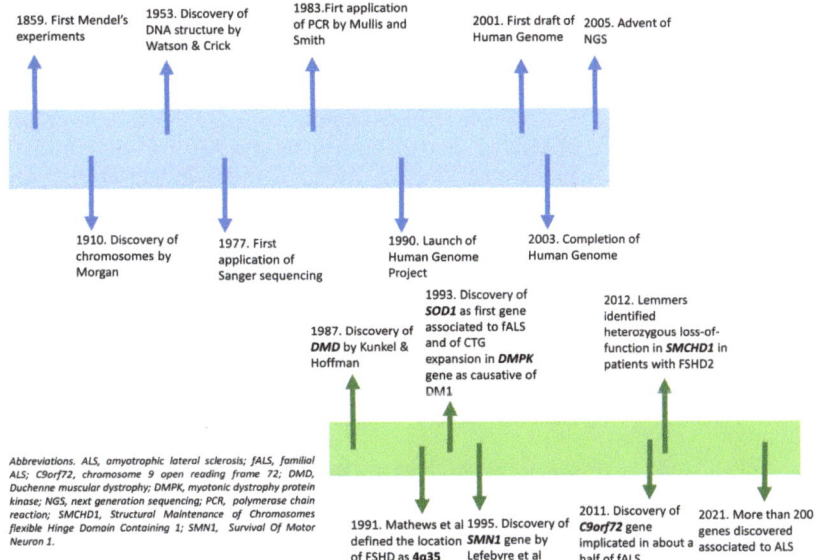

Figure 1. Timeline representing the main genetic discoveries (**top**) and the main genes discovered in Neuromuscular disorders (NMDs) (**below**).

Depending on the extent of genetic sequences to be analyzed, testing may be designed to sequence a set of genes associated with clinically related syndromes (gene panel sequencing, GPS), the protein encoding regions of the genome (whole-exome sequencing, WES), or even the whole genome of a patient (whole-genome sequencing, WGS) [23]; the method, therefore, makes possible the screening of many genes/genomic regions simultaneously, in a far more cost- and time-effective manner. Concerning NMDs, there are still examples where single gene testing (e.g., Sanger sequencing, multiple ligation probe analysis-MLPA) should be considered as a standard and first test; this is especially true if the majority of disease causing mutations for a given disease entity are quantitative rather than qualitative (e.g., DMD or SMA), or if the pathology of interest is caused by a single gene (monogenic) or by repeat expansions (e.g., spinocerebellar ataxias, SCAs) [24]. Certainly, NGS has revolutionized the diagnostic approach of many NMDs, being the most commonly used method in clinical practice for first-line diagnosis of diseases for which a wide range of genetic aberrations might be responsible for a similar phenotype, including congenital muscular dystrophies and congenital myopathies, limb girdle muscular dystrophies, congenital myasthenic syndromes, hereditary neuropathies, mitochondrial myopathies and motor neuron diseases such as ALS [25]. Additionally, allowing a better depth and coverage of gene, NGS improves discovery power by identifying novel gene variants not previously associated with a disease [7]; in nine years, NGS has resulted in a near doubling of the number of genes implicated in NMDs, from 290 in 2010 to 535 in 2019 [25]. One typical example is represented by ALS, whose field continues to develop rapidly with multiple disease gene discoveries per year. Ten years ago, its commercial genetic testing was limited to sequencing of SOD1, the first ALS-associated gene identified in 1993 [26]; actually, about 200 genes have been discovered as associated to this pathology [27], with a consequent obvious relevance for diagnosis and genetic counselling.

5. NGS and Its Hurdles

With the advent of NGS approaches a growing number of causative variants can be identified [28–30]. Even so, the majority of patients with NMDs still remain undiagnosed with variable success rates, mainly depending on the selected patient population and the applied method [31–39]. It is, therefore, a major challenge facing clinicians and geneticists to further enhance the application of NGS techniques. For example, it is a subject of ongoing debate which exact NGS approach is optimal from a diagnostic and cost-point perspective [40].

Detailed phenotyping obtained from a complete and accurate clinical evaluation is certainly important to begin the diagnostic work-up and it is increasingly recognized as a prerequisite for NGS-based diagnostics and research. In addition, the effective use of NGS in diagnostics, regardless of the approach chosen (GPS, WES or WGS), should take into account information regarding the workflows relevance, such as analysis, coverage and sequencing depth to understand each specific clinical application and diagnostic capabilities.

All NGS approaches, even GPS, generate a large volume of sequencing data which have to be processed by proper bioinformatics pipelines: the larger the genomic region to investigate (from GPS to WGS), the smaller the average sequence depth [41], and the greater the number of variants identified. Analysis of such sequencing data requires an important computational effort and needs skilled bioinformaticians able to use and choose the different tools available in each sequencing analysis step [42].

5.1. GPS Panel Sequencing

GPS test consists of multiple genes sequenced at the same time and secures that all coding exons of the genes of interest are targeted and sufficiently high covered; the majority of panels are probably custom-made, although for some more common diseases, commercially panels are available; both custom-made panels can include a single very long gene up to several hundreds genes of interest. Genes usually are grouped together based on producing the same phenotype when mutated, and for such reasons, the procedure is especially indicated as a first-tier diagnostic method if clinical diagnosis of a heterogeneous disorder does not lead to a particular gene [24]. GPS are frequently used in routine diagnostics since are cheaper then WES and WGS due to fewer genes targeted and require less data processing, analysis and storage. Since the analyzed region is smaller, deeper coverage is obtained, allowing a better detection of some copy number variations (CNVs) (e.g., PMP22 duplication/deletion [43]) and mosaicism, compared to WES [44]. In addition GPS do not reveal findings unrelated to the phenotype being investigated, avoiding incidental findings and ethical problems [44].

While these genomic tools are not capable of isolating genes associated with novel diseases, they are successfully used in the field of clinical diagnosis of NMDs [45,46], especially of those characterized by clinical overlap and oligogenic inheritance. For example, NGS panel of 56 putative candidate genes codifying for proteins involved in excitability, excitation-contraction coupling, and metabolism of muscle fibers has been demonstrated to be a useful approach in the molecular diagnosis of skeletal muscle channelopathies [47]. Moreover, in an Italian study focused on molecular analysis of familial ALS patients, the detection rate of pathogenic variants using GPS (45%) was higher respect to Sanger sequencing (23.8%), due to the mutations found in minor ALS genes [48], thus demonstrating the usefulness of targeted sequencing in ALS molecular diagnostics.

The biggest challenge of a gene panel for a given disease consists in its design; attention should be paid to which genes to include in order to maximize the diagnostic yield, and simultaneously minimize costs and volume of sequencing data obtained. A periodic update of the genes list in panels is needed, due to the frequent and continuous identification of novel causative genes.

5.2. Whole-Exome Sequencing (WES)

WES is able to encompass the entire coding regions of the genome where an estimated 85% of disease-causing variants are believed to occur [3]; it is often performed in unsolved cases after a GPS approach, in patients affected by unknown diseases [4] or in cases where no reasonable hypothesis about which gene is causing the NMD can be made [7]. Therefore, WES has the inherent potential to identify novel disease genes and allows a diagnostic re-evaluation at a later time.

Concerning the isolation of disease-causing genes, two main approaches are usually used. The first consists in the analysis of WES (and WGS) of a group of patients characterized by the same clinical features and consecutive filtering of variants located in a common gene for all or some of the members of the studied group. The second one is represented by the analysis of isolated patients in conjunction with parents (trio analysis) and/or informative members of their family, and filtering of variants by different mode of inheritance [44].

The first proof-of-principle study for exome sequencing in NMD was performed for Charcot–Marie–Tooth neuropathies: WES was applied in a large family and a causative mutation in GJB1 was identified in two affected individuals [49].

Over time, the diagnostic value of WES in NMDs has been demonstrated in several studies. Haskell et al. (2018) performed WES in 93 NMDs pediatric and adult patients with overall diagnostic yield of 12.9%, and only 63% prior phenotyping testing, including invasive muscle biopsy, was informative to reach the diagnosis [39]. Waldrop et al. (2019) performed trios-WES in 31 pediatric patients yielding a diagnostic rate of 39%; two rare genetic cases, Vici syndrome associated with EGP5, infantile hypotonia with psychomotor retardation, and characteristic facies—three caused by TBCK pathogenic variants, were identified. With positive genetic diagnosis and proper surveillance, treatment could be provided [50]. The diagnostic utility of comprehensive GPS and WES has been considered to be comparable in practice [24,51]. In contrast, it is still unclear whether the widely used small-scale panels, as often mandated by national health care providers, achieve similar results [40,50]. Another issue requiring refinement is the correct identification of causative variants against the abundance of irrelevant background variation. The widely used guidelines of the American College of Medical Genetics and Genomics (ACMG) consider various strands of genetic and clinical evidence for variant classification [52]. Whilst some variants can reliably be classified as benign or pathogenic right away, the causative effect often remains uncertain after genetic testing (variants of unknown significance, VUSs) [53]. It has already been shown that uncertain findings can be successfully reclassified using clinical reconsideration, complementary family genotyping or supporting functional data [54–56]. Such approaches have the ability to reveal minor and initially overlooked clinical features, bringing to light specific phenotypic fits potentially underpinning the pathogenic relevance of variants. The WES approach was also able to discover a wide range of phenotypes associated with some disease genes, finding a connection between what had previously considered distinct clinical entities. In congenital myopathies, the traditional classification based on histopathological findings is now flanked by genetic classification [57]. For example, the term "congenital titinopathy" is now suggested to describe a group of titin (TTN)-related diseases [58], as the term "ryanodine receptor (RYR)-related myopathies" similarly includes a wide phenotypic range [59]. Although WES is considered a powerful tool in molecular diagnostics, it suffers from some limitations: short-read WES is of limited usefulness for detecting variants other than single nucleotide variants (SNVs) and small insertions/deletions (indels), such CNVs, expansions, or contractions in repetitive regions, chromosomal rearrangements and deep intronic variants. CNVs such as exon deletion in SMN1 in SMA, exon deletion or duplication in dystrophinopathy, PMP22 duplication in Charcot–Marie–Tooth diseases could be evaluated by MLPA, specific GPS or WGS. Expansion or contraction in repetitive regions including CTG triplet repeats in DM and contraction of the D4Z4 macrosatellite repeat in DUX4 in FSHD could be evaluated by fragment analysis. Correct clinical diagnosis of these distinctive NMDs guiding the appropriate target gene study would avoid unnecessary WES that could not detect these variants. WES may also miss the variants outside the exome that arise in the deep intronic or untranslated regions (UTR); it is estimated that 15% of variants potentially causative of mendelian traits are localized in non-coding regions of the genome and all these variants would be missed performing WES [60].

5.3. Whole-Genome Sequencing (WGS)

The limitations discussed above can be overcome by the use of WGS; this approach is characterized by an uniform coverage in coding and non-coding regions and is able to detect CNVs, gross chromosomal abnormalities and deep intronic variants [4]. WGS represents a powerful tool for genomic research, since it may solve WES-negative results obtained in patients affected by a NMD.

In the neurogenetics field, WGS was first successfully applied to a recessive form of CMT disease with an unknown genetic basis: thanks to this approach, variants in the novel SH3TC2 associated gene were identified and a genetics diagnosis was made [61].

In literature, there are some other examples of NMDs diagnosed with WGS. Such approach identified truncating mutations in RBCK gene in a family quartet with two children, both affected with a previously unreported disease, characterized by progressive muscular weakness and cardiomyopathy [62]. Recently, a novel insertion in PMP22 gene was linked with a clinical diagnosis of CMT3 thanks to WGS, supporting the heterogeneity of PMP22 related to CMT [63].

Rapid WGS is a faster approach of NGS which can return results in as little as 26 h with high precision and sensitivity. Usually, analysis is focused on ~6000 genes causative of the known monogenic disorders, and is further limited to variants in genes that ranked high in correspondence to the phenotype of the affected infant/child. If a single, likely causative variant is identified for an autosomal recessive condition, the entire coding region is manually inspected [64]. Often, rapid WGS of parent–infant trios are conducted since the approach is critical for recognition of de novo variants. Petrikin et al. (2015) applied a rapid WGS approach to a select a population of ill infants in a Level IV neonatal intensive care unit ($n = 35$), reaching a diagnosis of a causative genetic disease in 57% of patients (20% of neurological findings). Moreover, since WGS also provides good coverage of the mitochondrial genome, one maternally inherited diagnosis in the 35 cases was obtained [64]. The major limits in using WGS today in daily routine diagnostics consist in costs and interpretation: computational infrastructures suited to store and analyze terabytes of data are necessary, as well as experience in variant interpretation [3,4]. In addition, since WGS reveals about 3 to 5 million variants per individual [65], it may also return incidental findings that may be relevant to the patients current or future health yet unrelated to the initial line of questioning. Moreover, a study conducted by Alfares et al. (2018) reported that diagnostic yield from WGS was only 7% higher than WES, recommending the reanalysis of WES raw data before performing WGS [66] (Figure 2).

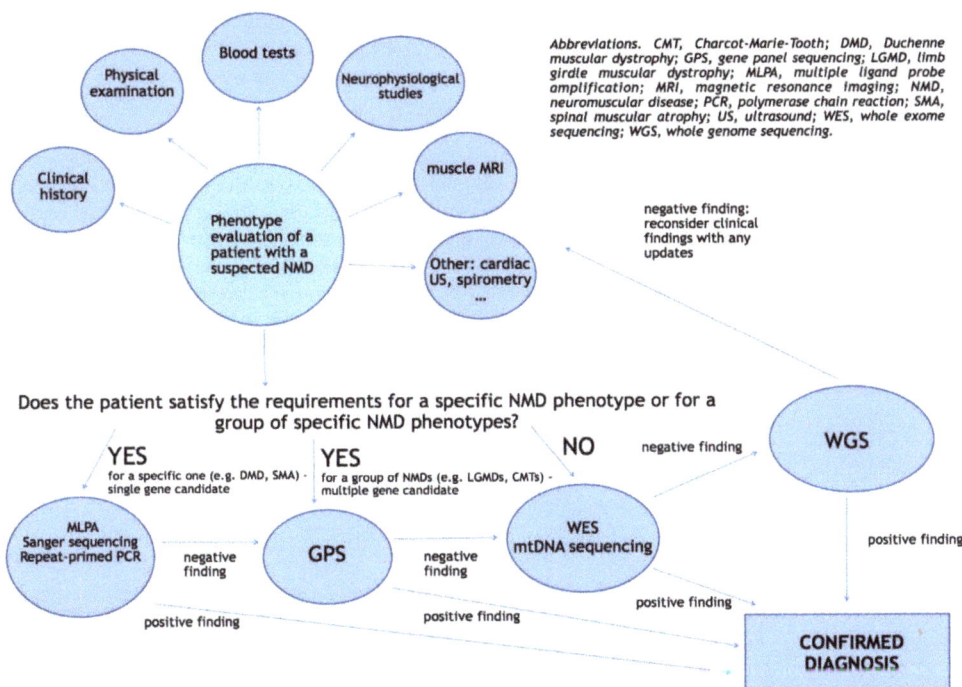

Figure 2. Proposal for a diagnostic algorithm of genetic testing in NMDs.

5.4. Mitochondrial Genome Sequencing

The clinical diagnosis of mitochondrial disorders has always been challenging. Although several well-defined clinical syndromes are easily recognized (such as chronic progressive external ophthalmoplegia, CPEO; and mitochondrial encephalomyopathy with lactic acidosis and stroke-like episodes, MELAS), many patients or families do not manifest all the canonical symptoms and signs; so this clinical heterogeneity, together with the vast genetic heterogeneity, often makes the diagnosis of mitochondrial diseases difficult [67].

The genetic basis of mitochondrial disorders is indeed complex: the mitochondrial proteome shows a dual genetic origin and therefore pathogenetic variants can reside in both nuclear and mitochondrial DNA. Moreover, any mode of inheritance (maternal, autosomal recessive, autosomal dominant, and X-linked) are described and can lead to both familial and sporadic cases. However, the majority of adult patients with mitochondrial diseases have mutations in mitochondrial DNA (mtDNA). Pathogenic deletions or SNVs of mtDNA usually affect a proportion of mtDNA molecules (heteroplasmy) [67]. Since the first discovery of mitochondrial disease-causing variant in the mtDNA in 1988 [68], technologies for genetic testing have evolved from the targeted mtDNA and candidate gene Sanger sequencing, to the more unbiased and systematic technologies based on the NGS. Although candidate gene and mtDNA sequencing remain fast and cost-effective methods for genetically and phenotypically well-defined syndromes, such as the Leber's hereditary optic neuropathy (LHON), the genetic heterogeneity of mitochondrial disorders, together with often unspeficic biochemical and metabolic findings, makes the choice of feasible number of candidate genes difficult. Indeed, screening of 64 candidate genes through Sanger sequencing established a diagnosis in just 11% of cases [69].

The use of NGS-based approaches has enabled analysis of nuclear genes simultaneously with mtDNA. WES particurarly has been successfully used to detect both nuclear and mtDNA variants in mitochondrial disorders. Given the cost constraints and additional complexity of WES, it is more commonly used only after obtaining negative results from targeted analysis such as mtDNA sequencing.

On the other hand, the NGS era caused a revolution in genetics of mitochondrial disease. Apart from diagnostic rates and expanding the genotype-phenotype association, it accelerated discovery of novel disease genes, which is over 20 per year since 2012 [70]. Starting with the more targeted approaches, application of NGS to sequence mtDNA is a routine first step in many diagnostic centers, especially for the cases with adult onset and where phenotype is highly evocative of a mtDNA etiology [71]. Apart form providing variant discovery, it also allows exact measurement of heteroplasmy levels [72]. Considering that in pediatric-onset cases, analysis is usually performed in urine and blood, instead in adult-onset ones it is usually performed in muscle, as the affected tissue is the most informative and causative variants may be undetected in blood due to tissue-heteroplasmy. In fact, as observed in CPEO, single large-scale mtDNA deletions are mostly affecting the post-mitotic skeletal muscle.

Expanding the diagnostic focus to the nuclear genes, GPS provide a targeted, deep sequencing of the predefined sets of mitochondrial disease genes, as well as candidate genes encoding for the proteins involved in essential mitochondrial function, whose disruption is thus likely to cause a disease. Available panels range from 100 genes associated with complex I efficiency to the "MitoExome", targeting the predicted mitochondrial proteome: the success rate varies from 7% to 31% [73–76]. GPS offer advantages in the higher coverage of targeted regions, as well as easier data interpretation; however the constant updates of reported disease genes, the often low phenotype–genotype correlation, the inability to surely define a mitochondrial disease by clinical symptoms, and the lower diagnostic yield of GPS compared to WES have made the latter the more preferable choice [71]. In modern diagnostics, WES has become a desired first-tier tool of investigation, especially in the cases of early-onset mitochondrial disease, where the cause of disease likely lies in the nuclear DNA [77] and because it also allows the analysis of mtDNA in the given tissue [78]. Within rare disease-diagnostic cohorts, mitochondrial diseases sit at the upper end of the WES diagnostic rate [79], ranging from 35% to 70% [80–82].

Limitations of WES regarding the genome coverage can be overcome with whole genome sequencing (WGS). Recently, trio-WGS was performed in an Australian cohort of 40 pediatric patients with clinical features suggestive of mitochondrial disease reaching a definitive molecular diagnosis in 55% of cases; moreover, three potential novel genes (ARX, NBAS and SKIV2L) associated to mitochondrial disease were identified [83].

5.5. Data Analysis and Challenges

Despite its enormous strengths and potentialities, NGS has also limitations and challenges, especially in the diagnostic field in which reaching a molecular diagnosis is fundamental: troubles regard especially the bioinformatic analysis and data interpretation.

NGS needs a bioinformatic workflow which is extremely complex: output signals generated by the NGS platform are converted in short sequences of nucleotides (short reads, ≈100–200 bp) to which base quality scores are then assigned. Reads are aligned to the reference genome and genetic variants are called, filtered and then subjected to interpretation: this step is more and more difficult going to increase the extension of the analyzed genomic regions.

Computational algorithms are used at all stages (alignment, variant calling, annotation, interpretation) and are still subject to final optimization. Different software packages are available and may result in different final interpretations; the use of different thresholds for statistical significance and variant calling would produce a different final list of putative genes.

In a typical pipeline, raw sequence data are aligned to the reference sequence using an aligner software, with the resulting alignments typically store in binary alignment map (BAM) file format; BAM files represent the standard format for storing and sharing NGS data. Prior to variant calling, routine quality control of analysis-ready BAMs should be performed with the aim to evaluate key sequencing metrics, verify the achievement of a sufficient coverage and check samples for the possible presence of contamination [41]. Incorrect mapping of reads can readily lead to erroneous identification of sequence variants, highlighting the importance of alignment accuracy; the most common alignment problem arises from reads that map to multiple locations on the reference sequence (multireads) and their correct assignment to the original sites remains challenging and fundamental. For SNVs/indels detection, the choice of a single variant caller is usually sufficient, since their detection tools have demonstrated high accuracy. However, combining the results of different callers, may offer a slight sensitivity advantage; without a "gold standard" calling algorithm, one may focus on those variants that are called by two or more callers to ensure a better chance of validation [84].

NGS, providing horizontal coverage and accuracy rates < 100%, could result in false positive results and missing variants (false negatives). Artifactual variant calls are often related to errors in short-read alignment and can be systematically filtered without significantly compromising sensitivity. For clinically relevant variants, a visual review of the alignment is recommended in order to identify false-positive variant calls that slip past automated filters. Several frequently occurring artifacts that can be identified by manual review are represented by low-quality base calls, read-end artifacts due to local misalignment near indels, strand bias artifacts, erroneous alignments in low-complexity regions and paralogous alignments of reads not well represented in the reference.

Concerning de novo variants, in addition to filtering for artifactual calls, they should be queried against public databases of genome variation, such as the gnomAD database [41].

There is significant debate within the diagnostics community regarding the necessity of confirming NGS variant calls by Sanger sequencing, considering that numerous laboratories report having 100% specificity from the NGS data alone [85]; probably, the burden of additional confirmatory testing is likely to decrease as technologies continue to evolve.

While pipelines have been primarily focused on the removal of false positives, less attention has been paid to the characterization of the fraction of false negatives, whose rate is strongly dependent on calling pipeline parameters, and especially, on read coverage. Since false negatives rate has been shown to be higher (~6–18%) than that of false positives (<3%) [86], missing mutations have to be considered a significant feature of genomic datasets and demand additional fine-tuning of bioinformatics pipelines.

Another critical point of bioinformatic workflow is represented by the variant classification and interpretation, mainly for effect of VUSs. It is incredibly difficult to prove causality for variants never reported, or located in a gene that has never been associated with disease or in a gene previously associated to a different phenotype: functional studies, segregation studies, additional families and other genetic analysis are essential to support the link [44].

A process that today is considered useful for a possible reclassification of previously identified VUSs or, more generally, for an increase in the diagnostic yield of non-diagnostic NGS is represented by the periodic "reanalysis" of archived NGS data: since annually ~250 gene-disease and ~9200 variant-disease associations are reported, this increase in information helps to establish additional diagnoses and maximize the diagnostic performance. Wenger et al. (2017) comprehensively reanalyzed 40 unsolved WES cases for which a nondiagnostic exome report was issued, on average, 20 months before reanalysis; a definitive diagnosis was identified in 10% (4/40) of cases [87] showing that a "negative" nondiagnostic result from NGS sequencing does not always mean that the disease etiology lies outside of the data already produced.

Although notable improvements in molecular analysis and bioinformatics are continually described, the technical limitations of short-read NGS are well known. Approximately 8.5% of the genome is extremely resistant to SNVs/small indels calling due to repetitive sequence or segmental duplications, causing poor variant detection in some clinically relevant genes [44]; this also have an effect in the detection of expansions or variants within NEB and TTN triplicated regions [43]. Moreover, in terms of capture efficiency, an important subset of GC-rich exons of coding genes is missed; accordingly, causative disease mutations present in these regions will be missed. Finally, the presence of highly homologous regions could generate coverage deficiency. Although these regions are captured and covered by multiple reads, quality control filters discard them because the same read can be aligned in multiple different regions, and therefore, coverage drops and variants present in those regions may be missed [44].

To overcome such technical limits, novel sequencing (e.g., long-read sequencing) and informatics are needed to find genetic variants that may be resistant to detection with the current standard NGS procedures.

5.6. Emerging Technologies

An innovative research sequencing that could provide opportunities to solve many complex problems linked to short-read NGS is long-read sequencing, also called third-generation technology. It can achieve read lengths as high as 15 kb (average of 3 kb) [88], well beyond Sanger or short-read NGS technologies, and therefore, it enables an improved detection of large indels, structural variations, haplotyping and repeat expansions [89].

Such technology in a research context has been shown to be able to capture clinically relevant variations, such as the D4Z4 repeat expansion responsible for FSHD with an estimated sequence accuracy of the total repeat region of 99.8% based on a comparison with the reference sequence [90].

Several long-read sequencing technologies have been successfully tested also for the detection of the exanucleotide repeat expansion in C9orf72 gene [91,92] which is the most common genetic cause of ALS and frontotemporal dementia (FTD) [93]. The technology endeed can span the entire C9orf72 GGGGCC expansion facilitating reliable estimation of expansion sizes and shows the ability to evaluate sequence content; this might help to determine the presence of interruptions in C9orf72 expansions [91] which is highly relevant since interruptions act as disease modifiers in other repeat expansion disorders [94].

The use of short-read or long-read sequencing depends on the research or clinical application [89]; however, as the technology and bioinformatic tools continue to improve, long-read sequencing will likely become a regular feature in the rare disease genomics tools kit [43].

Despite the tremendous impact, the diagnostic yield of all technologies described is far from complete: short- and long-sequencing enables the detection of very numerous coding and non-coding variants, but equally enormous advances in characterizing especially the non-coding alterations have not been met. RNA-sequencing (RNA-seq, also called transcriptome sequencing) analysis is able to add crucial functional evidence to the genetic information obtained by WES and WGS, and enables an increase in the diagnostic yield of different pathologies.

RNA-seq applies NGS technologies to qualitatively and quantitatively profile the full set of transcripts (transcriptome), including mRNAs, small RNAs and other non-coding RNA [84]. The procedure involves isolation of total RNA from tissues or cells of interest; RNAs are purified, fragmented and reverse transcribed into cDNA molecules which then are enriched by PCR. Following quality control and quantification, libraries are finally subjected to sequencing [65]. Similar to DNA-Seq analysis, RNA-seq data analysis involves base calling, reads mapping, transcriptome reconstruction, and also expression quantification and differential expression analysis [95].

This technique provides an opportunity to evaluate the real effect of the variation in the DNA as it undergoes transcription and is valuable as a complementary diagnostic tool; it not only permits the detection of genetic variants at the mRNA sequence level, but allows direct probing of the effect of genetic variants by assessing altered expression levels, aberrant splicing, or gene fusions [96]. Therefore, observing changes at the mRNA level can point towards the pathogenetic variant that might have otherwise been ignored (e.g., cryptic splice site) or not to be observed with WES or WGS (e.g., large structural change) [65].

RNA-seq analysis is also a useful approach in providing crucial functional evidence for pathological relevance in aberrant splicing of some VUSs or synonymous variants that previously evaded variant prioritization through NGS applied to DNA [65].

RNA-seq approach is widely used in the cancer field for its ability to detect gene fusions [65] and as a prognostic outcome measure, e.g., by assessing the expression of certain gene sets aiding treatment decisions for breast cancer or leukemia, and for monitoring immune responses hinting at possible rejections following organ transplantation [96]. However, different studies reported on RNA-seq performed on NMDs. Cummings et al. (2017) studied with this approach a cohort of 50 patients with NMDs: RNA-seq enabled validation of candidate splice-disrupting mutations and identified splice-altering variants in both exonic and deep intronic regions, yielding an overall diagnosis rate of 35%, and resulting in the discovery of a recurrent de novo intronic mutation in COL6A1 [97] which is now known to be a common cause of collagen VI-related dystrophies [98]. A similar approach applied to patients' fibroblasts resulted in molecular diagnosis in 5/48 patients (10%) affected by mitochondrial disease previously undiagnosed by WES. This technique detected aberrantly expressed genes, aberrant splicing events, and monoallelically expressed rare variants as the molecular cause in patient-derived fibroblasts, and identified a novel mitochondriopathy disease associated gene (TIMMDC1) [99]. A third study conducted by Gonorazky et al. (2019) used RNA-seq in 25 NGS-negative patients affected by monogenetic NMDs and found a genetic cause in 36% of them; moreover they establish that blood-based RNA-seq is not adequate for neuromuscular diagnostics, whereas myotubes generated by transdifferentiation from fibroblasts accurately reflect the muscle transcriptome and faithfully reveal disease-causing mutations [100]. Taken together, all these studies clearly demonstrate the power of RNA-seq to reliably detect pathogenic RNA defects in NMDs diagnosis that were not evident solely from genetic information.

Potential disease-causing variations in non-coding DNA can be successfully scanned applying NGS to DNA and RNA simultaneously. RNA-seq of leukocytes of a patient with sporadic atypical SMA identified a highly significant and atypical ASAH1 isoform not explained by a missense mutation previously found by DNA sequencing providing a molecular diagnosis of autosomal-recessive SMA with progressive myoclonic epilepsy [101]. Again, a combining WGS and RNAseq analysis was applied to a large consanguineous family in which members displayed autosomal recessively inherited SCA: homozygosity mapping, rare variant search, and comparison of the transcriptomes of affected and unaffected family members led to the detection of a causative homozygous point mutation in non-coding RNA RNU12 [102].

Finally, RNA-seq can also help to determine relative abundance and stability of transcripts that might correlate with disease severity and prognosis [25].

6. Discussion

Providing patients with a genetic diagnosis is nowadays mandatory. Diagnosis gives a chance for these patients to be recruited in clinical trials and it also helps in their care. It provides the mode of inheritance and can help define the prognosis, progression, and critical comorbidities for screening [1]. The American Association of Neuromuscular and Electrodiagnostic Medicine (AANEM) recognized the importance of genetic testing in NMDs and produced a consensus statement regarding its clinical utility, pointing out its fundamental role in the diagnosis and management because of cost effectiveness, disease management, quality of life, and family planning [103]. Moreover genetic testing allows access to therapy or enrollment in novel clinical trials or disease registries. This is even more true given the availability of personalized therapies; examples are the new drugs used in SMA [104,105], or the identification of the presence of the C9orf72 hexanucleotide repeat expansion or SOD1 mutations in ALS as a necessary criterion for enrollment into clinical trials for antisense oligonucleotide (ASO) therapy [7]. Establishing a specific molecular diagnosis is important for several reasons: (1) for disease management and treatment; (2) to decrease psychosocial burden because management and prevention protocols may be adopted; (3) to prevent unnecessary treatments and diagnostic procedures for other family members and for the patients in case symptoms may be related to the disease process itself without needing further investigations (e.g., liver biopsies for increase in liver enzymes which are to be interpreted in the muscle disease process itself); (4) to identify recurrence risk and genetic counselling to family planning and (5) to participate in clinical trials and patient registries [106]. Referring physicians should be very clear on the limitations of genetic testing during counselling and the following "points" should be emphasized: (a) a negative result does not exclude a genetic basis or contribution to the condition; (b) the test may be uninformative if a VUS is identified; and (c) positive results do not uniformly allow prediction of penetrance or disease course. Families who are not ready to undergo genetic testing may consider DNA banking to permit future testing [107]. As treatment options become available the approach to genetic testing in children will need to be revisited especially thinking that experience from previous trials and real-world data for example in SMA [108,109] strongly supports and provides evidence that the earlier the treatment, the better the outcome.

7. Conclusions

Genetics in neuromuscular disorders is extremely complex. The clinical evaluation is fundamental to target the appropriate genetic testing. A negative result should direct clinicians towards other single gene analysis or towards wider sequencing approach such as GPS, WES and WGS. Uncertain findings (such as VUS) still remain a challenge for clinicians in this "diagnostic odyssey". Pursuing the genetic diagnosis should always take into account the benefits that the patients can obtain in terms of therapeutic offer or trial enrollment.

Author Contributions: Conceptualization, A.B.; Writing, A.B., L.M., V.A.S.; Original Draft Preparation, A.B., L.M.; Resources, L.M.; Supervision, V.A.S.; Review and Editing, V.A.S. All authors have read and agreed to the published version of the manuscript.

Funding: This research received no external funding.

Acknowledgments: A.B. and V.A.S. are members of the European Reference Network (ERN) Euro-NMD.

Conflicts of Interest: The authors declare no conflict of interest.

References

1. Zatz, M.; Passos-Bueno, M.R.; Vainzof, M. Neuromuscular disorders: Genes, genetic counseling and therapeutic trials. *Genet. Mol. Biol.* **2016**, *39*, 339–348. [CrossRef] [PubMed]
2. Amato, A.A.; Russel, J.A. *Neuromuscular Disorders*, 2nd ed.; McGraw-Hill Education: New York, NY, USA, 2016; pp. 2–21.
3. Efthymiou, S.; Manole, A.; Houlden, H. Next-generation sequencing in neuromuscular diseases. *Curr. Opin. Neurol.* **2016**, *29*, 527–536. [CrossRef] [PubMed]
4. Di Resta, C.; Pipitone, G.B.; Carrera, P.; Ferrari, M. Current scenario of the genetic testing for rare neurological disorders exploiting next generation sequencing. *Neural. Regen. Res.* **2021**, *16*, 475–481. [CrossRef] [PubMed]
5. Fogel, B.L. Genetic and genomic testing for neurologic disease in clinical practice. *Handb. Clin. Neurol.* **2018**, *147*, 11–22. [CrossRef]
6. Toft, M. Advances in genetic diagnosis of neurological disorders. *Acta Neurol. Scand. Suppl.* **2014**, *198*, 20–25. [CrossRef]
7. Orengo, J.P.; Murdock, D.R. Genetic Testing in Neuromuscular Disorders. Understanding ordering and interpretation of genetic tests is paramount for clinical management. *Pract. Neurol.* **2019**, 35–41.
8. D'Amico, A.; Catteruccia, M.; Baranello, G.; Politano, L.; Govoni, A.; Previtali, S.C.; Pane, M.; D'Angelo, M.G.; Bruno, C.; Messina, S.; et al. Diagnosis of Duchenne Muscular Dystrophy in Italy in the last decade: Critical issues and areas for improvements. *Neuromuscul. Disord.* **2017**, *27*, 447–451. [CrossRef]
9. Pera, M.C.; Coratti, G.; Berti, B.; D'Amico, A.; Sframeli, M.; Albamonte, E.; de Sanctis, R.; Messina, S.; Catteruccia, M.; Brigati, G.; et al. Diagnostic journey in Spinal Muscular Atrophy: Is it still an odyssey? *PLoS ONE* **2020**, *15*, e0230677. [CrossRef]
10. Hilbert, J.E.; Johnson, N.E.; Moxley, R.T., 3rd. New insights about the incidence, multisystem manifestations, and care of patients with congenital myotonic dystrophy. *J. Pediatr* **2013**, *163*, 12–14. [CrossRef]
11. Hilbert, J.E.; Ashizawa, T.; Day, J.W.; Luebbe, E.A.; Martens, W.B.; McDermott, M.P.; Tawil, R.; Thornton, C.A.; Moxley, R.T., 3rd. Diagnostic odyssey of patients with myotonic dystrophy. *J. Neurol.* **2013**, *260*, 2497–2504. [CrossRef]

12. Zampatti, S.; Colantoni, L.; Strafella, C.; Galota, R.M.; Caputo, V.; Campoli, G.; Pagliaroli, G.; Carboni, S.; Mela, J.; Peconi, C.; et al. Facioscapulohumeral muscular dystrophy (FSHD) molecular diagnosis: From traditional technology to the NGS era. *Neurogenetics* **2019**, *20*, 57–64. [CrossRef]
13. Martínez-Molina, M.; Argente-Escrig, H.; Polo, M.F.; Hervás, D.; Frasquet, M.; Cortés, V.; Sevilla, T.; Vázquez-Costa, J.F. Early Referral to an ALS Center Reduces Several Months the Diagnostic Delay: A Multicenter-Based Study. *Front. Neurol.* **2020**, *11*, 604922. [CrossRef]
14. Peterlin, B.; Gualandi, F.; Maver, A.; Servidei, S.; van der Maarel, S.M.; Lamy, F.; Mejat, A.; Evangelista, T.; Ferlini, A. Genetic testing offer for inherited neuromuscular diseases within the EURO-NMD reference network: A European survey study. *PLoS ONE* **2020**, *15*, e0239329. [CrossRef]
15. Arnold, W.D.; Flanigan, K.M. A practical approach to molecular diagnostic testing in neuromuscular diseases. *Phys. Med. Rehabil. Clin. N. Am.* **2012**, *23*, 589–608. [CrossRef]
16. Vgontzas, A.; Renthal, W. Introduction to neurogenetics. *Am. J. Med.* **2019**, *132*, 142–152. [CrossRef]
17. Vivekanandam, V.; Männikkö, R.; Matthews, E.; Hanna, M.G. Improving genetic diagnostics of skeletal muscle channelopathies. *Expert Rev. Mol. Diagn.* **2020**, *20*, 725–736. [CrossRef]
18. Durmaz, A.A.; Karac, E.; Demkow, U.; Toruner, G.; Schoumans, J.; Cogulu, O. Evolution of Genetic Techniques: Past, Present, and Beyond. *Biomed. Res. Int.* **2015**, *2015*, 461524. [CrossRef]
19. Watson, J.D.; Crick, F.H. The structure of DNA. *Cold Spring Harb. Symp Quant. Biol.* **1953**, *18*, 123–131. [CrossRef]
20. Mullis, K.; Faloona, F.; Scharf, S.; Saiki, R.; Horn, G.; Erlich, H. Specific enzymatic amplification of DNA in vitro: The polymerase chain reaction. *Cold Spring Harb. Symp Quant. Biol.* **1986**, *51*, 263–273. [CrossRef]
21. Sanger, F.; Nicklen, S.; Coulson, A.R. DNA sequencing with chain-terminating inhibitors. *Proc. Natl. Acad. Sci. USA* **1977**, *74*, 5463–5467. [CrossRef]
22. Marian, A.J. Clinical Interpretation and Management of Genetic Variants. *JACC Basic Transl. Sci.* **2020**, *5*, 1029–1042. [CrossRef] [PubMed]
23. Shieh, P.B. Advances in the Genetic Testing of Neuromuscular Diseases. *Neurol. Clin.* **2020**, *38*, 519–528. [CrossRef] [PubMed]
24. Volk, A.E.; Kubisch, C. The rapid evolution of molecular genetic diagnostics in neuromuscular diseases. *Curr. Opin. Neurol.* **2017**, *30*, 523–528. [CrossRef] [PubMed]
25. Thompson, R.; Spendiff, S.; Roos, A.; Bourque, P.R.; Warman Chardon, J.; Kirschner, J.; Horvath, R.; Lochmüller, H. Advances in the diagnosis of inherited neuromuscular diseases and implications for therapy development. *Lancet Neurol.* **2020**, *19*, 522–532. [CrossRef]
26. Rosen, D.R.; Siddique, T.; Patterson, D.; Figlewicz, D.A.; Sapp, P.; Hentati, A.; Donaldson, D.; Goto, J.; O'Regan, J.P.; Deng, H.X.; et al. Mutations in Cu/Zn superoxide dismutase gene are associated with familial amyotrophic lateral sclerosis. *Nature* **1993**, *362*, 59–62. [CrossRef]
27. Shatunov, A.; Al-Chalabi, A. The genetic architecture of ALS. *Neurobiol. Dis.* **2021**, *147*, 105156. [CrossRef]
28. Yang, Y.; Muzny, D.M.; Reid, J.G.; Bainbridge, M.N.; Willis, A.; Ward, P.A.; Braxton, A.; Beuten, J.; Xia, F.; Niu, Z.; et al. Clinical whole-exome sequencing for the diagnosis of mendelian disorders. *N. Engl. J. Med.* **2013**, *369*, 1502–1511. [CrossRef]
29. Lee, H.; Deignan, J.L.; Dorrani, N.; Strom, S.P.; Kantarci, S.; Quintero-Rivera, F.; Das, K.; Toy, T.; Harry, B.; Yourshaw, M.; et al. Clinical exome sequencing for genetic identification of rare Mendelian disorders. *JAMA* **2014**, *312*, 1880–1887. [CrossRef]
30. Yavarna, T.; Al-Dewik, N.; Al-Mureikhi, M.; Ali, R.; Al-Mesaifri, F.; Mahmoud, L.; Shahbeck, N.; Lakhani, S.; AlMulla, M.; Nawaz, Z.; et al. High diagnostic yield of clinical exome sequencing in Middle Eastern patients with Mendelian disorders. *Hum. Genet.* **2015**, *134*, 967–980. [CrossRef]
31. Ankala, A.; da Silva, C.; Gualandi, F.; Ferlini, A.; Bean, L.J.; Collins, C.; Tanner, A.K.; Hegde, M.R. A comprehensive genomic approach for neuromuscular diseases gives a high diagnostic yield. *Ann. Neurol.* **2015**, *77*, 206–214. [CrossRef]
32. Klein, C.J.; Middha, S.; Duan, X.; Wu, Y.; Litchy, W.J.; Gu, W.; Dyck, P.J.; Gavrilova, R.H.; Smith, D.I.; Kocher, J.P.; et al. Application of whole exome sequencing in undiagnosed inherited polyneuropathies. *J. Neurol. Neurosurg. Psychiatry* **2014**, *85*, 1265–1272. [CrossRef]
33. Chae, J.H.; Vasta, V.; Cho, A.; Lim, B.C.; Zhang, Q.; Eun, S.H.; Hahn, S.H. Utility of next generation sequencing in genetic diagnosis of early onset neuromuscular disorders. *J. Med. Genet.* **2015**, *52*, 208–216. [CrossRef]
34. Ghaoui, R.; Cooper, S.T.; Lek, M.; Jones, K.; Corbett, A.; Reddel, S.W.; Needham, M.; Liang, C.; Waddell, L.B.; Nicholson, G.; et al. Use of Whole-Exome Sequencing for Diagnosis of Limb-Girdle Muscular Dystrophy: Outcomes and Lessons Learned. *JAMA Neurol.* **2015**, *72*, 1424–1432. [CrossRef]
35. Gorokhova, S.; Cerino, M.; Mathieu, Y.; Courrier, S.; Desvignes, J.P.; Salgado, D.; Béroud, C.; Krahn, M.; Bartoli, M. Comparing targeted exome and whole exome approaches for genetic diagnosis of neuromuscular disorders. *Appl. Transl. Genom.* **2015**, *7*, 26–31. [CrossRef]
36. Tian, X.; Liang, W.C.; Feng, Y.; Wang, J.; Zhang, V.W.; Chou, C.H.; Huang, H.D.; Lam, C.W.; Hsu, Y.Y.; Lin, T.S.; et al. Expanding genotype/phenotype of neuromuscular diseases by comprehensive target capture/NGS. *Neurol. Genet.* **2015**, *1*, e14. [CrossRef]
37. Evilä, A.; Arumilli, M.; Udd, B.; Hackman, P. Targeted next-generation sequencing assay for detection of mutations in primary myopathies. *Neuromuscul. Disord.* **2016**, *26*, 7–15. [CrossRef]

38. Fattahi, Z.; Kalhor, Z.; Fadaee, M.; Vazehan, R.; Parsimehr, E.; Abolhassani, A.; Beheshtian, M.; Zamani, G.; Nafissi, S.; Nilipour, Y.; et al. Improved diagnostic yield of neuromuscular disorders applying clinical exome sequencing in patients arising from a consanguineous population. *Clin. Genet.* **2017**, *91*, 386–402. [CrossRef]
39. Haskell, G.T.; Adams, M.C.; Fan, Z.; Amin, K.; Guzman Badillo, R.J.; Zhou, L.; Bizon, C.; Chahin, N.; Greenwood, R.S.; Milko, L.V.; et al. Diagnostic utility of exome sequencing in the evaluation of neuromuscular disorders. *Neurol. Genet.* **2018**, *4*, e212. [CrossRef]
40. Schofield, D.; Alam, K.; Douglas, L.; Shrestha, R.; MacArthur, D.G.; Davis, M.; Laing, N.G.; Clarke, N.F.; Burns, J.; Cooper, S.T.; et al. Cost-effectiveness of massively parallel sequencing for diagnosis of paediatric muscle diseases. *NPJ Genom. Med.* **2017**, *2*, 4. [CrossRef]
41. Koboldt, D.C. Best practices for variant calling in clinical sequencing. *Genome. Med.* **2020**, *12*, 91. [CrossRef]
42. Strande, N.T.; Brnich, S.E.; Roman, T.S.; Berg, J.S. Navigating the nuances of clinical sequence variant interpretation in Mendelian disease. *Genet. Med.* **2018**, *20*, 918–926. [CrossRef]
43. Beecroft, S.J.; Yau, K.S.; Allcock, R.J.N.; Mina, K.; Gooding, R.; Faiz, F.; Atkinson, V.J.; Wise, C.; Sivadorai, P.; Trajanoski, D.; et al. Targeted gene panel use in 2249 neuromuscular patients: The Australasian referral center experience. *Ann. Clin. Transl. Neurol.* **2020**, *7*, 353–362. [CrossRef]
44. Fernandez-Marmiesse, A.; Gouveia, S.; Couce, M.L. NGS Technologies as a Turning Point in Rare Disease Research, Diagnosis and Treatment. *Curr. Med. Chem.* **2018**, *25*, 404–432. [CrossRef]
45. Todd, E.J.; Yau, K.S.; Ong, R.; Slee, J.; McGillivray, G.; Barnett, C.P.; Haliloglu, G.; Talim, B.; Akcoren, Z.; Kariminejad, A.; et al. Next generation sequencing in a large cohort of patients presenting with neuromuscular disease before or at birth. *Orphanet. J. Rare Dis.* **2015**, *10*, 148. [CrossRef]
46. Lévesque, S.; Auray-Blais, C.; Gravel, E.; Boutin, M.; Dempsey-Nunez, L.; Jacques, P.E.; Chenier, S.; Larue, S.; Rioux, M.F.; Al-Hertani, W.; et al. Diagnosis of late-onset Pompe disease and other muscle disorders by next-generation sequencing. *Orphanet J. Rare Dis.* **2016**, *11*, 8. [CrossRef]
47. Brugnoni, R.; Maggi, L.; Canioni, E.; Verde, F.; Gallone, A.; Ariattik, A.; Filosto, M.; Petrelli, C.; Logullo, F.O.; Esposito, M.; et al. Next-generation sequencing application to investigate skeletal muscle channelopathies in a large cohort of Italian patients. *Neuromuscul. Disord.* **2020**. [CrossRef]
48. Lamp, M.; Origone, P.; Geroldi, A.; Verdiani, S.; Gotta, F.; Caponnetto, C.; Devigili, G.; Verriello, L.; Scialò, C.; Cabona, C.; et al. Twenty years of molecular analyses in amyotrophic lateral sclerosis: Genetic landscape of Italian patients. *Neurobiol. Aging* **2018**, *66*, 179.e5–179.e16. [CrossRef]
49. Montenegro, G.; Powell, E.; Huang, J.; Speziani, F.; Edwards, Y.J.; Beecham, G.; Hulme, W.; Siskind, C.; Vance, J.; Shy, M.; et al. Exome sequencing allows for rapid gene identification in a Charcot-Marie-Tooth family. *Ann. Neurol.* **2011**, *69*, 464–470. [CrossRef]
50. Waldrop, M.A.; Pastore, M.; Schrader, R.; Sites, E.; Bartholomew, D.; Tsao, C.Y.; Flanigan, K.M. Diagnostic Utility of Whole Exome Sequencing in the Neuromuscular Clinic. *Neuropediatrics* **2019**, *50*, 96–102. [CrossRef]
51. LaDuca, H.; Farwell, K.D.; Vuong, H.; Lu, H.M.; Mu, W.; Shahmirzadi, L.; Tang, S.; Chen, J.; Bhide, S.; Chao, E.C. Exome sequencing covers >98% of mutations identified on targeted next generation sequencing panels. *PLoS ONE* **2017**, *12*, e0170843. [CrossRef]
52. Richards, S.; Aziz, N.; Bale, S.; Bick, D.; Das, S.; Gastier-Foster, J.; Grody, W.W.; Hegde, M.; Lyon, E.; Spector, E.; et al. Standards and guidelines for the interpretation of sequence variants: A joint consensus recommendation of the American College of Medical Genetics and Genomics and the Association for Molecular Pathology. *Genet. Med.* **2015**, *17*, 405–424. [CrossRef] [PubMed]
53. Petersen, B.S.; Fredrich, B.; Hoeppner, M.P.; Ellinghaus, D.; Franke, A. Opportunities and challenges of whole-genome and -exome sequencing. *BMC Genet.* **2017**, *18*, 14. [CrossRef] [PubMed]
54. Shashi, V.; McConkie-Rosell, A.; Schoch, K.; Kasturi, V.; Rehder, C.; Jiang, Y.H.; Goldstein, D.B.; McDonald, M.T. Practical considerations in the clinical application of whole-exome sequencing. *Clin. Genet.* **2016**, *89*, 173–181. [CrossRef] [PubMed]
55. Baldridge, D.; Heeley, J.; Vineyard, M.; Manwaring, L.; Toler, T.L.; Fassi, E.; Fiala, E.; Brown, S.; Goss, C.W.; Willing, M.; et al. The Exome Clinic and the role of medical genetics expertise in the interpretation of exome sequencing results. *Genet. Med.* **2017**, *19*, 1040–1048. [CrossRef]
56. Tsai, G.J.; Rañola, J.M.O.; Smith, C.; Garrett, L.T.; Bergquist, T.; Casadei, S.; Bowen, D.J.; Shirts, B.H. Outcomes of 92 patient-driven family studies for reclassification of variants of uncertain significance. *Genet. Med.* **2019**, *21*, 1435–1442. [CrossRef]
57. Ravenscroft, G.; Laing, N.G.; Bönnemann, C.G. Pathophysiological concepts in the congenital myopathies: Blurring the boundaries, sharpening the focus. *Brain* **2015**, *138*, 246–268. [CrossRef]
58. Oates, E.C.; Jones, K.J.; Donkervoort, S.; Charlton, A.; Brammah, S.; Smith, J.E., 3rd; Ware, J.S.; Yau, K.S.; Swanson, L.C.; Whiffin, N.; et al. Congenital Titinopathy: Comprehensive characterization and pathogenic insights. *Ann. Neurol.* **2018**, *83*, 1105–1124. [CrossRef]
59. Jungbluth, H.; Dowling, J.J.; Ferreiro, A.; Muntoni, F. RYR1 Myopathy Consortium. 217th ENMC International Workshop: RYR1-related myopathies, Naarden, The Netherlands, 29–31 January 2016. *Neuromuscul. Disord.* **2016**, *26*, 624–633. [CrossRef]
60. Mazzarotto, F.; Olivotto, I.; Walsh, R. Advantages and Perils of Clinical Whole-Exome and Whole-Genome Sequencing in Cardiomyopathy. *Cardiovasc. Drugs* **2020**, *34*, 241–253. [CrossRef]

61. Lupski, J.R.; Reid, J.G.; Gonzaga-Jauregui, C.; Rio Deiros, D.; Chen, D.C.; Nazareth, L.; Bainbridge, M.; Dinh, H.; Jing, C.; Wheeler, D.A.; et al. Whole-genome sequencing in a patient with Charcot-Marie-Tooth neuropathy. *N. Engl. J. Med.* **2010**, *362*, 1181–1191. [CrossRef]
62. Wang, K.; Kim, C.; Bradfield, J.; Guo, Y.; Toskala, E.; Otieno, F.G.; Hou, C.; Thomas, K.; Cardinale, C.; Lyon, G.J.; et al. Whole-genome DNA/RNA sequencing identifies truncating mutations in RBCK1 in a novel Mendelian disease with neuromuscular and cardiac involvement. *Genome. Med.* **2013**, *5*, 67. [CrossRef]
63. Han, L.; Huang, Y.; Nie, Y.; Li, J.; Chen, G.; Tu, S.; Shen, P.; Chen, C. A novel PMP22 insertion mutation causing Charcot-Marie-Tooth disease type 3: A case report. *Medicine* **2021**, *100*, e25163. [CrossRef] [PubMed]
64. Petrikin, J.E.; Willig, L.K.; Smith, L.D.; Kingsmore, S.F. Rapid whole genome sequencing and precision neonatology. *Semin Perinatol.* **2015**, *39*, 623–631. [CrossRef]
65. Kremer, L.S.; Wortmann, S.B.; Prokisch, H. "Transcriptomics": Molecular diagnosis of inborn errors of metabolism via RNA-sequencing. *J. Inherit. Metab. Dis.* **2018**, *41*, 525–532. [CrossRef]
66. Alfares, A.; Aloraini, T.; Al Subaie, L.; Alissa, A.; Al Qudsi, A.; Alahmad, A.; Al Mutairi, F.; Alswaid, A.; Alothaim, A.; Eyaid, W.; et al. Whole-genome sequencing offers additional but limited clinical utility compared with reanalysis of whole-exome sequencing. *Genet. Med.* **2018**, *20*, 1328–1333. [CrossRef] [PubMed]
67. Schon, K.R.; Ratnaike, T.; van den Ameele, J.; Horvath, R.; Chinnery, P.F. Mitochondrial Diseases: A Diagnostic Revolution. *Trends Genet.* **2020**, *36*, 702–717. [CrossRef]
68. Wallace, D.C.; Singh, G.; Lott, M.T.; Hodge, J.A.; Schurr, T.G.; Lezza, A.M.; Elsas, L.J., 2nd; Nikoskelainen, E.K. Mitochondrial DNA mutation associated with Leber's hereditary optic neuropathy. *Science* **1988**, *242*, 1427–1430. [CrossRef]
69. Neveling, K.; Feenstra, I.; Gilissen, C.; Hoefsloot, L.H.; Kamsteeg, E.J.; Mensenkamp, A.R.; Rodenburg, R.J.; Yntema, H.G.; Spruijt, L.; Vermeer, S.; et al. A post-hoc comparison of the utility of sanger sequencing and exome sequencing for the diagnosis of heterogeneous diseases. *Hum. Mutat.* **2013**, *34*, 1721–1726. [CrossRef]
70. Frazier, A.E.; Thorburn, D.R.; Compton, A. G Mitochondrial energy generation disorders: Genes, mechanisms, and clues to pathology. *J. Biol. Chem.* **2019**, *294*, 5386–5395. [CrossRef]
71. Gusic, M.; Prokisch, H. Genetic basis of mitochondrial diseases. *FEBS Lett.* **2021**. [CrossRef]
72. Tang, S.; Wang, J.; Zhang, V.W.; Li, F.Y.; Landsverk, M.; Cui, H.; Truong, C.K.; Wang, G.; Chen, L.C.; Graham, B.; et al. Transition to next generation analysis of the whole mitochondrial genome: A summary of molecular defects. *Hum. Mutat.* **2013**, *34*, 882–893. [CrossRef] [PubMed]
73. Calvo, S.E.; Tucker, E.J.; Compton, A.G.; Kirby, D.M.; Crawford, G.; Burtt, N.P.; Rivas, M.; Guiducci, C.; Bruno, D.L.; Goldberger, O.A.; et al. High-throughput, pooled sequencing identifies mutations in NUBPL and FOXRED1 in human complex I deficiency. *Nat. Genet.* **2010**, *42*, 851–858. [CrossRef] [PubMed]
74. Vasta, V.; Ng, S.B.; Turner, E.H.; Shendure, J.; Hahn, S.H. Next generation sequence analysis for mitochondrial disorders. *Genome Med.* **2009**, *1*, 100. [CrossRef]
75. DaRe, J.T.; Vasta, V.; Penn, J.; Tran, N.T.B.; Hahn, S.H. Targeted exome sequencing for mitochondrial disorders reveals high genetic heterogeneity. *BMC Med. Genet.* **2013**, *14*, 118. [CrossRef]
76. Legati, A.; Reyes, A.; Nasca, A.; Invernizzi, F.; Lamantea, E.; Tiranti, V.; Garavaglia, B.; Lamperti, C.; Ardissone, A.; Moroni, I.; et al. New genes and pathomechanisms in mitochondrial disorders unravelled by NGS technologies. *BBA-Bioenergetics* **2016**, *1857*, 1326–1335. [CrossRef]
77. Wortmann, S.B.; Mayr, J.A.; Nuoffer, J.M.; Prokisch, H.; Sperl, W. A guideline for the diagnosis of pediatric mitochondrial disease: The value of muscle and skin biopsies in the genetics era. *Neuropediatrics* **2017**, *48*, 309–314. [CrossRef]
78. Wagner, M.; Berutti, R.; Lorenz-Depiereux, B.; Graf, E.; Eckstein, G.; Mayr, J.A.; Meitinger, T.; Ahting, U.; Prokisch, H.; Strom, T.M.; et al. Mitochondrial DNA mutation analysis from exome sequencing-A more holistic approach in diagnostics of suspected mitochondrial disease. *J. Inherit. Metab. Dis.* **2019**, *42*, 909–917. [CrossRef]
79. Wolf, N.I.; Smeitink, J.A. Mitochondrial disorders: A proposal for consensus diagnostic criteria in infants and children. *Neurology* **2002**, *59*, 1402–1405. [CrossRef]
80. Pronicka, E.; Piekutowska-Abramczuk, D.; Ciara, E.; Trubicka, J.; Rokicki, D.; Karkucinska-Wieckowska, A.; Pajdowska, M.; Jurkiewicz, E.; Halat, P.; Kosinska, J.; et al. New perspective in diagnostics of mitochondrial disorders: Two years' experience with whole-exome sequencing at a national paediatric centre. *J. Transl. Med.* **2016**, *14*, 174. [CrossRef]
81. Puusepp, S.; Reinson, K.; Pajusalu, S.; Murumets, U.; Oiglane-Shlik, E.; Rein, R.; Talvik, I.; Rodenburg, R.J.; Ounap, K. Effectiveness of whole exome sequencing in unsolved patients with a clinical suspicion of a mitochondrial disorder in Estonia. *Mol. Genet. Metab. Rep.* **2018**, *15*, 80–89. [CrossRef]
82. Theunissen, T.E.J.; Nguyen, M.; Kamps, R.; Hendrickx, A.T.; Sallevelt, S.; Gottschalk, R.W.H.; Calis, C.M.; Stassen, A.P.M.; de Koning, B.; Mulder-Den Hartog, E.N.M.; et al. Whole exome sequencing is the preferred strategy to identify the genetic defect in patients with a probable or possible mitochondrial cause. *Front. Genet.* **2018**, *9*, 400. [CrossRef] [PubMed]
83. Riley, L.G.; Cowley, M.J.; Gayevskiy, V.; Minoche, A.E.; Puttick, C.; Thorburn, D.R.; Rius, R.; Compton, A.G.; Menezes, M.J.; Bhattacharya, K.; et al. The diagnostic utility of genome sequencing in a pediatric cohort with suspected mitochondrial disease. *Genet. Med.* **2020**, *22*, 1254–1261. [CrossRef] [PubMed]
84. Xuan, J.; Yu, Y.; Qing, T.; Guo, L.; Shi, L. Next-generation sequencing in the clinic: Promises and challenges. *Cancer Lett.* **2013**, *342*, 284–295. [CrossRef] [PubMed]

85. Mu, W.; Lu, H.M.; Chen, J.; Li, S.; Elliott, A.M. Sanger Confirmation Is Required to Achieve Optimal Sensitivity and Specificity in Next-Generation Sequencing Panel Testing. *J. Mol. Diagn.* **2016**, *18*, 923–932. [CrossRef]
86. Bobo, D.; Lipatov, M.; Rodriguez-Flores, J.L.; Auton, A.; Henn, B.M. False Negatives Are a Significant Feature of Next Generation Sequencing Callsets. *Biorxiv* **2016**. [CrossRef]
87. Wenger, A.M.; Guturu, H.; Bernstein, J.A.; Bejerano, G. Systematic reanalysis of clinical exome data yields additional diagnoses: Implications for providers. *Genet. Med.* **2017**, *19*, 209–214. [CrossRef]
88. Rhoads, A.; Au, K.F. PacBio Sequencing and Its Applications. *Genom. Proteom. Bioinform.* **2015**, *13*, 278–289. [CrossRef]
89. Hu, T.; Chitnis, N.; Monos, D.; Dinh, A. Next-generation sequencing technologies: An overview. *Hum. Immunol.* **2021**. [CrossRef]
90. Mitsuhashi, S.; Nakagawa, S.; Takahashi Ueda, M.; Imanishi, T.; Frith, M.C.; Mitsuhashi, H. Nanopore-based single molecule sequencing of the D4Z4 array responsible for facioscapulohumeral muscular dystrophy. *Sci. Rep.* **2017**, *7*, 14789. [CrossRef]
91. Ebbert, M.T.W.; Farrugia, S.L.; Sens, J.P.; Jansen-West, K.; Gendron, T.F.; Prudencio, M.; McLaughlin, I.J.; Bowman, B.; Seetin, M.; DeJesus-Hernandez, M.; et al. Long-read sequencing across the C9orf72 'GGGGCC' repeat expansion: Implications for clinical use and genetic discovery efforts in human disease. *Mol. Neurodegener.* **2018**, *13*, 46. [CrossRef]
92. Giesselmann, P.; Brändl, B.; Raimondeau, E.; Bowen, R.; Rohrandt, C.; Tandon, R.; Kretzmer, H.; Assum, G.; Galonska, C.; Siebert, R.; et al. Analysis of short tandem repeat expansions and their methylation state with nanopore sequencing. *Nat. Biotechnol.* **2019**, *37*, 1478–1481. [CrossRef]
93. Masrori, P.; Van Damme, P. Amyotrophic lateral sclerosis: A clinical review. *Eur. J. Neurol.* **2020**, *27*, 1918–1929. [CrossRef]
94. Van der Ende, E.L.; Jackson, J.L.; White, A.; Seelaar, H.; van Blitterswijk, M.; Van Swieten, J.C. Unravelling the clinical spectrum and the role of repeat length in C9ORF72 repeat expansions. *J. Neurol. Neurosurg. Psychiatry* **2021**. [CrossRef]
95. Ji, F.; Sadreyev, R.I. RNA-seq: Basic Bioinformatics Analysis. *Curr. Protoc. Mol. Biol.* **2018**, *124*, e68. [CrossRef]
96. Byron, S.A.; Van Keuren-Jensen, K.R.; Engelthaler, D.M.; Carpten, J.D.; Craig, D.W. Translating RNA sequencing into clinical diagnostics: Opportunities and challenges. *Nat. Rev. Genet.* **2016**, *17*, 257–271. [CrossRef]
97. Cummings, B.B.; Marshall, J.L.; Tukiainen, T.; Lek, M.; Donkervoort, S.; Foley, A.R.; Bolduc, V.; Waddell, L.B.; Sandaradura, S.A.; O'Grady, G.L.; et al. Improving genetic diagnosis in Mendelian disease with transcriptome sequencing. *Sci. Transl. Med.* **2017**, *9*, eaal5209. [CrossRef]
98. Bolduc, V.; Foley, A.R.; Solomon-Degefa, H.; Sarathy, A.; Donkervoort, S.; Hu, Y.; Chen, G.S.; Sizov, K.; Nalls, M.; Zhou, H.; et al. A recurrent COL6A1 pseudoexon insertion causes muscular dystrophy and is effectively targeted by splice-correction therapies. *JCI Insight* **2019**, *4*, e124403. [CrossRef]
99. Kremer, L.S.; Bader, D.M.; Mertes, C.; Kopajtich, R.; Pichler, G.; Iuso, A.; Haack, T.B.; Graf, E.; Schwarzmayr, T.; Terrile, C.; et al. Genetic diagnosis of Mendelian disorders via RNA sequencing. *Nat. Commun.* **2017**, *8*, 15824. [CrossRef]
100. Gonorazky, H.D.; Naumenko, S.; Ramani, A.K.; Nelakuditi, V.; Mashouri, P.; Wang, P.; Kao, D.; Ohri, K.; Viththiyapaskaran, S.; Tarnopolsky, M.A.; et al. Expanding the Boundaries of RNA Sequencing as a Diagnostic Tool for Rare Mendelian Disease. *Am. J. Hum. Genet.* **2019**, *104*, 1007. [CrossRef]
101. Kernohan, K.D.; Frésard, L.; Zappala, Z.; Hartley, T.; Smith, K.S.; Wagner, J.; Xu, H.; McBride, A.; Bourque, P.R.; Consortium, C.R.C.; et al. Whole-transcriptome sequencing in blood provides a diagnosis of spinal muscular atrophy with progressive myoclonic epilepsy. *Hum. Mutat.* **2017**, *38*, 611–614. [CrossRef]
102. Elsaid, M.F.; Chalhoub, N.; Ben-Omran, T.; Kumar, P.; Kamel, H.; Ibrahim, K.; Mohamoud, Y.; Al-Dous, E.; Al-Azwani, I.; Malek, J.A.; et al. Mutation in noncoding RNA RNU12 causes early onset cerebellar ataxia. *Ann. Neurol.* **2017**, *81*, 68–78. [CrossRef]
103. Kassardjian, C.D.; Amato, A.A.; Boon, A.J.; Boon, A.J.; Childers, M.K.; Klein, C.J.; AANEM Professional Practice Committee. The utility of genetic testing in neuromuscular disease: A consensus statement from the AANEM on the clinical utility of genetic testing in diagnosis of neuromuscular disease. *Muscle Nerve* **2016**, *54*, 1007–1009. [CrossRef]
104. Finkel, R.S.; Mercuri, E.; Darras, B.T.; Connolly, A.M.; Kuntz, N.L.; Kirschner, J.; Chiriboga, C.A.; Saito, K.; Servais, L.; Tizzano, E.; et al. Nusinersen versus sham control in infantile-onset spinal muscular atrophy. *N. Engl. J. Med.* **2017**, *377*, 1723–1732. [CrossRef]
105. Mercuri, E.; Darras, B.T.; Chiriboga, C.A.; Day, J.W.; Campbell, C.; Connolly, A.M.; Iannaccone, S.T.; Kirschner, J.; Kuntz, N.L.; Saito, K.; et al. Nusinersen versus sham control in later-onset spinal muscular atrophy. *N. Engl. J. Med.* **2018**, *378*, 625–635. [CrossRef]
106. Ravi, B.; Antonellis, A.; Sumner, C.J.; Lieberman, A.P. Genetic approaches to the treatment of inherited neuromuscular diseases. *Hum. Mol. Genet.* **2019**, *28*, R55–R64. [CrossRef]
107. Roggenbuck, J.; Quick, A.; Kolb, S.J. Genetic testing and genetic counseling for amyotrophic lateral sclerosis: An update for clinicians. *Genet. Med.* **2017**, *19*, 267–274. [CrossRef]
108. De Vivo, D.C.; Bertini, E.; Swoboda, K.J.; Hwu, W.L.; Crawford, T.O.; Finkel, R.S.; Kirschner, J.; Kuntz, N.L.; Parsons, J.A.; Ryan, M.M.; et al. Nusinersen initiated in infants during the presymptomatic stage of spinal muscular atrophy: Interim efficacy and safety results from the Phase 2 NURTURE study. *Neuromuscul. Disord.* **2019**, *29*, 842–856. [CrossRef]
109. Pane, M.; Coratti, G.; Sansone, V.A.; Messina, S.; Catteruccia, M.; Bruno, C.; Sframeli, M.; Albamonte, E.; Pedemonte, M.; D'Amico, A.; et al. Type I SMA "new natural history": Long-term data in nusinersen-treated patients. *Ann. Clin. Transl. Neurol.* **2021**, *8*, 548–557. [CrossRef] [PubMed]

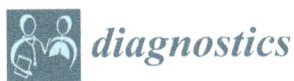

Article

Next-Generation Molecular Investigations in Lysosomal Diseases: Clinical Integration of a Comprehensive Targeted Panel

Bénédicte Sudrié-Arnaud [1], Sarah Snanoudj [1,2], Ivana Dabaj [2,3], Hélène Dranguet [1,2], Lenaig Abily-Donval [2,3], Axel Lebas [4], Myriam Vezain [5], Bénédicte Héron [6,7], Isabelle Marie [8], Marc Duval-Arnould [9], Stéphane Marret [2,3], Abdellah Tebani [1,2] and Soumeya Bekri [1,2,*]

1. Department of Metabolic Biochemistry, Rouen University Hospital, 76000 Rouen, France; b.sudrie-Arnaud@chu-rouen.fr (B.S.-A.); sarah.snanoudj@chu-rouen.fr (S.S.); helene.dranguet@chu-rouen.fr (H.D.); abdellah.tebani@chu-rouen.fr (A.T.)
2. Normandie Univ, UNIROUEN, CHU Rouen, INSERM U1245, 76000 Rouen, France; ivana.dabaj@chu-rouen.fr (I.D.); lenaig.donval@gmail.com (L.A.-D.); stephane.marret@chu-rouen.fr (S.M.)
3. Department of Neonatal Pediatrics, Intensive Care and Neuropediatrics, Rouen University Hospital, 76000 Rouen, France
4. Department of Neurophysiology, Rouen University Hospital, 76031 Rouen, France; axel.lebas@chu-rouen.fr
5. Normandie Univ, UNIROUEN, INSERM U1245, Department of Genetics and Reference Center for Developmental Disorders, Rouen University Hospital, Normandy Center for Genomic and Personalized Medicine, 76000 Rouen, France; myriam.vezain@inserm.fr
6. Centre de Référence des Maladies Lysosomales, Service de Neurologie Pédiatrique, CHU Armand Trousseau-La Roche Guyon, GHUEP, APHP, 75000 Paris, France; benedicte.heron@aphp.fr
7. Center for Lysosomal Diseases, Pediatric Neurology Department, UH Armand Trousseau-La Roche Guyon, APHP, GUEP, 75000 Paris, France
8. Department of Internal Medicine, Rouen University Hospital, 76000 Rouen, France; isabelle.marie@chu-rouen.fr
9. Department of Pediatrics, Bicetre Hospital, APHP, 75000 Paris, France; marc.duval-arnould@aphp.fr
* Correspondence: soumeya.bekri@chu-rouen.fr

Abstract: Diagnosis of lysosomal disorders (LDs) may be hampered by their clinical heterogeneity, phenotypic overlap, and variable age at onset. Conventional biological diagnostic procedures are based on a series of sequential investigations and require multiple sampling. Early diagnosis may allow for timely treatment and prevent clinical complications. In order to improve LDs diagnosis, we developed a capture-based next generation sequencing (NGS) panel allowing the detection of single nucleotide variants (SNVs), small insertions and deletions, and copy number variants (CNVs) in 51 genes related to LDs. The design of the LD panel covered at least coding regions, promoter region, and flanking intronic sequences for 51 genes. The validation of this panel consisted in testing 21 well-characterized samples and evaluating analytical and diagnostic performance metrics. Bioinformatics pipelines have been validated for SNVs, indels and CNVs. The clinical output of this panel was tested in five novel cases. This capture-based NGS panel provides an average coverage depth of 474× which allows the detection of SNVs and CNVs in one comprehensive assay. All the targeted regions were covered above the minimum required depth of 30×. To illustrate the clinical utility, five novel cases have been sequenced using this panel and the identified variants have been confirmed using Sanger sequencing or quantitative multiplex PCR of short fluorescent fragments (QMPSF). The application of NGS as first-line approach to analyze suspected LD cases may speed up the identification of alterations in LD-associated genes. NGS approaches combined with bioinformatics analyses, are a useful and cost-effective tool for identifying the causative variations in LDs.

Keywords: NGS; next generation sequencing; inborn errors of metabolism; lysosomal disorders

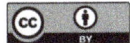

1. Introduction

The lysosome is an intracellular organelle characterized by its acidic pH, and its main function consists in degradation of intra or extracellular macromolecules into monomers. This metabolic process is carried out by more than fifty lysosomal enzymes. Additionally, over a hundred structural proteins and carriers essential for lysosomal function have been identified [1]. "Lysosomal storage disorders" (LSD) was the conventional term used to describe the group of inborn errors of metabolism (IEMs) related to the absence or failure of substrate degradation or transport, and their subsequent accumulation in the lysosome [2]. However, in recent years, the lysosome is being viewed as a dynamic structure with multiple roles in nutrient sensing, autophagy, apoptosis, and cellular response to environmental cues. It is also a signaling hub that interacts with other organelles [3]. In this context, the chosen term has shifted to lysosomal disorders (LDs) instead of LSD to better reflect the complexity of these diseases. In LDs, the inheritance pattern is autosomal recessive except for three disorders (Fabry, Danon, and Hunter diseases) which are X-linked. Clinical presentations of LDs vary greatly, and age at onset ranges from the antenatal period all the way to adulthood. However, in some cases, cardinal signs may steer clinical physicians towards a particular disorder, such as specific dysmorphic features, ocular or articular involvement, organomegaly, multiple dysostosis, valvulopathy, neurological defects or psychomotor delay. An early diagnosis allows an appropriate medical care, as many specific treatments have recently been developed, and thus reduces morbidity [4,5]. Currently, biological diagnosis relies on a three-phase process: (i) characterization of accumulated metabolites, (ii) enzyme activity assessment, and (iii) molecular investigations. Additionally, in some cases, molecular study as first-line exploration is mandatory to reach the diagnosis. For instance, in case of X-linked pathologies such as Fabry disease, the measurement of enzyme activity may fail to identify heterozygous females due to X inactivation process. Besides, in some autosomal disorders, such as most of neuronal ceroid lipofuscinosis (NCL), no biological tests are available and molecular approaches are the only diagnostic option.

The rise of "omics-based" approaches and the tremendous technological shift, in both multiscale biological information capture and data management, offer a remarkable opportunity to change the ways we screen, diagnose, treat, and monitor inherited metabolic diseases [5–7]. Next generation sequencing (NGS) technologies represent an essential tool for rapid and effective diagnosis of these diseases and may be used in some complex situations prior to multiple and often sequential functional studies. Recent studies highlighted the clinical utility of NGS approach for LD genetic diagnosis [8–11]. Here we report on the design, validation and testing of an NGS panel for genes involved in LDs named LysoGene.

2. Materials and Methods

2.1. Patients

Twenty-one well-characterized LD patients have been included for validation purposes (Supplementary Table S1). Twenty-seven disease-causing variations and 50 benign variations have been previously identified by Sanger sequencing and were used for validation of the single nucleotide variants (SNVs) and small insertions/deletions (indels) sequencing process and the bioinformatics pipeline (Supplementary Tables S1 and S2). To illustrate the clinical utility of this panel, five LD patients are reported.

Case 1: A female child presented at 3 months of age with severe organomegaly (hepatomegaly at 6 cm and splenomegaly at 9 cm), associated with severe malnutrition, without diarrhea. No dysmorphy was noted. The liver biopsy was in favor of a storage disease.

Case 2: This female child was born at term from a non-consanguineous couple, eutrophic after a normal pregnancy, and with a good adaptation to extra-uterine life. At the age of two and a half years old, she presented with a speech delay and a flat tympanogram and transtympanic ventilation tube was inserted. At 3 years old, she was hospitalized for seizures with predominantly right occipital spikes on the electroencephalogram (EEG) wake and sleep patterns. A second episode of seizures induced by hyperthermia occurred a few months later. She had a disturbed sleep pattern with repeated awakenings, agitation and crying, sensory dysregulation including severe agitation and intolerance to loud noises, and poor communication. Brain MRI showed a retrocerebellar arachnoid cyst and cerebellar atrophy. Based on these elements, late infantile neuronal ceroid lipofuscinosis (CLN2, CLN5, CLN6 or CLN7) was suspected.

Case 3: This was the third child of a couple, born prematurely at 35 weeks of gestation by caesarean section for abnormal fetal heart rhythm. She was hospitalized at 3 months of age for psychomotor regression with decrease of focus and ocular following of objects and persons, as well as axial hypotonia. High blood pressure was diagnosed in the emergency department, and the child was put on calcium channel blocker. The MRI and the EEG showed no anomalies. A cherry red macula was found on ophthalmological examination. A LysoGene panel was requested.

Case 4: The patient was the second child of healthy non-consanguineous parents. Pregnancy was without particularity with a birth weight of 2830 g, a birth length of 47 cm and a head circumference of 34 cm. He was hospitalized in the neonatal intensive care for amniotic fluid aspiration associated with patent ductus arteriosus and suspicion of neonatal infection. This child acquired walking at around 12 months old, day and night cleanliness at 4 years old. At two and a half years old, he was treated for bilateral serous otitis media revealed by a hoarse voice and difficulties understanding. At three years old, he did not pronounce words properly and only formed simple sentences. He had a behavioral disorder with aggressiveness, concentration difficulties and disabling headaches. At 5 years old, he had a height and weight at + 1SD and presented with signs of storage such as square face, skin thickening, and enlarged joints and bone. At the metabolic level, elevated urinary excretion of heparan sulfate and a decreased activity in Heparan-alpha-glucosaminide N-acetyltransferase were consistent with Sanfilippo type C (Mucopolysaccharidosis type IIIC) diagnosis. The *HGSNAT* gene was analyzed using Sanger sequencing and two pathogenic variants were identified in the heterozygous state: a splicing variant (NM_152419.2:c.234+1G>A-p.?) resulting in a modification of the exon 2 splicing, and a missense variant NM_152419.2:c.710C>A-p.(Pro237Gln). Both variants are reported in the Human Gene Mutation Database (HGMD) and have been published [12]. However, allelic segregation analysis showed that both variants were inherited from the mother who was clinically healthy. Of note, the DNA sample from the father was not available to us. We decided to investigate this case using the LysoGene panel to unveil the alteration inherited from the father.

Case 5: A 31-year-old patient presented with diffuse myalgia. He had progressive exercise intolerance during the last 5 years. He also suffered from sleep apnea. The patient had been hospitalized several times and underwent many explorations without any diagnosis having been reached. Classical neuromuscular work up was normal, including electromyogram (EMG) and creatine phosphokinase (CPK).

Written informed consents were obtained from the parents when the patient is under 18 or from the adult patient in order to perform any investigation related to their pathology.

2.2. NGS Sequencing

DNA extraction: for NGS analysis, blood genomic DNAs were extracted using a silica-membrane-based DNA purification method (QIAamp DNA Blood Mini Kit, QIAGEN). NGS sequencing was performed in the IRIB-Rouen University Hospital Facility (Service Commun de Génomique).

Gene panel design: our approach aimed to capture, and sequence 51 genes implicated in LD (Table 1, Supplementary Table S3). Five additional genes were included for identity monitoring of patients (*CCDC88C, NIPBL, MLH1, APC, PTEN*). The design of the LysoGene panel covered the coding regions, the promoter region and the flanking intronic sequences for 43 genes. In addition, 3′ untranslated sequences were included for 2 genes (*AGA* and *ARSA*), and the entire gene sequences were covered for 6 genes (*ARSB, CLN3, CLN8, IDS, SGSH*, and *NAGLU*). In total, 708 regions were targeted including 506 exonic regions.

Custom primers were designed using the SureDesign software (Agilent Technologies, Santa Clara, CA, USA).

Library preparation and sequencing: the library preparation protocol was set up using the QXT SureSelect enrichment kit from Agilent. Library construction was done using enzymatic fragmentation and the SureSelectQXT kit (Agilent Technologies, Santa Clara, CA, USA) to capture targeted sequences. Patients' libraries were pooled after the enrichment step. The protocol was either performed manually or automated on a Sciclone NGSx workstation (PerkinElmer, Waltham, MA, USA). Libraries were sequenced on a MiSeq or a NextSeq 500 platform (Illumina, San Diego, CA, USA) using 2×150 bp paired-end sequencing.

Bioinformatics pipelines: for the detection of SNVs, indels and copy number variants (CNVs), a double bioinformatics pipeline was used with complementary algorithms in order to optimize the disease-causing variant detection rate:

(i) The bcl2fastq conversion software (Illumina, v2.20) was used for reads demultiplexing and generation of Fastq files. Sequenced reads were mapped to the human reference sequence (GRCh37, Hg19) using the Burrows–Wheeler Aligner (BWA v.0.7.17). Read duplicates were marked with Picard tools (v2.18.0), local realignments around indels, base-quality-score recalibration and variant calling were performed with the Genome Analysis Toolkit (GATK 4.0.6.0). Single-nucleotide variants and small indels were identified with the GATK HaplotypeCaller (v4.0.6.0), VarScan2 (v2.4.3) and Vardict (v1.5.1). Variants were then annotated with SnpEff (v.4.2) and Alamut-batch (v.1.12).

(ii) The second pipeline, large-scale rearrangements and the related CNVs were detected using the CANOES and GRIDSS software [13–15].

For each sequencing run, PDF quality reports integrating the number of clusters/mm^2, percentage of bases with a Qscore > 30, FastQC reports, percentage of mapped, reads, on- and off-targets percentages, percentage of covered bases and mean sequencing depth were automatically generated using the in-house tool PyQua (Python Qualitics).

Data analysis: An in-house software, CanDiD allowed for the prioritization and filtration of variants using defined criteria such as minor allele frequency in public databases or consequences of the variant (missense, synonym, nonsense, splicing). The filtered variants were compared to variant databases including dbSNP (https://www.ncbi.nlm.nih.gov/snp/ (accessed on 10 January 2021)), GnomAD (https://gnomad.broadinstitute.org/ (accessed on 10 January 2021)), HGMD (http://www.hgmd.cf.ac.uk/ (accessed on 10 January 2021)), LOVD (https://databases.lovd.nl/shared/genes (accessed on 10 January 2021)), and gene specific databases such as NPC-db2 (https://medgen.medizin.uni-tuebingen.de/NPC-db2/ (accessed on 10 January 2021)), Pompe variant database (http://www.pompevariantdatabase.nl/ (accessed on 10 January 2021)), and dbFGP (http://www.dbfgp.org/dbFgp/fabry/Mutation.html (accessed on 10 January 2021)).

The analysis of the captured sequence takes into account the clinical context. In this perspective, we defined five overlapping sub-panels for sequence analysis (Figure 1): Organomegaly (27 genes), neurological impairment (38 genes), bone abnormalities (23 genes), neuronal ceroid lipofuscinoses (10 genes), and cherry red spots (8).

Evaluation of the pathogenicity of the variants were analyzed with in silico tools such as SIFT [16], PolyPhen2 [17] or MutationTaster [18] and M-CAP [19] to predict potential deleterious effect on protein function, and HumanSplicingFinder 2.4.1 [20], MaxEntScan [21], NNSPLICE [22], GeneSplicer [23], SpliceSiteFinder [24], and ESEFinder [25] for possible effect on splicing. Variant classification was done according to the recommendations of the American College of Medical Genetics [26].

The control of the sample identity was performed using a multiplex SNaPshot analysis comparing five SNPs located within the captured regions of 5 genes unrelated to LDs included in the panel. To validate the panel in a diagnostic context, analytical accuracy, intra-assay and inter-assay reproducibility were assessed.

Table 1. Included genes in the LysoGene panel.

Disease	Inheritance	Gene	NM_
α-glucosidase deficiency	AR	GAA	NM_000152.3
α-mannosidase deficiency	AR	MAN2B1	NM_000528.3
Aspartylglucosaminidase deficiency	AR	AGA	NM_000027.3
β-mannosidase deficiency	AR	MANBA	NM_005908.3
α-fucosidase deficiency	AR	FUCA1	NM_000147.4
Cathepsin A deficiency	AR	CTSA	NM_000308.2
α-N-acetylgalactosaminidase deficiency	AR	NAGA	NM_000262.2
α-neuraminidase deficiency	AR	NEU1	NM_000434.3
Cystinosin deficiency	AR	CTNS	NM_004937.2
Lysosome-associated membrane protein 2 deficiency	XL	LAMP2	NM_002294.2
Niemann-Pick disease type C1	AR	NPC1	NM_000271.4
Niemann-Pick disease type C2	AR	NPC2	NM_006432.3
Sialin deficiency	AR	SLC17A5	NM_012434.4
Mucolipin 1 deficiency	AR	MCOLN1	NM_020533.2
Lysosomal acid lipase deficiency	AR	LIPA	NM_000235.2
Cathepsin K deficiency	AR	CTSK	NM_000396.3
UDP-N-acetylglucosamine-2-epimerase/N-acetylmannosamine kinase deficiency	AR	GNE	NM_005476.5
UDP-N-acetylglucosamine-1-phosphotransferase α/β subunit deficiency	AR	GNPTAB	NM_024312.4
α-iduronidase deficiency	AR	IDUA	NM_000203.3
Iduronate sulfatase deficiency	XLR	IDS	NM_000202.5
Heparan N-sulfatase deficiency	AR	SGSH	NM_000199.3
N-acetylglucosaminidase deficiency	AR	NAGLU	NM_000263.3
Heparan-α-glucosaminide N-acetyltransferase deficiency	AR	HGSNAT	NM_152419.2
N-acetylglucosamine 6-sulfatase deficiency	AR	GNS	NM_002076.3
N-acetylgalactosamine 6-sulfatase deficiency	AR	GALNS	NM_000512.4
Hyaluronidase deficiency	AR	HYAL1	NM_153281.1
N-acetylgalactosamine 4-sulfatase deficiency	AR	ARSB	NM_000046.3
β-glucuronidase deficiency	AR	GUSB	NM_000181.3
Palmitoyl-protein thioesterase 1 deficiency	AR	PPT1	NM_000310.3
Cathepsin D deficiency	AR	CTSD	NM_001909.4
Progranulin deficiency	AD, AR	GRN	NM_002087.2
Tripeptidyl-peptidase 1 deficiency	AR	TPP1	NM_000391.3
CLN3 disease	AR	CLN3	NM_001042432.1
CLN4 disease	AD	DNAJC5	NM_025219.2
CLN5 disease	AR	CLN5	NM_006493.2
CLN6 disease	AR	CLN6	NM_017882.2
CLN7 disease	AR	MFSD8	NM_152778.2
CLN8 disease	AR	CLN8	NM_018941.3
Osteopetrosis	AR	OSTM1	NM_014028.3
Formyl-glycine generating enzyme deficiency	AR	SUMF1	NM_182760.3
GM2 activator protein deficiency	AR	GM2A	NM_000405.4
Arylsulfatase A deficiency	AR	ARSA	NM_000487.5
Acid ceramidase deficiency, inflammatory phenotype	AR	ASAH1	NM_177924.3
α-Galactosidase A deficiency	XL	GLA	NM_000169,2
Glucocerebrosidase deficiency	AR	GBA	NM_001005741.2
β-galactosylceramidase deficiency	AR	GALC	NM_000153.3
Acid sphingomyelinase deficiency	AR	SMPD1	NM_000543.4
β-hexosaminidase β-subunit deficiency	AR	HEXB	NM_000521.3
β-hexosaminidase α-subunit deficiency	AR	HEXA	NM_000520.4
β-galactosidase deficiency, GM1 gangliosidosis phenotype	AR	GLB1	NM_000404.2
Atypical Gaucher disease due to saposin C deficiency	AR	PSAP	NM_002778.2

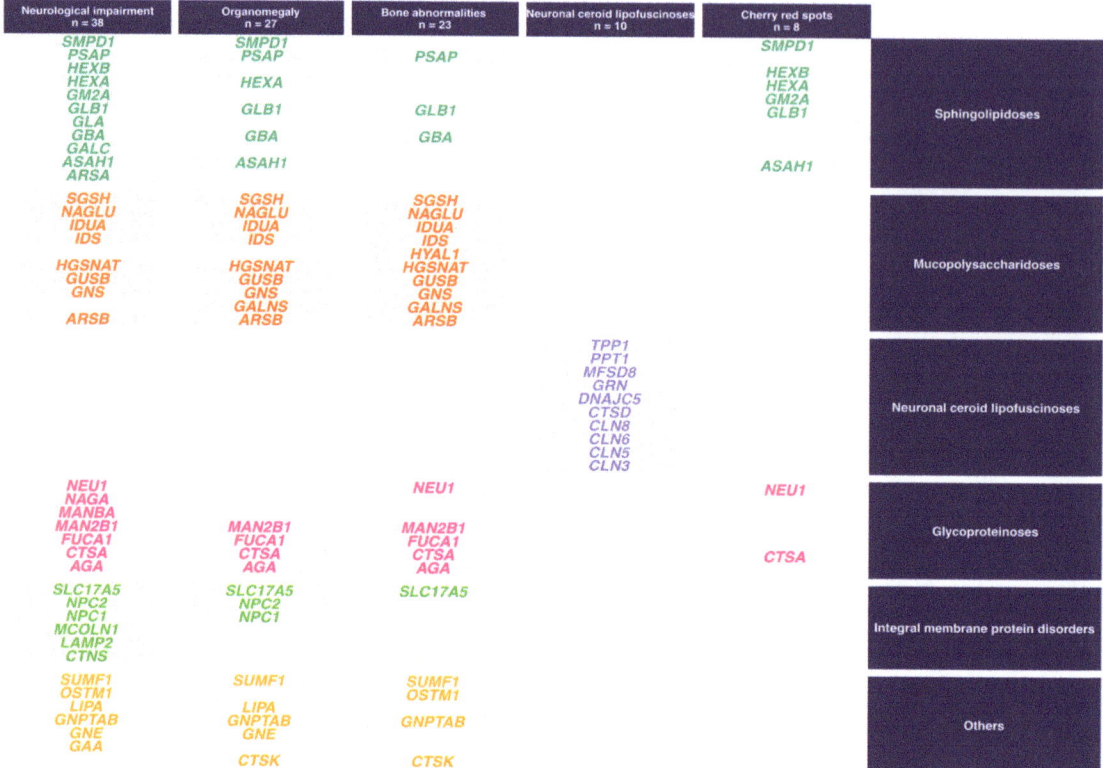

Figure 1. Overview of the genes included in the different LysoGene sub-panels.

3. Results

3.1. Quality Metrics

The NGS assay provided an average read depth of 474×. This deep coverage allowed for simultaneous detection of SNVs and CNVs in one comprehensive analysis. All the targeted regions were covered above the minimum depth required of 30×.

3.2. Panel Performances for the Detection of SNVs and Indels

Accuracy: The concordance between this panel results and the reference data was 100% for all 77 variants. Thus, the detection of these variants has been achieved with 100% analytic sensitivity.

Intra- and inter-assay reproducibility: the ratios between the values obtained for all metrics measured in the samples used for intra- and interassay reproducibility tests were equal or close to 1 (Supplementary Tables S4 and S5) demonstrating the consistency of the results.

3.3. Panel Performances for the Detection of CNVs

For CNVs, the performances of the in-house bioinformatics tool, CANOES, for assessing the read depth from capture-based NGS data were evaluated. The validation of this workflow has been published recently and highlighted very high sensitivity and positive predictive value for NGS gene panels [27].

3.4. Clinical Utility Assessment

To illustrate the clinical utility of this panel, we report 5 cases in which the NGS approach proved to be significantly more efficient than traditional Sanger sequencing. All the variants identified through the NGS workflow have been confirmed using Sanger sequencing (SNVs and indels) or quantitative multiplex PCR of short fluorescent fragments-QMPSF (CNVs).

Case 1: The LysoGene panel enabled the characterization of 2 pathogenic heterozygous variants in *NPC2* gene. The variant NM_006432.3:c.58G>T-p.(Glu20 *) has been reported in HGMD and has been published [28]. The second frameshift variant, c.87del-p.(Val30Trpfs*5) is novel. The presence of these variants was consistent with the diagnosis of Niemann Pick C type 2 disease. Sanger sequencing of *NPC2* in the parents confirmed allelic segregation.

Case 2: The analysis of the neuronal lipofuscinosis ceroid sub-panel allowed the characterization of two pathogenic heterozygous variants in the *TPP1* gene in this patient. Both variants, NM_000391.3:c.196C>T-p.(Gln66 *) and c.622C>T; p.(Arg208 *), have been reported in HGMD and previously published [29,30]. Allelic segregation was confirmed by the study of the parents' DNA.

Case 3: Given the clinical picture, priority was given to the analysis of genes involved in pathologies with macular cherry-red spots (Figure 1). Two pathogenic variants were identified in *HEXB*, NM_000521.3:c.1165dup-p.(Gln389Profs*22) which has never been described before, and c.1417+5G>A-p.? predicted to abolish the splicing donor site [31]. Enzymatic activities of hexosaminidase A and total hexosaminidases were greatly reduced in leukocytes and plasma. All these results pointed to Sandhoff disease.

Case 4: NGS sequencing of *HGSNAT* gene succeeded in retrieving the variants inherited from the mother (NM_152419.2:c.234+1G>A-p.? and c.710C>A-p.(Pro237Gln)) and enabled the identification of a heterozygous deletion of exon 15 (NM_152419.2:c.(1464+1_1465-1)_(1542+1_1543-1)del-p.?) which is carried by the paternal allele. This finding made it possible to confirm on a molecular basis the diagnosis of Sanfilippo type C in this patient.

Case 5: Rapid *GAA* gene sequencing using the LysoGene panel enabled the characterization of two pathogenic heterozygous variants: NM_000152.2:c.-32-13T>G-p.? in intron 1 which has previously been reported in adult form of Pompe disease [32], and c.2238G>C-p.(Trp746Cys) in exon 16 [33]. Sanger sequencing of the parents' DNA confirmed allelic segregation. Metabolic work up showed a reduced acid maltase activity.

4. Discussion

Diagnostic difficulties in LDs arise from the wide clinical, biochemical and molecular heterogeneity observed in these pathologies and highlight the crucial need of multidisciplinary collaboration for the diagnosis and management of these diseases [34,35]. LDs, like other IEMs, are primarily due to monogenic alteration, but a large number of genetic and environmental factors modulate their phenotypic expression and underlie the wide range of clinical severity associated with LDs. This concept has been extended to connect IEMs to common diseases as part of a metabolic disease spectrum. All these pathologies imply necessarily several genes and represent a continuum. Indeed, in IEMs, the influence of one gene is dominant and in common diseases an equivalent contribution of several gene alterations might be observed [36]. In addition, some LDs display phenotypic overlaps that often lead to misdiagnosis. Testing several hypotheses sequentially may result in a delay or failure to succeed in reaching the diagnosis. Of note, some lysosomal hydrolases may have reduced in vitro activity in clinically healthy individuals, referred to as pseudodeficiency. A set of variants known to cause pseudodeficiency has been characterized in the sequences of the corresponding genes that leads to an in vitro instability of the enzyme while the enzyme remains functionally active in vivo [37].

To smooth out and speed up LD screening and diagnosis, a paradigm shift is urgently needed to move from hypothesis-driven to data-driven strategies. Omics approaches along with bioinformatics tools offer a great opportunity to establish a validated workflow enabling the assessment of a large panel of diseases. Subsequently, targeted approach technologies may be used to confirm the identified abnormalities.

Here, we describe the analytical validation of an NGS-based sequencing panel encompassing 51 genes implicated in LDs. The assay demonstrated a high sensitivity and reliability and was efficient in characterizing both variants involving a small number of nucleotides (SNVs/indels) and large-scale rearrangements (CNVs). By multiplexing patient samples and several genes on a single platform, the limitations related to Sanger sequencing were addressed. This approach allowed for both lowering the costs and enhancing the diagnostic effectiveness. Recent studies reported NGS-based analyses in LD genetic diagnosis [8–11]. CNV detection was reported in only one study that included 28 LD genes [11]. Of note, the present work enabled the analysis of CNVs, not reachable by Sanger sequencing, for all the included 51 LD-related genes. This markedly broadens the scope of this panel for LD genetic investigations.

To illustrate the clinical integration of our panel, we reported 5 LD patients for which NGS analysis provided with fast and accurate results.

The NGS panel allowed us to guide the diagnosis toward of Niemann-Pick type C in Case 1, Sandhoff disease in Case 3 and Pompe disease in Case 5 while the clinical pictures were unspecific. In Case 2, the clinical presentation was suggestive of a ceroid lipofuscinosis. A fast molecular diagnosis was critical as a clinical trial for TPP1 deficiency based on intraventricular enzyme replacement therapy was ongoing. To be efficient, this treatment had to be implemented before psychomotor regression [38]. NGS analysis helped in identifying pathogenic variants in *TPP1* gene and the patient was successfully included in the ongoing clinical trial. The clinical utility of simultaneous CNV characterization is exemplified in Case 4. Indeed, the NGS workflow allowed the retrieval of the SNVs located on the maternal allele as well as the characterization of a CNV inherited from the father. Thus, NGS approach enabled the confirmation of this diagnosis on a molecular basis.

5. Conclusions

Clinical heterogeneity, phenotypic overlap, and variable age at onset are still major hurdles for fast and effective diagnosis of LDs. Combining NGS-based technology capabilities with efficient bioinformatics workflows offer a promising opportunity to enhance LD characterization through high throughput molecular profiling. Two main driving diagnosis situations stand out: (i) in typical clinical presentation, targeted biochemical profiling is the gold standard informative way to go with a subsequent molecular confirmation; (ii) in challenging clinical situation, first-tier NGS-based molecular profiling seems to be more informative to parse the clinical puzzle. In addition, conventional biochemical profiling confirmation is strongly recommended whenever possible.

Supplementary Materials: The following are available online at https://www.mdpi.com/2075-4418/11/2/294/s1, Table S1: cohort molecular data, Table S2: variant effect, Table S3: panel gene classification, Table S4: intra-assay variation assessment, Table S5: inter-assay variation assessment.

Author Contributions: Conceptualization, S.B.; formal analysis, B.S.-A., H.D. and M.V.; data curation, B.S.-A., S.S., I.D., L.A.-D., A.L., B.H., I.M., M.D.-A., S.M., A.T., and S.B.; writing—original draft preparation, B.S.-A., S.B.; writing—review and editing, A.T., S.M. and S.B.; visualization, A.T.; supervision, S.B.; project administration, S.B. All authors have read and agreed to the published version of the manuscript.

Funding: This research received no external funding.

Institutional Review Board Statement: The study was conducted according to the guidelines of the Declaration of Helsinki, and approved by the Institutional Review Board of Rouen University Hospital N° E2021-09.

Informed Consent Statement: Informed written consent was obtained from all subjects involved in the study.

Data Availability Statement: All the data that support the findings are presented in the manuscript and the Supplementary Materials.

Acknowledgments: The authors would like to thank the patients and the family members for their participation in this research.

Conflicts of Interest: The authors declare no conflict of interest.

References

1. Coutinho, M.F.; Alves, S. From rare to common and back again: 60years of lysosomal dysfunction. *Mol. Genet. Metab.* **2016**, *117*, 53–65. [CrossRef]
2. de Duve, C. The lysosome turns fifty. *Nat. Cell Biol.* **2005**, *7*, 847–849. [CrossRef]
3. Parenti, G.; Andria, G.; Ballabio, A. Lysosomal storage diseases: From pathophysiology to therapy. *Annu. Rev. Med.* **2015**, *66*, 471–486. [CrossRef]
4. Schultz, M.L.; Tecedor, L.; Chang, M.; Davidson, B.L. Clarifying lysosomal storage diseases. *Trends Neurosci.* **2011**, *34*, 401–410. [CrossRef]
5. Tebani, A.; Afonso, C.; Marret, S.; Bekri, S. Omics-based strategies in precision medicine: Toward a Paradigm shift in inborn errors of metabolism investigations. *Int. J. Mol. Sci.* **2016**, *17*, 1555. [CrossRef] [PubMed]
6. Sudrié-Arnaud, B.; Marguet, F.; Patrier, S.; Martinovic, J.; Louillet, F.; Broux, F.; Charbonnier, F.; Dranguet, H.; Coutant, S.; Vezain, M.; et al. Metabolic causes of nonimmune hydrops fetalis: A next-generation sequencing panel as a first-line investigation. *Clin. Chim. Acta.* **2018**, *481*, 1–8. [CrossRef] [PubMed]
7. Tebani, A.; Abily-Donval, L.; Afonso, C.; Marret, S.; Bekri, S. Clinical metabolomics: The new metabolic window for inborn errors of metabolism investigations in the post-genomic era. *Int. J. Mol. Sci.* **2016**, *17*, 1167. [CrossRef] [PubMed]
8. Encarnação, M.; Coutinho, M.F.; Silva, L.; Ribeiro, D.; Ouesleti, S.; Campos, T.; Santos, H.; Martins, E.; Cardoso, M.T.; Vilarinho, L.; et al. Assessing lysosomal disorders in the NGS era: Identification of novel rare variants. *Int. J. Mol. Sci.* **2020**, *21*, 6355. [CrossRef] [PubMed]
9. Gheldof, A.; Seneca, S.; Stouffs, K.; Lissens, W.; Jansen, A.; Laeremans, H.; Verloo, P.; Schoonjans, A.S.; Meuwissen, M.; Barca, D.; et al. Clinical implementation of gene panel testing for lysosomal storage diseases. *Mol. Genet. Genom. Med.* **2019**, *7*, e00527. [CrossRef]
10. Málaga, D.R.; Brusius-Facchin, A.C.; Siebert, M.; Pasqualim, G.; Saraiva-Pereira, M.L.; Souza, C.F.M.; Schwartz, I.V.D.; Matte, U.; Giugliani, R. Sensitivity, advantages, limitations, and clinical utility of targeted next-generation sequencing panels for the diagnosis of selected lysosomal storage disorders. *Genet. Mol. Biol.* **2019**, *42*, 197–206. [CrossRef]
11. Muñoz, G.; García-Seisdedos, D.; Ciubotariu, C.; Piris-Villaespesa, M.; Gandía, M.; Martín-Moro, F.; Gutiérrez-Solana, L.G.; Morado, M.; López-Jiménez, J.; Sánchez-Herranz, A.; et al. Early detection of lysosomal diseases by screening of cases of idiopathic splenomegaly and/or thrombocytopenia with a next-generation sequencing gene panel. *JIMD Rep.* **2020**, *51*, 53–61. [CrossRef]
12. Hrebícek, M.; Mrázová, L.; Seyrantepe, V.; Durand, S.; Roslin, N.M.; Nosková, L.; Hartmannová, H.; Ivánek, R.; Cízkova, A.; Poupetová, H.; et al. Mutations in TMEM76 * cause mucopolysaccharidosis IIIC (Sanfilippo C syndrome). *Am. J. Hum. Genet.* **2006**, *79*, 807–819. [CrossRef] [PubMed]
13. Backenroth, D.; Homsy, J.; Murillo, L.R.; Glessner, J.; Lin, E.; Brueckner, M.; Lifton, R.; Goldmuntz, E.; Chung, W.K.; Shen, Y. CANOES: Detecting rare copy number variants from whole exome sequencing data. *Nucleic Acids Res.* **2014**, *42*, e97. [CrossRef] [PubMed]
14. Muller, E.; Brault, B.; Holmes, A.; Legros, A.; Jeannot, E.; Campitelli, M.; Rousselin, A.; Goardon, N.; Frébourg, T.; Krieger, S.; et al. Genetic profiles of cervical tumors by high-throughput sequencing for personalized medical care. *Cancer Med.* **2015**, *4*, 1484–1493. [CrossRef] [PubMed]
15. Cameron, D.L.; Schröder, J.; Penington, J.S.; Do, H.; Molania, R.; Dobrovic, A.; Speed, T.P.; Papenfuss, A.T. GRIDSS: Sensitive and specific genomic rearrangement detection using positional de Bruijn graph assembly. *Genome Res.* **2017**, *27*, 2050–2060. [CrossRef]
16. Ng, P.C.; Henikoff, S. Predicting deleterious amino acid substitutions. *Genome Res.* **2001**, *11*, 863–874. [CrossRef]
17. Adzhubei, I.A.; Schmidt, S.; Peshkin, L.; Ramensky, V.E.; Gerasimova, A.; Bork, P.; Kondrashov, A.S.; Sunyaev, S.R. A method and server for predicting damaging missense mutations. *Nat. Methods* **2010**, *7*, 248–249. [CrossRef]
18. Schwarz, J.M.; Rödelsperger, C.; Schuelke, M.; Seelow, D. MutationTaster evaluates disease-causing potential of sequence alterations. *Nat. Methods* **2010**, *7*, 575–576. [CrossRef] [PubMed]
19. Jagadeesh, K.A.; Wenger, A.M.; Berger, M.J.; Guturu, H.; Stenson, P.D.; Cooper, D.N.; Bernstein, J.A.; Bejerano, G. M-CAP eliminates a majority of variants of uncertain significance in clinical exomes at high sensitivity. *Nat. Genet.* **2016**, *48*, 1581–1586. [CrossRef] [PubMed]
20. Desmet, F.O.; Hamroun, D.; Lalande, M.; Collod-Béroud, G.; Claustres, M.; Béroud, C. Human Splicing Finder: An online bioinformatics tool to predict splicing signals. *Nucleic Acids Res.* **2009**, *37*, e67. [CrossRef]
21. Yeo, G.; Burge, C.B. Maximum entropy modeling of short sequence motifs with applications to RNA splicing signals. *J. Comput. Biol.* **2004**, *11*, 377–394. [CrossRef]
22. Reese, M.G.; Eeckman, F.H.; Kulp, D.; Haussler, D. Improved splice site detection in Genie. *J. Comput. Biol.* **1997**, *4*, 311–323. [CrossRef]

23. Pertea, M.; Lin, X.; Salzberg, S.L. GeneSplicer: A new computational method for splice site prediction. *Nucleic Acids Res.* **2001**, *29*, 1185–1190. [CrossRef]
24. Leman, R.; Gaildrat, P.; Le Gac, G.; Ka, C.; Fichou, Y.; Audrezet, M.P.; Caux-Moncoutier, V.; Caputo, S.M.; Boutry-Kryza, N.; Léone, M.; et al. Novel diagnostic tool for prediction of variant spliceogenicity derived from a set of 395 combined in silico/in vitro studies: An international collaborative effort. *Nucleic Acids Res.* **2018**, *46*, 7913–7923. [CrossRef] [PubMed]
25. Cartegni, L.; Wang, J.; Zhu, Z.; Zhang, M.Q.; Krainer, A.R. ESEfinder: A web resource to identify exonic splicing enhancers. *Nucleic Acids Res.* **2003**, *31*, 3568–3571. [CrossRef] [PubMed]
26. Richards, S.; Aziz, N.; Bale, S.; Bick, D.; Das, S.; Gastier-Foster, J.; Grody, W.W.; Hegde, M.; Lyon, E.; Spector, E.; et al. Standards and guidelines for the interpretation of sequence variants: A joint consensus recommendation of the american college of medical genetics and genomics and the association for molecular pathology. *Genet. Med.* **2015**, *17*, 405–424. [CrossRef]
27. Quenez, O.; Cassinari, K.; Coutant, S.; Lecoquierre, F.; Le Guennec, K.; Rousseau, S.; Richard, A.C.; Vasseur, S.; Bouvignies, E.; Bou, J.; et al. Detection of copy-number variations from NGS data using read depth information: A diagnostic performance evaluation. *Eur. J. Hum. Genet.* **2020**. [CrossRef]
28. Naureckiene, S.; Sleat, D.E.; Lackland, H.; Fensom, A.; Vanier, M.T.; Wattiaux, R.; Jadot, M.; Lobel, P. Identification of HE1 as the second gene of Niemann-Pick C disease. *Science* **2000**, *290*, 2298–2301. [CrossRef]
29. Sleat, D.E.; Donnelly, R.J.; Lackland, H.; Liu, C.G.; Sohar, I.; Pullarkat, R.K.; Lobel, P. Association of mutations in a lysosomal protein with classical late-infantile neuronal ceroid lipofuscinosis. *Science* **1997**, *277*, 1802–1805. [CrossRef] [PubMed]
30. Sleat, D.E.; Gin, R.M.; Sohar, I.; Wisniewski, K.; Sklower-Brooks, S.; Pullarkat, R.K.; Palmer, D.N.; Lerner, T.J.; Boustany, R.M.; Uldall, P.; et al. Mutational analysis of the defective protease in classic late-infantile neuronal ceroid lipofuscinosis, a neurodegenerative lysosomal storage disorder. *Am. J. Hum. Genet.* **1999**, *64*, 1511–1523. [CrossRef] [PubMed]
31. Maegawa, G.H.; Tropak, M.; Buttner, J.; Stockley, T.; Kok, F.; Clarke, J.T.; Mahuran, D.J. Pyrimethamine as a potential pharmacological chaperone for late-onset forms of GM2 gangliosidosis. *J. Biol. Chem.* **2007**, *282*, 9150–9161. [CrossRef]
32. Huie, M.L.; Chen, A.S.; Tsujino, S.; Shanske, S.; DiMauro, S.; Engel, A.G.; Hirschhorn, R. Aberrant splicing in adult onset glycogen storage disease type II (GSDII): Molecular identification of an IVS1 ($-13T \longrightarrow G$) mutation in a majority of patients and a novel IVS10 (+1GT$\longrightarrow$CT) mutation. *Hum. Mol. Genet.* **1994**, *3*, 2231–2236. [CrossRef]
33. Wan, L.; Lee, C.C.; Hsu, C.M.; Hwu, W.L.; Yang, C.C.; Tsai, C.H.; Tsai, F.J. Identification of eight novel mutations of the acid alpha-glucosidase gene causing the infantile or juvenile form of glycogen storage disease type II. *J. Neurol.* **2008**, *255*, 831–838. [CrossRef] [PubMed]
34. Coutinho, M.F.; Matos, L.; Alves, S. From bedside to cell biology: A century of history on lysosomal dysfunction. *Gene* **2015**, *555*, 50–58. [CrossRef] [PubMed]
35. Mehta, A.B.; Winchester, B. *Lysosomal Storage Disorders—A Practial Guide*, 1st ed.; Wiley-Blackwell: Hoboken, NJ, USA, 2012; pp. 20–28.
36. Argmann, C.A.; Houten, S.M.; Zhu, J.; Schadt, E.E. A next generation multiscale view of inborn errors of metabolism. *Cell Metab.* **2016**, *23*, 13–26. [CrossRef]
37. Olkhovych, N.V.; Gorovenko, N.G. Determination of frequencies of alleles, associated with the pseudodeficiency of lysosomal hydrolases, in population of Ukraine. *Ukr. Biochem. J.* **2016**, *88*, 96–106. [CrossRef]
38. Schulz, A.; Ajayi, T.; Specchio, N.; de Los Reyes, E.; Gissen, P.; Ballon, D.; Dyke, J.P.; Cahan, H.; Slasor, P.; Jacoby, D.; et al. Study of intraventricular cerliponase alfa for CLN2 disease. *N. Engl. J. Med.* **2018**, *378*, 1898–1907. [CrossRef] [PubMed]

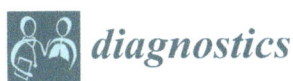

Article

Early Onset Ataxia with Comorbid Dystonia: Clinical, Anatomical and Biological Pathway Analysis Expose Shared Pathophysiology

Deborah A. Sival [1,*,†], Martinica Garofalo [1,†], Rick Brandsma [1], Tom A. Bokkers [1], Marloes van den Berg [1], Tom J. de Koning [2,3], Marina A. J. Tijssen [2] and Dineke S. Verbeek [3]

1 Department of Paediatric Neurology, Beatrix Children's Hospital, University Medical Center Groningen, University of Groningen, 9700 RB Groningen, The Netherlands; m.garofalo@student.rug.nl (M.G.); R.Brandsma-3@umcutrecht.nl (R.B.); tombokkers@live.nl (T.A.B.); m.van.den.berg.21@student.rug.nl (M.v.d.B.)
2 Department of Neurology, Beatrix Children's Hospital, University Medical Center Groningen, University of Groningen, 9700 RB Groningen, The Netherlands; t.j.de.koning@umcg.nl (T.J.d.K.); m.a.j.de.koning-tijssen@umcg.nl (M.A.J.T.)
3 Department of Genetics, Beatrix Children's Hospital, University Medical Center Groningen, University of Groningen, 9700 RB Groningen, The Netherlands; d.s.verbeek@umcg.nl
* Correspondence: d.a.sival@umcg.nl
† These authors fulfill requirements for first authorship.

Received: 7 October 2020; Accepted: 16 November 2020; Published: 24 November 2020

Abstract: In degenerative adult onset ataxia (AOA), dystonic comorbidity is attributed to one disease continuum. However, in early adult onset ataxia (EOA), the prevalence and pathogenesis of dystonic comorbidity (EOAD$^+$), are still unclear. In 80 EOA-patients, we determined the EOAD$^+$-prevalence in association with MRI-abnormalities. Subsequently, we explored underlying biological pathways by genetic network and functional enrichment analysis. We checked pathway-outcomes in specific EOAD$^+$-genotypes by comparing results with non-specifically (in-silico-determined) shared genes in up-to-date EOA, AOA and dystonia gene panels (that could concurrently cause ataxia and dystonia). In the majority (65%) of EOA-patients, mild EOAD$^+$-features concurred with extra-cerebellar MRI abnormalities (at pons and/or basal-ganglia and/or thalamus ($p = 0.001$)). Genetic network and functional enrichment analysis in EOAD$^+$-genotypes indicated an association with organelle- and cellular-component organization (important for energy production and signal transduction). In non-specifically, in-silico-determined shared EOA, AOA and dystonia genes, pathways were enriched for Krebs-cycle and fatty acid/lipid-metabolic processes. In frequently occurring EOAD$^+$-phenotypes, clinical, anatomical and biological pathway analyses reveal shared pathophysiology between ataxia and dystonia, associated with cellular energy metabolism and network signal transduction. Insight in the underlying pathophysiology of heterogeneous EOAD$^+$-phenotype-genotype relationships supports the rationale for testing with complete, up-to-date movement disorder gene lists, instead of single EOA gene-panels.

Keywords: clinical genetics; early onset ataxia; dystonia; neurodevelopment; network analysis; bioinformatics; ataxia; phenotype; child

1. Introduction

The diagnosis "early onset ataxia" refers to a group of rare, genetically inheritable diseases with an estimated prevalence of 14.6 per 100,000 individuals, initiated before the 25th year of life. These "ataxic syndromes" involve a heterogeneous group of underlying disorders that may phenotypically involve: (a) pure ataxic features; (b) predominant ataxic features in combination with other comorbid movement disorder features; (c) mild ataxic features in combination with other primary movement disorder features; (d) hardly discernible, disputable or even absent ataxic features, but with an underlying diagnosis that is phenotypically described as ataxic in the Online Mendelian Inheritance in Man (OMIM) database [1]. Depending on the age of the patient at disease presentation, patients are categorized as 'early onset ataxia' (EOA, i.e., initiation before 25 years of age) or degenerative 'adult onset ataxia' (AOA, i.e., initiation after 25 years of age) [2]. Both disease groups are distinctly different. Beside the age of onset, EOA and AOA groups are also different regarding: motor phenotype, genes involved, genetic mode of inheritance, nature of associated genetic mutations and patterns of disease progression.

Previous studies in patients with AOA have shown that the presence of ataxia with comorbid dystonia (AOAD$^+$) concerns a relatively frequently observed clinical phenotype in adulthood-onset ataxias [3–5]. Depending on the underlying AOA gene mutation, the percentage of comorbid dystonia (AOAD$^+$) may vary between 0% up and 53% [5]. In AOA, the exact pathogenic mechanism for dystonic comorbidity is not fully characterized, yet. Considering the degenerative nature of AOA disease courses, one could assume that extra-cerebellar degeneration may be involved when disorders progress [5]. However, there are also AOA phenotypes that can initially present with dystonia instead of ataxia [6–8]. In a previous study, we have explored the converging biological pathways for dystonia and AOA by determining the "shared genetics" between spinocerebellar ataxias (SCA)- and dystonia genes [3]. Forthcoming results indicated that there was a marked over-representation of shared genes involved in GABA-ergic signalling and in neurodevelopment [3]. This implicates that, at least in addition to extra-cerebellar neurodegenerative damage, aberrations in neurotransmission and developmental regulated genes must be involved in the pathogenesis. In line with our previous findings in AOAD$^+$, we now aimed to explore the prevalence and underlying pathogenesis in paediatric and young adult patients with EOA, with the underlying hypothesis that EOAD$^+$ could be associated with abnormal regulation of developmental genes and aberrations of neurotransmitter pathways as well. In mixed dystonic and ataxic EOAD$^+$-phenotypes, we anticipated that pathogenetic insight would contribute to an insightful diagnostic approach.

In the present EOA study, we therefore aimed to elucidate the underlying key biological pathways of dystonic comorbidity (EOAD$^+$). We hypothesized that EOAD$^+$-phenotypes could be associated with: (1) extra-cerebellar neuro-degenerative alterations determinable by MRI; (2) identifiable shared genetic/molecular pathways determinable by gene co-expression networks in specific EOAD$^+$ genotypes; and (3) non-specifically (in-silico) determinable genetic/molecular pathways in shared genes between AOA, EOA and dystonia gene panels, that may induce ataxia and dystonia in a concurrent way. We hypothesized that if comorbid dystonia could be explained by neurodegenerative processes, we would expect an association between the prevalence of comorbid dystonia and disease duration and/or age of the patient, both in our cohort, as well as in literature. This could also implicate a higher prevalence of comorbid dystonia in adult patients with AOA than in young patients with EOA. When the comorbid occurrence of dystonia in EOA would rather be attributable to shared molecular pathways and pathogenetic mechanisms, one would expect potentially corresponding results between two different "genetic-network-analyses" groups: (1) in EOAD$^+$ genotypes, with specifically identified dystonic comorbidity; and (2) in non-specifically (in-silico-determined) shared genes in up-to-date with EOA, AOA and dystonia gene panels, that could theoretically cause ataxia and dystonia in a concurrent way [3].

In perspective of the above, we conducted this study in two parts: Part I: in a cohort of 80 EOA-patients, we investigated: (1) the prevalence of EOAD$^+$, (2) the association between prevalent EOAD$^+$ comorbidity and disease duration and/or age of the patient, and (3) the association between EOAD$^+$ comorbidity and patterns of extra-cerebellar MRI abnormalities.

Part II: By genetic network and functional enrichment analysis, we investigated: (1) the shared underlying pathways by determining co-expression networks in the identified EOAD$^+$ genotypes;

(2) the shared underlying pathways by determining co-expression networks in (in-silico-determined) shared genes between AOA, EOA and dystonia gene lists (panels); and (3) comparative outcomes between specifically identified EOAD+ genotypes (from our database) and non-specifically (in-silico determined) shared genes in up-to-date EOA, AOA and dystonia gene lists (panels).

To the best of our knowledge, this is the first study providing a comprehensive approach to explore the prevalence and pathogenesis of EOAD+.

2. Patients and Methods

The study was carried out following the rules of the Declaration of Helsinki of 1975 (revised in 2013), in accordance with the research and integrity codes of the University Medical Center Groningen (UMCG). The Medical Ethical Committee of UMCG had approved the study (study no. UMCG research register METc 2015/01053, METc approval date 11 July 2012). According to Dutch medical ethical law, both parents and children older than 12 years provided informed consent whereas children younger than 12 years of age provided informed assent for phenotypic assessment.

2.1. Phenotypic Assessment of Dystonic Comorbidity in a Cohort of EOA Patients

2.1.1. EOA Database

We included the video-recordings from a cohort of 80 EOA-patients that had visited the paediatric neurology outpatient clinic at UMCG over the last 10 years. Included patients fulfilled the criteria for "EOA", implicating: symptomatic initiation of ataxia before the 25th year of life or an underlying genetic diagnosis associated with a primary ataxic phenotype, as indicated by the OMIM database (Online Mendelian Inheritance in Man, OMIM. McKusick-Nathans Institute of Genetic Medicine, Johns Hopkins University (Baltimore, MD, USA), 24 December 2016. WorldWide Web: http://omim.org/). In accordance with international criteria for EOA databases, we included patients with congenital, developmental, metabolic, degenerative, and/or unknown causes of ataxia starting before the 25th year of life [9]. Patients were excluded when they exhibited iatrogenic causes, such as underlying infectious, traumatic, intoxicative, cerebrovascular, para- and/or neoplastic pathology [10]. For the underlying diagnosis, age of onset and disease duration of the included patients, see Table 1. The genetic diagnosis of the patients was made using targeted gene panels for either early onset ataxia or dystonia.

Table 1. Early onset ataxia (EOA) patient information.

Case	Age of Onset (Year)	Duration (Full Years)	Age at Assessment (Year)	Gene Name *	Mutation Type	Neurological Diagnosis
1	0	14	14	RELN	VUS	cerebel cort dyspl, hypopl pons
2	0	17	17	LAMA1A	MM	Poretti Boltzhausen syndrome
3	0	13	13	-	-	Dandy Walker malformation
4	0	14	14	Unknown	-	Unknown
5	0	9	9	SOX 10	MM	Shah-Waardenburg syndrome
6	0	22	22	CHD7	MM	CHARGE Syndrome
7	7	6	14	Unknown	-	Unknown
8	0	7	7	KIAA0586	MM	Joubert Syndrome 23
9	11	0	11	-	-	Cediak Higashi
10	0	12	12	SPTBN2	Del, MM	SCA5
11	3	7	11	Unknown	-	Unknown
12	2	8	10	FXN	GAArepeat	Friedreich's ataxia
13	0	10	10	CTNNB1-gen	MM	AD MR 19
14	0	8	9	KCNC3	MM	SCA13
15	0	9	10	Unknown	-	Unknown
16	1	7	8	HSD17B10	MM	MHBD-deficiency
17	4	5	9	FXN	GAA repeat	Friedreich's ataxia
18	3	4	7	EBF3 mutation	MM	HADDS syndrome
19	4	1	5	FXN	GAA repeat	Friedreich's ataxia
20	0	0	1	INPPE5	MM	Joubert syndrome type 1

Table 1. Cont.

Case	Age of Onset (Year)	Duration (Full Years)	Age at Assessment (Year)	Gene Name *	Mutation Type	Neurological Diagnosis
21	14	1	16	Unknown	-	Unknown
22	5	6	11	GOSR2	MM	Northsea progr myocl
23	2	4	6	Unknown	-	Unknown
24	0	5	5	Unknown	-	Unknown
25	2	8	10	Unknown	-	Unknown
26	13	2	15	CACNA1A	MM	Episodic Ataxia type 2
27	4	7	11	FXN	GAA repeat	Friedreich's ataxia
28	2	5	7	KCND3	MM	SCA19
29	6	8	14	CACNA1A	MM	Episodic Ataxia type 2
30	1	2	3	CAMTA1	MM	CAMTA1
31	0	13	13	Unknown	-	Unknown
32	2	7	9	TITF1	MM	Benign Hereditary Chorea
33	4	2	6	ZMYND11	MM	AD, MR type 30
34	1	12	13	ITPR1	MM	SCA 29
35	3	9	12	ITPR1	MM	SCA29
36	4	11	15	ITPR1	MM	SCA29
37	12	0	12	Unknown	-	Unknown
38	1	1	2	Unknown	-	Unknown
39	6	3	9	SPTBN2	Del, MM	SCA5
40	1	7	8	ATP1A3	MM	RDP-AHC-Atax
41	2	5	8	ATP1A3	MM	AHC
42	9	23	32	TTPA	MM	AVED
43	4	11	15	FXN	GAA repeat	Friedreich's Ataxia
44	12	3	15	NPC	MM	Niemann Pick
45	12	22	34	TTPA	MM	AVED
46	1	25	26	T8993G	MM	NARP
47	16	11	28	TTPA	MM	AVED
48	5	11	16	HTT	CAG repeat	Juvenile Huntington
49	1	18	19	ATM	MM	Ataxia Telangiectasia
50	5	3	8	FXN	GAA repeat	Friedreich's Ataxia
51	0	5	5	-	-	cong malf fossa pos
52	11	6	18	mtDNA	MM	Kearns Sayre Syndrome
53	10	2	13	FXN	GAA repeat	Friedreich's ataxia
54	14	3	18	SPG-11	MM	HSP
55	1	17	18	GOSR2	MM	Northsea progr myocl
56	2	23	25	GOSR2	MM	Northsea progr myocl
57	0	6	6	Unknown	-	Unknown
58	3	13	16	CACNA1A	CAG repeat	Episodic Ataxia type 1
59	0	15	15	KIAA0586	MM	Joubert Syndrome 23
60	3	3	6	GOSR2	MM	Northsea progr myocl
61	3	13	16	CACNA1A	CAG repeat	Episodic Ataxia type 1
62	13	9	22	TTPA	MM	AVED
63	2	0	3	GOSR2	MM	Northsea progr myocl
64	2	18	20	GOSR2	MM	Northsea progr myocl
65	2	1	3	ALDH3A2	MM	SjogrenLarsson
66	8	5	13	SPG11	MM	Spastic paraplegia 11
67	6	13	19	FXN	GAA repeat	Friedreich's Ataxia
68	7	14	21	FXN	GAA repeat	Friedreich's Ataxia
69	9	13	22	FXN	GAA repeat	Friedreich's Ataxia
70	6	10	17	FXN	GAA repeat	Friedreich's Ataxia
71	4	10	14	FXN	GAA repeat	Friedreich's Ataxia
72	5	7	12	FXN	GAA repeat	Friedreich's Ataxia
73	2	9	11	TUBB2A	MM	CDCBM5
74	1	1	3	ATP1A3	MM	FIPWE
75	1	11	12	CACNA1A	CAG repeat	Episodic Ataxia type 2
76	7	5	12	ATXN7	CAG repeat	SCA7
77	15	0	16	SLC2A1 gen	MM	Glut-1 def
78	0	3	3	Unknown	-	Unknown
79	5	4	9	FXN	GAA repeat	Friedreich's ataxia
80	6	10	16	FXN	GAA repeat	Friedreich's Ataxia

Gene name * = gene name, mutations are specified in the Suppl. Table S1; cerebel cort dyspl = cerebellar cortical hypoplasia; hypopl = hypoplasia; VUS = variant of unknown significance; MM = missense mutation; MHBD = 2-methyl-3-hydroxybutyryl-CoA-hydrogenase deficiency, HADDS = hypotonie; ataxie and delayed development syndrome; RDP-AHC-Atax = disease continuum of rapid onset parkinsonism (RDP); alternating hemiplegia of childhood (AHC); ataxia AVED = Ataxia with isolated vitamin E deficiency; NARP = neuropathy; ataxia and retinitis pigmentosa; cong malf fossa pos = congenital malformation fossa posterior; CDCBM5 = cortical dysplasia, complex, with other brain malformations; FIPWE = fever-induced paroxysmal weakness and encephalopathy.

2.1.2. Phenotypic Assessment

In accordance with previously described methodology [1], we included videotaped SARA (scale for assessment and rating of ataxia [11]) or ICARS (international cooperative ataxia rating scale [12]) performances, that had been video-taped at the outpatient clinic for patient surveillance reasons. Both scales have been shown to capture paediatric ataxic movement disorder features in a similarly reliable way [13,14]. Furthermore, SARA has been shown to capture other phenotypic features of comorbid movement disorders, as well [15]. We included previously video-taped motor performances of 80 patients fulfilling the criteria of EOA. When patients had been videotaped on several occasions, we systematically included the motor performances that had been performed at the shortest disease duration (i.e., youngest age) of the patient. This provided us the opportunity to assess the motor phenotypes at a relatively early, mostly ambulant disease stage, with the smallest chance of any potential ceiling effects (for instance by the inability to walk or stand). Two paediatric neurologists, specialized in movement disorders, independently phenotyped the videotapes. In accordance with previously described methods, the paediatric neurologists indicated the observed movement disorder features and estimated severity (Suppl. Figure S1 [1]). The assessors individually captured the "print screens" including the time frames from the video-fragments at which they observed dystonic posturing. Patients were assigned to the EOAD$^+$ study group when both assessors had indicated that comorbid dystonia was present. Patients were assigned to the EOAD$^-$ control group, when both assessors had indicated that comorbid dystonia was absent. In the remaining patients (neither belonging to the EOAD$^+$, nor to the EOAD$^-$ control group), both assessors explained their phenotypic choice in a separate after-session by play-back at the indicated time frames from the "print screens".

To allow subsequent statistical comparison on a sufficient number of genes in the study- and control-group, we had to supplement the EOAD$^-$ (control) group with additional ataxia genes that were reported without comorbid dystonia, in literature (PubMed and OMIM). For genes included in the EOAD$^+$ study and EOAD$^-$ control group, see Suppl. Table S2.

2.1.3. MRI Abnormalities in EOAD$^+$ and EOAD$^-$ Subgroups

We subdivided the local cohort of 80 EOA patients into phenotypes with and without comorbid dystonia (i.e., the EOAD$^+$ study-group and EOAD$^-$ control group, respectively). In both groups, we subsequently associated the underlying genotypes with the corresponding brain abnormalities reported in literature (PubMed and OMIM databases). We characterized cerebral MRI abnormalities in EOAD$^+$ and EOAD$^-$ groups for: (1) the neuro-anatomical location and (2) the nature of cerebral abnormalities.

2.2. Network Analysis

2.2.1. Pathway and Network Analysis on the Study-Group (EOAD$^+$) and Control-Group (EOAD$^-$)

In the EOAD$^+$ study group and EOAD$^-$ control group, we related the associated genotypes with the patterns of MRI abnormalities. Subsequently, we performed a pathway and network analysis to evaluate the underlying biological processes and molecular pathways associated with the characterized genetic subgroups. For this purpose, we used the co-expression tool GeneNetwork (www.genenetwork.nl) to generate gene networks using the gene set enrichment feature. The pathway enrichment prediction of the clusters in the disease-specific networks was also performed by GeneNetwork and only the top significant gene ontology (GO) biological pathways were considered. In order to obtain sufficient genes for statistical analysis of the EAOD$^-$ control group, we added ataxia genes that were not reported with comorbid dystonia in literature (*ABHD12*; *IFRD1*; *KIAA0226*; *PHYH*; *TDP1*; *VWA3B*; *GTF2H5*; *FLVCR1*; *ACO2*; *HSD17B4*; *DNAJC3* gene mutations; PubMed and OMIM).

2.2.2. Pathway and Network Analysis in EOA, AOA and Dystonia Genes

In order to compare our specific pathway and network results (obtained ad IIa), with the non-specific outcomes derived from (in-silico-determined) shared genes between complete, up-to-date clinically applied gene panels (that could concurrently induce ataxia and dystonia), we compiled the most recent disease associated gene lists (used for clinical genetic diagnostics at the Department of Genetics of the UMCG, Groningen, the Netherlands), including EOA (n = 152 genes), AOA (n = 80 genes) and dystonia (n = 100 genes); see Suppl. Table S3. The biological pathways that were enriched in the EOA, AOA and dystonia genes were identified by the Toppfun feature of ToppGene Suite (https://toppgene.cchmc.org). The GO biological pathways were considered significant up to p-values 0.005 (Bonferroni, e.g., corrected for multiple testing). In accordance with previously published methods [3], we used GeneNetwork (www.genenetwork.nl) a co-expression tool by integrating 31,499 public RNA-seq samples [16] to generate the EOA, AOA and dystonia gene co-expression networks using the gene set enrichment feature. The pathway enrichment prediction of the clusters in the disease-specific networks was also performed by GeneNetwork and only the top significant GO biological pathways were considered for this work. GO biological pathways were considered significant up to p-values of 5×10^{-5}.

2.2.3. Comparison of Shared Pathways between EOAD$^+$ and EOA, AOA and Dystonia Gene Panels (2a versus 2b)

Finally, we compared the underlying shared pathways between: (1) specific EOAD$^+$ genotypes that were phenotyped with comorbid dystonia; and (2) (in silico determined) non-specifically shared pathways, derived from up-to-date EOA, and AOA, dystonia gene lists panels, that could concurrently induce ataxia and dystonia. For this purpose, we used the EOA, and AOA, dystonia gene lists that are included in the gene panels at the University Medical Center Groningen.

2.3. Statistics

The reliability of the agreement between the observers, was indicated by Cohen's kappa. Results were interpreted in accordance with Landis and Koch as: poor ($k < 0$); slight (k 0–0.20); fair (k 0.21–0.40); moderate (k 0.41–0.60); substantial (k 0.61–0.80) and almost perfect (k 0.81–1.00) [17]. We determined normality of disease duration and age of the patient by Shapiro Wilk test. We associated the presence of comorbid dystonia with both disease duration (at the time of the included video-recording) and age of the patient by Mann–Whitney U test. The significance level was set at $\alpha = 0.05$. Statistical analysis was performed using IBM SPSS statistics 23.0, Statistics for Windows, Version 23.0. Armonk, NY, USA: IBM Corp. In the study and control group, we combined and compared specific groups of genes according to the associated MRI patterns, using the Fisher-exact test.

3. Results

3.1. Prevalence of Comorbid Dystonia in 80 Patients with EOA

3.1.1. Clinical Characteristics of Included EOA-Patients

For the underlying diagnosis, age of onset, disease duration of the included patients, see Table 1. The disease duration and age of the patient (at video-assessment) were not normally distributed (Shapiro Wilk test ($p = 0.001$)). In 84% (67/80) EOA patients, the underlying association with the disease symptom ataxia was confirmed by genetic, metabolic and/or radiologic findings. In 78/80 (98%) of the recorded EOA-patients, either one of the two observers had recognized the presence of the symptom ataxia. In 76/80 (95%) of the recorded EOA-patients, both observers had recognized the presence of the symptom ataxia. The two patients in whom none of the observers had recognized ataxia, were diagnosed with an *ATP1A3* and *TUBB2A* mutation, respectively. Both patients had been described with ataxic features in the records of the outpatient clinic, but these features could apparently not be identified during the off-line video-assessment of the specific SARA video-recording. For rough scoring data and specific gene mutations, see Suppl. Table S1. Scored dystonic comorbidity is indicated in Suppl. Table S4a.

3.1.2. Evaluation of Comorbid Dystonia

In 52/80 (65%) of the EOA-patients, comorbid presence of dystonia was indicated by both observers, characterized by "comorbid dystonia". In 11/80 (14%) of the EOA-patients, the symptom dystonia was assessed by one observer and in 17/80 (21%) dystonia was assessed as absent by both observers. In 3/52 (6%) of the EOA-patients with comorbid dystonia (*TTPA*, *ATP1A3* and *TUBB2A* gene mutations), both observers had indicated that dystonia was severely present and that dystonia was presented as the main phenotype. In two of these patients (*ATP1A3* and *TUBB2A* gene mutations), ataxia had not been identified. In the other 49/52 (94%) of EOA-patients with comorbid dystonia, both observers had indicated that dystonia was (mostly mildly) present and that dystonia concerned the secondary phenotype. Either presence, or absence of comorbid dystonia was not significantly associated with EOA disease duration and/or age of the patient ($p = 0.645$ and $p = 0.103$, respectively; Mann–Whitney U test), see Suppl. Table S4b. In the patients with successive video-recordings, dystonic features did not longitudinally change from mild to severe (data not shown).

3.1.3. Association between Phenotype and Underlying Etiology

EOAD+ phenotypes were associated with genetic mutations ($n = 41$; 79%), congenital malformations of the fossa posterior ($n = 2$; 4%) and unknown causes ($n = 9$; 17%), see Table 2a. The EOA phenotypes without comorbid dystonia (28/80; 35%) were associated with genetic mutations (13; 81%); congenital malformations of the fossa posterior ($n = 1$; 6%), and unknown causes ($n = 2$; 13%), see Table 2b. The diagnoses Friedreich's ataxia, North Sea progressive myoclonus epilepsy, episodic ataxia type 2 and congenital malformations of the fossa posterior were both associated with presence and with absence of comorbid dystonia (EOAD$^+$ and EOAD$^-$ phenotypes); see Table 2a,b, respectively.

Table 2. EOA gene mutations with (**a**) and respectively without comorbid dystonia (**b**).

a. with comorbid dystonia		
Gene mutation		
TUBB2A ($n = 1$)	*ATXN7* ($n = 1$)	*LAMA1A* ($n = 1$)
FTX ($n = 9$)	*KCNC3* ($n = 1$)	*CHD7* ($n = 1$)
INPPE5 ($n = 1$)	*ATM* ($n = 1$)	*LYST* ($n = 1$)
ATP1A3 ($n = 3$)	*CAMTA1* ($n = 1$)	*HSD17B10* ($n = 1$)
TTPA ($n = 3$)	*NARP* ($n = 1$)	*HADDS* ($n = 1$)
CACNA1A ($n = 3$)	*ZMYND11* ($n = 1$)	*CTNNB1* ($n = 1$)
GOSR2 ($n = 2$)	*ALDH3A2* ($n = 1$)	*HTT* ($n = 1$)
SPTBN2 ($n = 2$)	*TITF1* ($n = 1$)	*SPG11* ($n = 1$)
KIAA0586 ($n = 2$)	*NPC* ($n = 1$)	* unknown ($n = 12$)
b. without comorbid dystonia		
Gene Mutation		
KCND3 ($n = 1$)		*CACNA1A* ($n = 2$)
FTX ($n = 3$)		*SPG11* ($n = 1$)
GOSR2 ($n = 3$)		** unknown ($n = 3$)
ITPR1 ($n = 3$)		

Legends: * unknown ($n = 12$) = unknown/absent gene mutation in association with malformation of fossa posterior ($n = 2$); *LYST* = Cediak Higashi syndrome ($n = 1$); no clinical diagnosis ($n = 9$); ** unknown (n=3) = unknown/absent gene mutation in association with malformation of fossa posterior ($n = 1$); no clinical diagnosis ($n = 2$). The gene mutations *CACNA1A*, *FTX* and *GOSR2* were present in clinical cases with and without comorbid dystonia. Cases with a congenital malformation of the fossa posterior were both associated with and without comorbid dystonia.

3.1.4. Reliability of Agreement between the Observers

The reliability of the agreement between the observers, was indicated by Cohen's kappa of 0.668 ($p < 0.001$). The kappa value was interpreted as sufficient to good in accordance with Landis and Koch [17]. In 69/80 (86%) patients, there was full agreement between the two observers on the presence or absence of comorbid dystonia. In 11/80 (14%) patients, the presence of comorbid dystonia was only indicated by one observer. In these 11 patients, the other observer had explained that the dystonic-like features were recognized, but that these features could not be discriminated from dystonic-like features due to physiologic immaturity of the central nervous system. These cases were therefore excluded from the subsequent analysis of EOAD$^+$ and the EOAD$^-$ groups.

3.1.5. EOAD$^+$ and EOAD$^-$ Groups and Associated MRI Abnormalities

In the investigated cohort, there were 25 genotypes in association with EOAD$^+$, 6 genotypes in association with EOAD$^-$ and 4 genotypes in association with both EOAD$^+$ and EOAD$^-$. In total, only 2 genotypes were included in the EOAD-control group. We, therefore, supplemented the EOAD-control group with ataxia genotypes that were not reported with comorbid dystonia in literature (including *ABHD12*; *IFRD1*; *KIAA0226*; *PHYH*; *TDP1*; *VWA3B*; *GTF2H5*; *FLVCR1*; *ACO2*; *HSD17B4*; *DNAJC3* gene mutations; PubMed and OMIM). For the included EOAD$^+$ and EOAD$^-$ groups and associated MRI abnormalities, see Suppl. Table S2. Reported MRI abnormalities were subdivided into hypoplasia; atrophy; and specifically described damage (see also Suppl. Table S2). Associating reported MRI abnormalities with EOAD$^+$ and EOAD$^-$ phenotypes, revealed a significant association between EOAD$^+$ phenotypes and abnormalities at the pons and/or basal ganglia and/or thalamus ($p = 0.001$), see Suppl. Table S5. Comparing the division of white and grey matter damage between EOAD$^+$ versus EOAD$^-$ groups, did not reveal statistical differences, see Suppl. Table S6.

3.2. Pathway and Network Analysis

3.2.1. EOAD$^+$ Genotypes

In the EOAD$^+$ gene group, pathway analysis revealed the strongest enrichment for GO biological processes involved in organelle organization ($p = 8.853 \times 10^{-17}$), and additionally in cellular component organization or biogenesis ($p = 2.315 \times 10^{-12}$), chromosome organization ($p = 7.158 \times 10^{-8}$) and cytoskeleton organization ($p = 3.441 \times 10^{-7}$). These are cellular processes resulting in the assembly, (re-) arrangement or disassembly of organelles, cellular components, chromosomes and cytoskeleton in a cell. For pathway and network analysis in EOAD$^+$ and EOAD$^-$ groups in association with allocated MRI damage, see Table 3.

Table 3. Top biological pathways in Early Onset Ataxia and Dystonia (EOAD$^+$) and (EOAD$^-$).

Subgroup	Most Significant Pathways	*p*-Value
EOA, Dystonia + (EOAD$^+$)	1. organelle organization 2. cellular component organization or biogenesis 3. cellular component organization 4. chromosome organization 5. cytoskeleton organization	8.853×10^{-17} 2.315×10^{-12} 1.767×10^{-11} 7.158×10^{-8} 3.441×10^{-7}
EOA, Dystonia − (EOAD$^-$)	1. small molecule metabolic process 2. cellular lipid metabolic process 3. lipid metabolic process 4. cellular lipid catabolic process 5. carboxylic acid metabolic process	1.091×10^{-17} 2.773×10^{-15} 2.866×10^{-15} 6.840×10^{-15} 1.376×10^{-14}
EOA, White Matter damage + (EOAW$^+$)	1. organelle organization 2. cellular component organization 3. cellular component organization or biogenesis 4. regulation of organelle organization 5. regulation of cellular component organization	4.102×10^{-8} 6.759×10^{-8} 8.330×10^{-8} 4.108×10^{-7} 6.354×10^{-6}

Table 3. Cont.

Subgroup	Most Significant Pathways	p-Value
EOA, White matter damage − (EOAW⁻)	1. ribonucleoprotein complex biogenesis	1.897×10^{-6}
	2. cellular nitrogen compound metabolic process	3.662×10^{-6}
	3. ribosome biogenesis	8.758×10^{-6}
	4. cellular component organization or biogenesis	9.220×10^{-5} *
	5. RNA processing	1.389×10^{-4} *
EOA, extracerebellar damage + (EOAX⁺)	1. carboxylic acid metabolic process	5.703×10^{-10}
	2. oxoacid metabolic process	9.228×10^{-9}
	3. organic acid metabolic process	1.635×10^{-8}
	4. cellular lipid catabolic process	1.742×10^{-6}
	5. vacuolar transport	3.896×10^{-6}
EOA, extracerebellar damage − (EOAX⁻)	1. RNA metabolic process	4.933×10^{-16}
	2. mRNA metabolic process	1.716×10^{-14}
	3. nucleic acid metabolic process	2.453×10^{-13}
	4. gene expression	9.775×10^{-13}
	5. mRNA processing	5.158×10^{-12}
EOA, cerebellar damage + (EOAC⁺)	1. cellular component organization	9.435×10^{-11}
	2. cellular component organization or biogenesis	1.286×10^{-10}
	3. organelle organization	9.573×10^{-10}
	4. cellular localization	3.517×10^{-7}
	5. vacuolar transport	3.177×10^{-6}
EOA, cerebellar damage − (EOAC⁻)	1. No statistical significant pathways could be found.	
EOA, dystonia+, White matter damage + (EOAD⁺W⁺)	1. organelle organization	9.603×10^{-15}
	2. cellular component organization or biogenesis	3.714×10^{-13}
	3. cellular component organization	1.062×10^{-12}
	4. cellular localization	2.485×10^{-8}
	5. microtubule-based process	1.631×10^{-7}

+ = comorbid sign is present; − = comorbid sign is absent; EOAD = EOA and comorbid dystonia; EOAW = EOA and white matter damage; EOAX = EOA and extra-cerebellar damage; EOAC = EOA and cerebellar damage; EOADW = EOA, dystonia and white matter damage. * Not significant. Statistical significance for pathway analysis: $p < 5 \times 10^{-5}$.

3.2.2. Shared Genes in EOA, AOA and Dystonia Gene-Lists (Panels)

In EAO, AOA and dystonia gene lists (Suppl. Table S3), we identified 54 shared genes between EAO and AOA, 13 between EAO and dystonia, and 8 between AOA and dystonia (Suppl. Figure S2 and Suppl. Table S7). The latter 8 genes were also shared between EAO and dystonia (i.e., shared between EOA, AOA and dystonia). These gene mutations included: *ATP1A3* (associated with the expanding phenotypic spectrum of alternating hemiplegia of childhood, rapid-onset dystonia-parkinsonism, *CAPOS* and *FIPWE*) [18], *POLG* (mitochondrial depletion syndrome), *NPC1* (Niemann–Pick disease, type C1), *TUBB4A* (DYT4), *MTTP* (abetalipoproteinemia), *SPG7* −(spastic paraplegia 7) and *SLC2A1* (GLUT1 deficiency syndrome). Two of these genes, *NPC1* and *MTTP*, are associated with plasma lipoprotein particle organization and cholesterol homeostasis.

3.2.3. Pathway Analysis in EOA, AOA and Dystonia Gene Lists (Panels)

We identified 90 significant GO biological pathways in EOA, 39 in AOA and 132 in dystonia genes (Suppl. Tables S8–S10). Of these pathways, 8 were shared between the three disorders, including cation- and ion transport, cation- and ion transmembrane transport, inorganic cation- and ion transmembrane transport, transmembrane transport, and locomotion pointing to an important role of cellular communication via synaptic transmission and movement in the underlying shared biology. For EOA, the most enriched GO pathways were locomotion, neurogenesis, myelination, and ion transport. For AOA, similar to EOA, pathways were associated with locomotion, ion- and trans-membrane transport, chemical- and synaptic transmission, and anterograde trans-synaptic signaling. For dystonia, pathways such as cellular respiration, oxidation-reduction process, respiratory- and electron transport chain, mitochondrial respiratory chain complex assembly and mitochondrion organization were identified. Overall, EOA and AOA are more similar in their underlying biological pathways compared to either one of them with dystonia, whereas dystonia shared only a few ($n = 5$) unique biological pathways with EOA but not with AOA.

3.2.4. Network Analysis in EOA, AOA, Dystonia

The EOA, AOA, dystonia networks comprised of 7, 3, and 4 clusters, respectively (Suppl. Figures S3–S5). We identified 472 shared genes between the three networks (Figure 1A and Supp. Table S11). The networks of EOA-AOA showed most overlap in genes ($n = 1210$), compared to EOA-dystonia ($n = 1004$) and AOA-dystonia ($n = 500$). The 472 shared genes between the three networks were enriched for GO pathways (top 10 ToppGene) involved in carboxylic acid—and organic acid metabolic process, fatty acid—and lipid metabolic process, and organic—and carboxylic acid catabolic process (Figure 1B). The 532 uniquely shared genes between EOA and dystonia were enriched for GO pathways involved in cellular respiration, drug metabolic process, ATP biosynthetic process, respiratory electron chain transport and purine ribonucleoside triphosphate biosynthetic process (Suppl. Table S12), whereas the 28 uniquely shared genes between AOA and dystonia were enriched in GO pathways involved in the release of calcium into the cytosol and calcium ion transport (Suppl. Table S13).

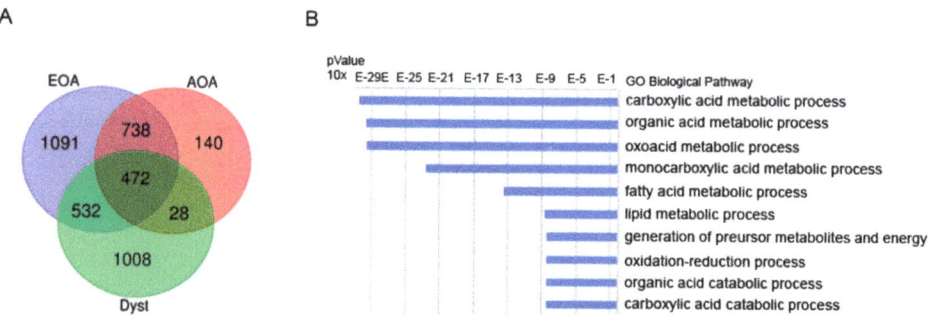

Figure 1. Shared genes and pathways between EAO, AOA and dystonia networks. Legend: (**A**) Venn diagram plot showing 472 common genes between EOA, AOA and dystonia. The gene networks of EOA—dystonia ($n = 1004$ (532 + 472)) reveal more overlap than the gene networks between AOA—dystonia ($n = 500$ (28 + 472)), suggesting that the gene networks of EOA is more similar to the dystonia network compared to the network of AOA—dystonia. (**B**) Top 10 of the most enriched pathways (top 10 ToppGene) of the common genes between EOA, AOA and dystonia. The most enriched pathways involved are involved in carboxylic acid—and organic acid metabolic process and fatty acid—and lipid metabolic process.

4. Discussion

To the best of our knowledge, this is the first study targeting at the underlying biological pathways in patients with EOA with comorbid dystonia (EOAD[+]-phenotypes). In the majority of EOA-patients, we observed only mildly dystonic features. The prevalence of dystonic comorbidity (65%) was apparently higher than previously reported prevalence in AOA-patients (0% to 53%, depending on the genotype) [5]. In addition to MRI abnormalities at the cerebellum, EOAD[+]-phenotypes revealed a strong association with MRI abnormalities at the basal ganglia and/or thalamus and/or pons (implicating disturbed signaling somewhere in the anatomical cortico-basal-ganglia-ponto-cerebellar network [19,20]). There was no association between the presence or absence of comorbid dystonia and EOA disease duration and/or age of the patient, implicating that other factors than ongoing neuro-degeneration are likely to play a role in the pathogenesis of comorbid dystonia. In our EOAD$^+$-study group, pathway and molecular co-expression network analysis indicated an underlying association with organelle and cellular organization (underlying energy production and signal transduction). As such pathways are not implicated in EOA alone, these findings are in line with previous studies demonstrating a pathophysiologic role for cytoskeletal reorganization in the underlying biology of dystonia [21]. Comparing these results with (in-silico-determined) network analysis in shared EOA, AOA and dystonia gene lists (panels), showed enrichment for Krebs-cycle (tricarboxylic acid cycle (TCA)) and fatty acid/lipid metabolic process, underlying the concept of hampered energy production and signal transduction. From these data, we conclude that both specifically (EOAD$^+$) and non-specifically (in silico determined) shared pathways and networks analyses implicate an underlying role for cellular energy production and network signal transduction in the pathogenesis of EOA with comorbid dystonia. This may have implications for genetic testing. Instead of testing with a single EOA gene panel, one may consider using Whole Exome Sequencing (WES), a complete movement disorder panel and copy number variation analysis, whereas diagnostics by Whole Genome Sequencing (WGS) may have a wider application, in the future. Previous studies in neuro-degenerative AOA disorders, have implicated that the comorbid presence of dystonia should be regarded as an expression of the same disease continuum [4,22,23]. Conversely, in adult patients, dystonic symptoms have also been associated with cerebellar pathology [24,25] and cerebellar symptoms, including action induced tremors [26], eye blink conditioning [27] and saccadic adaption [28]. However, in the presently studied cohort of 80 relatively young EOA patients, we observed comorbid dystonia (EOAD$^+$) in the majority (65%) of patients. This EOAD$^+$ subgroup revealed a large heterogeneity in genotype-phenotype relationships, reflected by: (1) identical genetic mutations that were associated with EOAD$^+$ and also with EOAD$^-$ phenotypes (in different patients), (2) absence of EOAD$^+$ features in genotypes that have been identified with comorbid dystonia in literature and (3) presence of EOAD$^+$ features in EOA genotypes that have not been reported with comorbid dystonic features, before. As expected, we observed that MRI abnormalities of the basal ganglia and/or pons and/or thalamus were associated with the EOAD$^+$ phenotype. In addition to the well-known association between abnormalities at the basal ganglia and thalamus with dystonia, the pedunculo-pontine tegmental nucleus (PPTg) at the pons has been shown to connect between the basal ganglia and cerebellar nuclei and thalamus [29] implicating that hampered signaling in the anatomical cortico-basal-ganglia-ponto-cerebellar network may be involved [19,20].

Comparing the dystonic prevalence in "early disease onset" EOA (EOAD$^+$; 65%) with previously reported "adult disease onset" AOA (AOAD$^+$; 0% to 53% depending on the genotype) [5,30–33], reveals a higher prevalence in the first group. This could be theoretically attributed to several factors. First, it is well known that dystonic-like features may physiologically appear in young children, due to the incomplete maturation of the central nervous system [34,35]. However, in EOA we observed no association between EOAD$^+$ and young age and/or shorter disease duration. Furthermore, the majority of patients were older than 10 years of age. After this age, physiologic dystonic-like features have mostly disappeared [34,35] and, finally, we had excluded all patients with doubtful minor developmental dystonic-like features from the study. Second, one could attribute the higher prevalence of dystonic comorbidity in EOA than in AOA to more advanced extra-cerebellar neuro-degeneration. However, considering the younger age of the EOA patients and the inclusion of the firstly recorded movement disorder performances, this appears unlikely, as well. Another, and much more likely explanation is provided by our non-specific, in silico pathway and network analysis, performed on shared genes between up-to-date EOA, AOA and dystonia gene panels. Comparing gene network similarities, revealed about twice as much overlapping gene networks between EAO- and dystonia-genes than between AOA- and dystonia-genes. From this molecular genetic perspective, it could be derived that dystonic comorbidity is also about twice as likely to concur with EOA than with AOA.

In the present study, we hypothesized that the underlying genetic mechanisms for EOAD$^+$ could both involve: (1) shared pathways inducing a specific EOAD$^+$ phenotype, and/or (2) non-specifically shared pathways by genes that may be concurrently expressed in EOA, AOA and dystonia, inducing comorbid features. Investigating shared pathways in the specific EOAD$^+$ group, revealed an association with organelle- and cellular- organization. Until now, these pathways have not been described in EOAD$^+$ before. Mitochondria are important organelles generating most of the cellular energy by the TCA (Krebs cycle). Pathways of cellular organizations are involved in the axonal cytoskeleton providing the basis for axonal transport and network signaling. This may imply that novel EOAD$^+$-phenotype related gene mutations could be found in association with these molecular pathways.

By investigating the non-specifically shared genes and pathways between EOA and AOA genes, we identified quite similar pathway enrichment for the EAO and AOA gene list, that was different from dystonia. The top biological pathways observed for EAO and AOA were involved in locomotion and neurogenesis. These biological pathways have also been implicated in the pathogenesis of ataxia syndromes [36,37]. The top biological pathways observed for dystonia were involved in cellular respiration and metabolism. Additionally, studies reported changes in cellular—and /or mitochondrial respiration in dystonia [38,39], supporting the validity of our in silico genetic analysis. Not surprisingly, none of the top pathways underlying either ataxia or dystonia were shared between EAO, AOA and dystonia. In fact, several pathways involved in cation and ion membrane transport were enriched in the common genes, pointing to an important role for neuronal communication that is also consistent with prior knowledge on the pathology of these mixed disorders [38,40,41]. Furthermore, we observed that carboxylic acid—and organic acid metabolic and catalytic processes were enriched in the common genes, pointing out to the tricarboxylic acid cycle (TCA), or Krebs cycle. The TCA cycle, is essential for mitochondrial ATP production and is fueled by fatty-acid–oxidation. Furthermore, the TCA cycle is crucial for the synthesis of gamma aminobutyric acid (GABA), the main neurotransmitter of Purkinje cells (PCs). In dystonic syndromes, it is reported that PCs are dysfunctional and in ataxic syndromes PCs are often also degenerative [25,42]. Of note, one of the clusters of the AOA network was enriched for genes involved in gamma-aminobutyric acid (GABA) signaling pathway, and altered GABA-ergic signaling has also been reported to play a role in patients with cervical dystonia [43]. Finally, cellular energy failure has been implicated in the pathogenesis of cerebral demyelination. Whether preferential loss of Myelin-associated glycoprotein is a feature of primary mitochondrial disorders [44], or due to mutations in nuclear genes is still unclear [45].

The enrichment for lipid and fatty acid homeostasis in the shared genes (Figure 1B) of the disease specific molecular networks further support the role for development of the central nervous system in the pathology of these disorders. Cholesterol is an essential lipid for mammalian cells, and is necessary for the numerous formations of efficient synapses, which stems from de novo synthesis [46]. Whereas fatty acids and their metabolites are required for normal brain development and the activation of gene transcription regulating long-chain polyunsaturated fatty acids formation. Many neurodegenerative diseases are associated with disrupted lipid- and cholesterol homeostasis, including such Niemann Pick type C disease, Smith Lemli Opitz, and SCA3 [46,47]. In neurodegenerative mouse models for spinocerebellar ataxia, it was shown that impaired cholesterol metabolism reduces the Purkinje cell number and induces motor coordination deficits [48]. Furthermore, it has been shown that that the cerebellum can modulate the basal ganglia activity [19,20] by input from the neurologic cerebello-thalamo-basal ganglia anatomical pathway [49]. In the central nervous system, oligodendrocytes generate multiple layers of myelin around axons of the central nervous system to enable fast and efficient nerve conduction. Until recently, saltatory nerve conduction was considered the only purpose of myelin, but myelinating oligodendrocytes can also provide metabolic support to neurons, and regulate ion and water homeostasis by adapting to activity-dependent neuronal signals [50]. Mutations in very long chain fatty acid elongase 4 and 5 (Elovl4 and ElovL5) are reported to cause spinocerebellar ataxia [51–53] and accumulation of the branched-chain acid fatty acid was reported to be associated with Refsum disease caused by mutations in Phytanic acid alpha-oxidation (in AOA gene panel) [54]. Additionally, MECR mutations cause a mitochondrial fatty-acid synthesis disorder and is characterized by a childhood-onset dystonia [55]. Altogether, these crucial biological pathways may thus support the hypothesis that they can concurrently underlie the initiation of ataxia and dystonia [4]. Nevertheless, this does not necessarily implicate that these pathways also play a specifically causative role in the pathogenesis of comorbid dystonia. However, investigating the pathway and network analysis in the specifically phenotyped EOAD$^+$ group, reveals a similar role for organelle and cellular organization in dystonic comorbidity. Although not identical, both specifically and non-specifically shared pathways may thus implicate an association with hampered cellular energy production and network signal transduction.

We are aware of some weaknesses to this study. In the first place, the presently studied EOA gene panel cannot be considered complete, since new genes are being, and will be added in the future. Furthermore, by using an EOA database from a single center, we cannot exclude local influences on the outcome data. For instance, we noticed that some of the EOAD$^+$ genes are not associated with dystonia in literature, and vice versa. However, considering the fact that (1) EOA is a rare disorder, (2) we were able to include a considerable cohort of 80 EOA patients, (3) the identified EOAD$^+$ phenotypes were linked with extra-cerebellar MRI alterations at the basal-ganglia-ponto-thalamic network, and (4) pathway- and network-analyses in both specific EOAD+ phenotypes and in silico determined shared genes reflected similarly underlying biological processes, we would suggest that the present results can be interpreted as indicative. Hopefully, future collaboration with European and even world-wide based ataxia databases will elucidate this.

In summary, in a local cohort of 80 EOA-patients, we observed dystonic comorbidity in the majority of patients. Exploration of the underlying clinical, anatomical and biological pathways revealed shared pathophysiology, despite genotype-phenotype heterogeneity. Both patient specific (in EOAD$^+$) and non-specific (in silico determined) pathway- and network-analyses implicated associated biological pathways involved in organelle and cellular organization, respectively in TCA cycle processes and lipid and fatty-acid homeostasis. Both outcomes suggest that hampered energy production and network signal transduction may play an underlying role in the pathophysiology of ataxia with comorbid dystonia.

These findings may have important implications for the diagnostic approach in mixed "EOA" comorbid dystonia movement disorders. Since network analyses in both specifically determined EOAD$^+$-genotypes and also in non-specifically, in silico, determined shared genes in EOA, AOA and dystonia panels both refer to similar underlying pathways, one may hypothesize the presence of a common pathogenesis. This would implicate that EOAD$^+$-phenotypes can be concurrently induced by shared genetic networks between EOA and dystonia genes. This could explain the heterogeneous genotype-phenotype relationships varying from predominant ataxia at one end of the spectrum, continuing with ataxia and comorbid dystonia, and, finally predominant dystonia at the other end of the spectrum.

Altogether, in perspective of: (1) the high prevalence of EOAD$^+$ phenotypes, (2) the heterogeneity of genotype-phenotype relationships, (3) the shared anatomical pathways and (4) the shared underlying biological pathways that contribute to the same disease continuum, it might be a rationalistic approach to test EOA patients with a complete, up to date movement disorder panel (including EOA and dystonia gene lists), instead of with a single EOA gene panel. In the future, we aim to investigate the pathogenesis of other mixed EOA phenotypes by determining shared pathways between EOA and other comorbid movement disorders, as well.

5. Conclusions

Comorbid dystonia is prevalent in the majority of EOA patients. The underlying biological pathways can be linked with energy depletion and hampered signal transduction involving the cortical-basal-ganglia-pontine-cerebellar network. Hopefully, future insight in the underlying processes causing the heterogeneous, mixed EOA phenotypes may contribute to the yield of diagnostic testing and innovative therapeutic strategies.

Supplementary Materials: The following are available online at http://www.mdpi.com/2075-4418/10/12/997/s1, Figures S1–S5: Figure S1: phenotypic assessment form, Figure S2: (A) Venn diagram plot comparing genes between EOA (N = 152 genes), AOA (N = 80 genes) and dystonia (N = 100 genes). (B) Venn diagram plot comparing GO biological pathways between EOA (N = 90 pathways), AOA (N = 39 pathways) and dystonia (N = 131 pathways), Figure S3: schematic representation of network of EOA genes comprised of 7 clusters generated by GeneNetwork (GeneNetwork.nl), Figure S4: schematic representation of network of AOA genes comprised of three clusters generated by GeneNetwork (GeneNetwork.nl), Figure S5: schematic representation of network of dystonia genes comprised of four clusters generated by GeneNetwork (GeneNetwork.nl). Tables S1–S13: Table S1: gene mutations and phenotypic assessment, Table S2: gene vs MRI database title, Table S3: EOA, AOA, dystonia gene panels, Table S4a: scored dystonic comorbidity, Table S4b: comorbid dystonia versus disease duration and age of the patients, Table S5: frequency table of allocated damage on MRI, Table S6: division of damage on MRI, Table S7: shared genes between EOA, AOA and dystonia gene panels, Table S8: enriched pathways of EOA genes, Table S9: enriched pathways of AOA genes, Table S10: enriched pathways of dystonia genes, Table S11: common genes between networks EOA, AOA and dystonia, Table S12: Top 10 GO biological pathways common genes networks EAO and dystonia, Table S13: Top 10 GO biological pathways common genes networks AOA and dystonia.

Author Contributions: Conceptualization, D.A.S., T.J.d.K., M.A.J.T. and D.S.V.; data curation, D.A.S., M.G. and M.v.d.B.; formal analysis, D.A.S., M.G., R.B., T.A.B., M.v.d.B. and D.S.V.; investigation, D.A.S., M.G., R.B., T.A.B., M.v.d.B. and D.S.V.; methodology, D.A.S., M.G., R.B., T.A.B., M.v.d.B. and D.S.V.; project administration, D.A.S.; supervision, D.A.S. and D.S.V.; validation, D.A.S., M.G., R.B., T.A.B. and D.S.V.; visualization, D.A.S., M.G., T.A.B. and D.S.V.; writing—original draft, D.A.S., M.G. and D.S.V.; writing—review and editing, D.A.S., T.J.d.K., M.A.J.T. and D.S.V. All authors have read and agreed to the published version of the manuscript.

Funding: This research received no external funding.

Acknowledgments: Deborah A. Sival, Tom J. de Koning, Marina A.J. Tijssen and Dineke S. Verbeek are member(s) of the European Reference Network for Rare Neurological Diseases—Project ID No 739510.

Conflicts of Interest: The authors declare no conflict of interest.

Abbreviations

EOA	early onset ataxia
EOAD+	early onset ataxia with dystonic comorbidity
EOAD−	early onset ataxia without dystonic comorbidity
TCA	tricarboxylic acid cycle
AOA	adult onset ataxia
AOAD+	adult onset ataxia with dystonic comorbidity
SCA	spino-cerebellar ataxia

References

1. Lawerman, T.F.; Brandsma, R.; Maurits, N.M.; Martinez-Manzanera, O.; Verschuuren-Bemelmans, C.C.; Lunsing, R.J.; Brouwer, O.F.; Kremer, H.P.; Sival, D. Paediatric motor phenotypes in early-onset ataxia, developmental coordination disorder, and central hypotonia. *Dev. Med. Child Neurol.* **2020**, *62*, 75–82. [CrossRef] [PubMed]
2. Harding, A.E. Clinical features and classification of inherited ataxias. *Adv. Neurol.* **1993**, *61*, 1–14. [PubMed]
3. Nibbeling, E.A.R.; Duarri, A.; Verschuuren-Bemelmans, C.C.; Fokkens, M.R.; Karjalainen, J.M.; Smeets, C.J.; De Boer-Bergsma, J.J.; Van Der Vries, G.; Dooijes, D.; Bampi, G.B.; et al. Exome sequencing and network analysis identifies shared mechanisms underlying spinocerebellar ataxia. *Brain* **2017**, *140*, 2860–2878. [CrossRef] [PubMed]
4. Prudente, C.N.; Hess, E.J.; Jinnah, H.A. Dystonia as a network disorder: What is the role of the cerebellum? *Neuroscience* **2014**, *260*, 23–35. [CrossRef] [PubMed]
5. Van Gaalen, J.; Giunti, P.; Van De Warrenburg, B.P. Movement disorders in spinocerebellar ataxias. *Mov. Disord.* **2011**, *26*, 792–800. [CrossRef] [PubMed]
6. Tewari, A.; Fremont, R.; Khodakhah, K. It's not just the basal ganglia: Cerebellum as a target for dystonia therapeutics. *Mov. Disord.* **2017**, *32*, 1537–1545. [CrossRef]

7. Muzaimi, M.B.; Wiles, C.M.; Robertson, N.P.; Ravine, D.; Compston, D.A.S. Task specific focal dystonia: A presentation of spinocerebellar ataxia type 6. *J. Neurol. Neurosurg. Psychiatry* **2003**, *74*, 1444–1445. [CrossRef]
8. Saunders-Pullman, R.; Raymond, D.; Stoessl, A.J.; Hobson, D.; Nakamura, T.; Pullman, S.; Lefton, D.; Okun, M.S.; Uitti, R.; Sachdev, R.; et al. Variant ataxia-telangiectasia presenting as primary-appearing dystonia in Canadian Mennonites. *Neurology* **2012**, *78*, 649–657. [CrossRef]
9. Vedolin, L.M.; González, G.; Souza, C.F.; Lourenço, C.; Barkovich, A.J. Inherited Cerebellar Ataxia in Childhood: A Pattern-Recognition Approach Using Brain MRI. *Am. J. Neuroradiol.* **2013**, *34*, 925–934. [CrossRef]
10. Lawerman, T.F.; Brandsma, R.; Van Geffen, J.T.; Lunsing, R.J.; Burger, H.; Tijssen, M.A.J.; De Vries, J.J.; De Koning, T.J.; Sival, D. Reliability of phenotypic early-onset ataxia assessment: A pilot study. *Dev. Med. Child Neurol.* **2016**, *58*, 70–76. [CrossRef]
11. Schmitz-Hübsch, T.; Du Montcel, S.T.; Baliko, L.; Berciano, J.; Boesch, S.; Depondt, C.; Giunti, P.; Globas, C.; Infante, J.; Kang, J.-S.; et al. Scale for the assessment and rating of ataxia: Development of a new clinical scale. *Neurology* **2006**, *66*, 1717–1720. [CrossRef] [PubMed]
12. Trouillas, P.; Takayanagi, T.; Hallett, M.; Currier, R.; Subramony, S.; Wessel, K.; Bryer, A.; Diener, H.; Massaquoi, S.; Gomez, C.; et al. International Cooperative Ataxia Rating Scale for pharmacological assessment of the cerebellar syndrome. *J. Neurol. Sci.* **1997**, *145*, 205–211. [CrossRef]
13. Brandsma, R.R.; Spits, A.A.; Kuiper, M.M.; Lunsing, R.R.; Burger, H.; Kremer, H.H.; Sival, D. The Childhood Ataxia and Cerebellar Group Ataxia rating scales are age-dependent in healthy children. *Dev. Med. Child Neurol.* **2014**, *56*, 556–563. [CrossRef]
14. Bürk, K.; Sival, D.A. Scales for the clinical evaluation of cerebellar disorders. *Handb. Clin. Neurol.* **2018**, *154*, 329–339. [CrossRef] [PubMed]
15. Brandsma, R.; Lawerman, T.F.; Kuiper, M.J.; Lunsing, R.J.; Burger, H.; Sival, D.A. Reliability and discriminant validity of ataxia rating scales in early onset ataxia. *Dev. Med. Child Neurol.* **2017**, *59*, 427–432. [CrossRef] [PubMed]
16. Pers, T.H.; Karjalainen, J.M.; Chan, Y.; Westra, H.-J.; Wood, A.R.; Yang, J.; Lui, J.C.; Vedantam, S.; Gustafsson, S.; Esko, T.; et al. Biological interpretation of genome-wide association studies using predicted gene functions. *Nat. Commun.* **2015**, *6*, 1–9. [CrossRef]
17. Landis, J.R.; Koch, G.G. The Measurement of Observer Agreement for Categorical Data. *Biometrics* **1977**, *33*, 159. [CrossRef] [PubMed]
18. Sweney, M.T.; Newcomb, T.M.; Swoboda, K.J. The expanding spectrum of neurological phenotypes in children with ATP1A3 mutations, Alternating Hemiplegia of Childhood, Rapid-onset Dystonia-Parkinsonism, CAPOS and beyond. *Pediatr. Neurol.* **2015**, *52*, 56–64. [CrossRef] [PubMed]
19. Schirinzi, T.; Sciamanna, G.; Mercuri, N.B.; Pisani, A. Dystonia as a network disorder. *Curr. Opin. Neurol.* **2018**, *31*, 498–503. [CrossRef] [PubMed]
20. Calderon, D.P.; Fremont, R.; Kraenzlin, F.; Khodakhah, K. The neural substrates of rapid-onset Dystonia-Parkinsonism. *Nat. Neurosci.* **2011**, *14*, 357–365. [CrossRef] [PubMed]
21. Atai, N.A.; Ryan, S.D.; Kothary, R.; Breakefield, X.O.; Nery, F.C. Untethering the Nuclear Envelope and Cytoskeleton: Biologically Distinct Dystonias Arising from a Common Cellular Dysfunction. *Int. J. Cell Biol.* **2012**, *2012*, 1–18. [CrossRef] [PubMed]
22. Nibbeling, E.A.R.; Delnooz, C.C.S.; De Koning, T.J.; Sinke, R.J.; Jinnah, H.A.; Tijssen, M.A.J.; Verbeek, D.S. Using the shared genetics of dystonia and ataxia to unravel their pathogenesis. *Neurosci. Biobehav. Rev.* **2017**, *75*, 22–39. [CrossRef] [PubMed]
23. Schreglmann, S.R.; Riederer, F.; Galovic, M.; Ganos, C.; Kägi, G.; Waldvogel, D.; Jaunmuktane, Z.; Schaller, A.; Hidding, U.; Krasemann, E.; et al. Movement disorders in genetically confirmed mitochondrial disease and the putative role of the cerebellum. *Mov. Disord.* **2018**, *33*, 146–155. [CrossRef] [PubMed]
24. Neychev, V.K.; Gross, R.E.; Lehéricy, S.; Hess, E.J.; Jinnah, H.A. The functional neuroanatomy of dystonia. *Neurobiol. Dis.* **2011**, *42*, 185–201. [CrossRef] [PubMed]
25. Zoons, E.; Tijssen, M. Pathologic changes in the brain in cervical dystonia pre- and post-mortem—A commentary with a special focus on the cerebellum. *Exp. Neurol.* **2013**, *247*, 130–133. [CrossRef] [PubMed]
26. Raethjen, J.; Deuschl, G. The oscillating central network of Essential tremor. *Clin. Neurophysiol.* **2012**, *123*, 61–64. [CrossRef]

27. Teo, J.T.; Van De Warrenburg, B.; Schneider, S.; Rothwell, J.; Bhatia, K. Neurophysiological evidence for cerebellar dysfunction in primary focal dystonia. *J. Neurol. Neurosurg. Psychiatry* **2009**, *80*, 80–83. [CrossRef]
28. Hubsch, C.; Vidailhet, M.; Rivaud-Péchoux, S.; Pouget, P.; Brochard, V.; Degos, B.; Pélisson, D.; Golmard, J.-L.; Gaymard, B.; Roze, E. Impaired saccadic adaptation in DYT11 dystonia. *J. Neurol. Neurosurg. Psychiatry* **2011**, *82*, 1103–1106. [CrossRef]
29. Mori, F.; Okada, K.-I.; Nomura, T.; Kobayashi, Y. The Pedunculopontine Tegmental Nucleus as a Motor and Cognitive Interface between the Cerebellum and Basal Ganglia. *Front. Neuroanat.* **2016**, *10*, 109. [CrossRef]
30. Schmitz-Hubsch, T.; Coudert, M.; Bauer, P.; Giunti, P.; Globas, C.; Baliko, L.; Filla, A.; Mariotti, C.; Rakowicz, M.; Charles, P.; et al. Spinocerebellar ataxia types 1, 2, 3, and 6: Disease severity and nonataxia symptoms. *Neurology* **2008**, *71*, 982–989. [CrossRef]
31. Mariotti, C.; Alpini, D.; Fancellu, R.; Soliveri, P.; Grisoli, M.; Ravaglia, S.; Lovati, C.; Fetoni, V.; Giaccone, G.; Castucci, A.; et al. Spinocerebellar ataxia type 17 (SCA17): Oculomotor phenotype and clinical characterization of 15 Italian patients. *J. Neurol.* **2007**, *254*, 1538–1546. [CrossRef]
32. Hagenah, J.M.; Zühlke, C.; Hellenbroich, Y.; Heide, W.; Klein, C. Focal dystonia as a presenting sign of spinocerebellar ataxia 17. *Mov. Disord.* **2004**, *19*, 217–220. [CrossRef]
33. Estrada, R.; Galarraga, J.; Orozco, G.; Nodarse, A.; Auburger, G. Spinocerebellar ataxia 2 (SCA2): Morphometric analyses in 11 autopsies. *Acta Neuropathol.* **1999**, *97*, 306–310. [CrossRef] [PubMed]
34. Kuiper, M.J.; Vrijenhoek, L.; Brandsma, R.; Lunsing, R.J.; Burger, H.; Eggink, H.; Peall, K.J.; Contarino, M.F.; Speelman, J.D.; Tijssen, M.A.J.; et al. The Burke-Fahn-Marsden Dystonia Rating Scale is Age-Dependent in Healthy Children. *Mov. Disord. Clin. Pr.* **2016**, *3*, 580–586. [CrossRef] [PubMed]
35. Kuiper, M.; Brandsma, R.; Vrijenhoek, L.; Tijssen, M.; Burger, H.; Dan, B.; Sival, D.A. Physiological movement disorder-like features during typical motor development. *Eur. J. Paediatr. Neurol.* **2018**, *22*, 595–601. [CrossRef] [PubMed]
36. Matilla-Dueñas, A.; Ashizawa, T.; Brice, A.; Magri, S.; McFarland, K.N.; Pandolfo, M.; Pulst, S.M.; Riess, O.; Rubinsztein, D.C.; Schmidt, T.H.; et al. Consensus Paper: Pathological Mechanisms Underlying Neurodegeneration in Spinocerebellar Ataxias. *Cerebellum* **2014**, *13*, 269–302. [CrossRef]
37. Smeets, C.; Verbeek, D.S. Cerebellar ataxia and functional genomics: Identifying the routes to cerebellar neurodegeneration. *Biochim. Biophys. Acta (BBA) Mol. Basis Dis.* **2014**, *1842*, 2030–2038. [CrossRef]
38. Jinnah, H.A.; Sun, Y.V. Dystonia genes and their biological pathways. *Neurobiol. Dis.* **2019**, *129*, 159–168. [CrossRef]
39. Casper, C.; Kalliolia, E.; Warner, T.T. Recent advances in the molecular pathogenesis of dystonia-plus syndromes and heredodegenerative dystonias. *Curr. Neuropharmacol.* **2013**, *11*, 30–40.
40. Sullivan, R.; Yau, W.Y.; O'Connor, E.; Houlden, H. Spinocerebellar ataxia: An update. *J. Neurol.* **2019**, *266*, 533–544. [CrossRef]
41. Synofzik, M.; Helbig, K.L.; Harmuth, F.; Deconinck, T.; Tanpaiboon, P.; Sun, B.; Guo, W.; Wang, R.; Palmaer, E.; Tang, S.; et al. De novo ITPR1 variants are a recurrent cause of early-onset ataxia, acting via loss of channel function. *Eur. J. Hum. Genet.* **2018**, *26*, 1623–1634. [CrossRef] [PubMed]
42. Xiao, R.; Zhong, H.; Li, X.; Ma, Y.; Zhang, R.; Wang, L.; Zang, Z.; Fan, X. Abnormal Cerebellar Development Is Involved in Dystonia-Like Behaviors and Motor Dysfunction of Autistic BTBR Mice. *Front. Cell Dev. Biol.* **2020**, *8*. [CrossRef] [PubMed]
43. Berman, B.D.; Pollard, R.T.; Shelton, E.; Karki, R.; Smith-Jones, P.M.; Miao, Y. GABAA Receptor Availability Changes Underlie Symptoms in Isolated Cervical Dystonia. *Front. Neurol.* **2018**, *9*, 188. [CrossRef] [PubMed]
44. Filosto, M.; Tomelleri, G.; Tonin, P.; Scarpelli, M.; Vattemi, G.; Rizzuto, N.; Padovani, A.; Simonati, A. Neuropathology of mitochondrial diseases. *Biosci. Rep.* **2007**, *27*, 23–30. [CrossRef] [PubMed]
45. Campbell, G.R.; Lax, N.Z.; Reeve, A.K.; Ohno, N.; Zambonin, J.L.; Blakely, E.L.; Taylor, R.W.; Bonilla, E.; Tanji, K.; DiMauro, S.; et al. Loss of Myelin-Associated Glycoprotein in Kearns-Sayre Syndrome. *Arch. Neurol.* **2012**, *69*, 490–499. [CrossRef]
46. Dietschy, J.M. Central nervous system: Cholesterol turnover, brain development and neurodegeneration. *Biol. Chem.* **2009**, *390*, 287–293. [CrossRef]
47. Nowaczyk, M.J.M.; Wassif, C.A. Smith-lemli-opitz syndrome. In *GeneReviews is a Registered Trademark of the University of Washington, Seattle*; Adam, M.P.; Ardinger, H.H.; Pagon, R.A., Eds.; University of Washington: Seattle, WA, USA, 1993.

48. Nóbrega, C.; Mendonça, L.; Marcelo, A.; Lamazière, A.; Tomé, S.; Despres, G.; Matos, C.A.; Mechmet, F.; Langui, D.; Dunnen, W.D.; et al. Restoring brain cholesterol turnover improves autophagy and has therapeutic potential in mouse models of spinocerebellar ataxia. *Acta Neuropathol.* **2019**, *138*, 837–858. [CrossRef]
49. Chen, C.H.; Fremont, R.; Arteaga-Bracho, E.E.; Khodakhah, K. Short latency cerebellar modulation of the basal ganglia. *Nat. Neurosci.* **2014**, *17*, 1767–1775. [CrossRef]
50. Stadelmann, C.; Timmler, S.; Barrantes-Freer, A.; Simons, M. Myelin in the Central Nervous System: Structure, Function, and Pathology. *Physiol. Rev.* **2019**, *99*, 1381–1431. [CrossRef]
51. Bourque, P.R.; Chardon, J.W.; Lelli, D.A.; Laberge, L.; Kirshen, C.; Bradshaw, S.H.; Hartley, T.; Boycott, K.M. Novel ELOVL4 mutation associated with erythrokeratodermia and spinocerebellar ataxia (SCA 34). *Neurol. Genet.* **2018**, *4*, e263. [CrossRef]
52. Deák, F.; Anderson, R.E.; Fessler, J.L.; Sherry, D.M. Novel Cellular Functions of Very Long Chain-Fatty Acids: Insight from ELOVL4 Mutations. *Front. Cell. Neurosci.* **2019**, *13*, 428. [CrossRef] [PubMed]
53. Gazulla, J.; Orduna-Hospital, E.; Benavente, I.; Rodríguez-Valle, A.; Osorio-Caicedo, P.; Andrés, S.A.-D.; García-González, E.; Fraile-Rodrigo, J.; Fernández-Tirado, F.J.; Berciano, J. Contributions to the study of spinocerebellar ataxia type 38 (SCA38). *J. Neurol.* **2020**, *267*, 2288–2295. [CrossRef] [PubMed]
54. Wanders, R.J.A.; Komen, J.; Ferdinandusse, S. Phytanic acid metabolism in health and disease. *Biochim. Biophys. Acta (BBA) Mol. Cell Biol. Lipids* **2011**, *1811*, 498–507. [CrossRef] [PubMed]
55. Heimer, G.; Kerätär, J.M.; Riley, L.G.; Balasubramaniam, S.; Eyal, E.; Pietikäinen, L.P.; Hiltunen, J.K.; Marek-Yagel, D.; Hamada, J.; Gregory, A.; et al. MECR Mutations Cause Childhood-Onset Dystonia and Optic Atrophy, a Mitochondrial Fatty Acid Synthesis Disorder. *Am. J. Hum. Genet.* **2016**, *99*, 1229–1244. [CrossRef]

Publisher's Note: MDPI stays neutral with regard to jurisdictional claims in published maps and institutional affiliations.

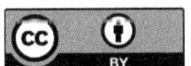

© 2020 by the authors. Licensee MDPI, Basel, Switzerland. This article is an open access article distributed under the terms and conditions of the Creative Commons Attribution (CC BY) license (http://creativecommons.org/licenses/by/4.0/).

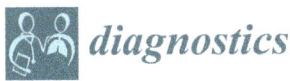 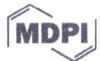

Case Report

Coexistence of Growth Hormone Deficiency and Pituitary Microadenoma in a Child with Unique Mosaic Turner Syndrome: A Case Report and Literature Review

Eu Gene Park [1], Eun-Jung Kim [2], Eun-Jee Kim [2], Hyun-Young Kim [2], Sun-Hee Kim [2] and Aram Yang [3,*]

1. Department of Pediatrics, Incheon St. Mary's Hospital, College of Medicine, The Catholic University of Korea, 56, Dongsu-ro, Bupyeong-gu, Incheon 21431, Korea; eugene.park@catholic.ac.kr
2. Samsung Medical Center, Department of Laboratory Medicine and Genetics, Sungkyunkwan University School of Medicine, 81 Irwon-ro, Gangnam-gu, Seoul 06351, Korea; ej1219.kim@samsung.com (E.-J.K.); eunjee.kim@samsung.com (E.-J.K.); hyuny.kim@samsung.com (H.-Y.K.); sunnyhk.kim@samsung.com (S.-H.K.)
3. Department of Pediatrics, Kangbuk Samsung Hospital, Sungkyunkwan University School of Medicine, 29 Saemunan-ro, Jongno-gu, Seoul 03181, Korea
* Correspondence: dkfkal0718@hanmail.net; Tel.: +82-2-2001-1980; Fax: +82-2-2001-1922

Received: 8 September 2020; Accepted: 2 October 2020; Published: 4 October 2020

Abstract: Turner syndrome (TS) is a genetic disorder with phenotypic heterogeneity caused by the monosomy or structural abnormalities of the X chromosome, and it has a prevalence of about 1/2500 females live birth. The variable clinical features of TS include short stature, gonadal failure, and skeletal dysplasia. The association with growth hormone (GH) deficiency or other hypopituitarism in TS is extremely rare, with only a few case reports published in the literature. Here, we report the first case of a patient with mosaic TS with complete GH deficiency and pituitary microadenoma, and we include the literature review. During the work-up of the patient for severe short stature, three GH provocation tests revealed peak GH levels of less than 5 ng/mL, which was compatible with complete GH deficiency. Sella magnetic resonance imaging showed an 8 mm non-enhancing pituitary adenoma with mild superior displacement of the optic chiasm. Karyotyping revealed the presence of ring chromosome X and monosomy X (46,X,r(X)/45,X/46,X,psu dic r(X;X)), which indicated a mosaic TS. It is important to consider not only chromosome analyses in females with short stature, but also the possibility of the coexistence of complete GH deficiency accompanying pituitary lesions in TS. In conclusion, the present study reports the first case of GH deficiency and pituitary adenoma in a patient with rare mosaic TS, which extends the genotype–phenotype spectrum for TS.

Keywords: Turner syndrome; mosaicism; ring chromosomes; growth hormone deficiency; pituitary microadenoma

---

1. Introduction

Turner syndrome (TS) is a genetic disorder occurring in females caused by the partial or complete absence of one of the X chromosomes. The condition affects approximately 1 in every 2500 females and requires a chromosomal analysis for definite diagnosis [1]. Short stature and hypergonadotropic hypogonadism are the principal features of TS [2,3]. Patients with TS are also susceptible to numerous other medical conditions, such as endocrine and metabolic disorders, autoimmune disease, and cardiovascular disease [4]. Multiple karyotypes including 45,X haploinsufficiency, 45,X with mosaicism, or X chromosome anomalies are associated with variable presentations along the TS phenotype spectrum; individuals with 45,X monosomy typically have the most severe phenotype [5].

Mosaic TS are subcategorized according to whether the second cell line contains a whole or part of a sex chromosome. In a study by Jacobs et al. [6], 16% of the 84 cases with TS had a standard karyotype of 45, X and a second cell line containing a ring chromosome X. The phenotypic variability of these mosaics is largely dependent on the size of the ring and the presence of a functioning *XIST*.

Patients with TS tend to have short stature and high body mass indices [7], but most often do not have growth hormone (GH) deficiency [4]. Females with TS make GH naturally in the pituitary gland, but their bodies do not use it appropriately. GH provocation tests are generally not indicated in TS unless the growth velocity is extremely low for the age and sex. Thus, the concurrent occurrence of GH deficiency and TS is a very rare condition. Moreover, the association of TS with hypopituitarism is also an uncommon finding [8].

To the best of our knowledge, there have been no previous reports of concomitant GH deficiency and structural pituitary abnormalities in TS. Here, we report the first case of the coexistence of GH deficiency and pituitary microadenoma in a TS patient.

2. Case Presentation

A female aged 13 years and 3 months visited the pediatric endocrinology clinic due to short stature. She was born at term via vaginal delivery weighing in at 2.5 kg and had no history of perinatal problems. The patient was the second child of non-consanguineous, healthy parents. Her medical history was unremarkable and did not include any head trauma, seizure, or infection of the central nervous system. No specific family history was found. The paternal and maternal heights were 169 and 163 cm, respectively, and the midparental height of 159.5 cm was within the normal range.

Ethics Statement: This study was approved by the Institutional Review Board of the Kangbuk Samsung Hospital and conducted according to the Declaration of Helsinki ethical principles (IRB 2019-11-051-001). Parental informed consent was obtained in accordance with institutional review board standards.

The patient was 133 cm (−3.4 standard deviation scores (SDS); 50th percentile in growth curves for TS (Figure S1)) in height with a growth velocity of less than 4 cm/year. She was 38.1 kg (10th percentile) in weight, and 21.6 kg/m^2 (79th percentile) in body mass index. The physical examination was unremarkable. The sexual maturity ratings of the breasts and pubic hair were Tanner stages 2 and 1, respectively. Bone age was 11 years, which was more than 2 years behind her chronological age. The skeletal survey was unremarkable except for a mild scoliosis. Biochemical tests revealed primary ovarian failure: follicle stimulating hormone (FSH) >190 mIU/mL (reference range (RR) 1.6–7); luteinizing hormone (LH) 50.3 mIU/mL (RR 1–7); estradiol <5 pg/mL (RR < 16). Other hormone levels were within normal range: insulin-like growth factor-1 (IGF-1) 325.66 ng/mL (RR 181–744); IGF-binding protein-3 (IGFBP-3) 2668.8 ng/mL (RR 1502–4427); prolactin 8.26 ng/mL (RR < 20); thyroid stimulating hormone (TSH) 7.7 µIU/mL (RR 0.5–4.5); free T4 1.65 ng/dL (RR 0.7–2.0) (Table S1). The results were normal for serum electrolyte, glucose, blood gases, hepatic and renal function, and routine urinalysis. Considering her severely short stature and growth deceleration, we performed a GH provocation test. The sampling for GH levels was carried out every 30 min for 120 min. The peak GH levels were 2.96 ng/mL, 3.63 ng/mL, and 3.06 ng/mL after the administration of arginine, L-dopa, and insulin, respectively. These results are indicative of complete GH deficiency.

Sella magnetic resonance imaging (MRI) analysis revealed a non-enhancing pituitary adenoma measuring 8 mm in diameter with a mild superior displacement of the optic chiasm (Figure 1).

A conventional chromosome study using peripheral blood showed the 98/177 (55.4%) cells with ring chromosome X, 75 (42.4%) cells with monosomy X, and 4 (2.2%) cells with pseudodicentric ring chromosome X: mos 46,X,r(X)(p22.2q23)(98)/45,X(75)/46,X,psu dic r(X;X)(p22.2q27;q25p11.2) [4] (Figure 2A,B), which indicated a mosaic TS. The subsequent fluorescence in situ hybridization (FISH) using an LSI KAL/CEP X probe (Vysis, Abbott Molecular Inc.) and a TelVysion Xq/Yq probe (Vysis) showed that r(X) lacked the *KAL* (*ANOS1*) gene on Xp22.3 and the Xq telomere (Figure 2C–E).

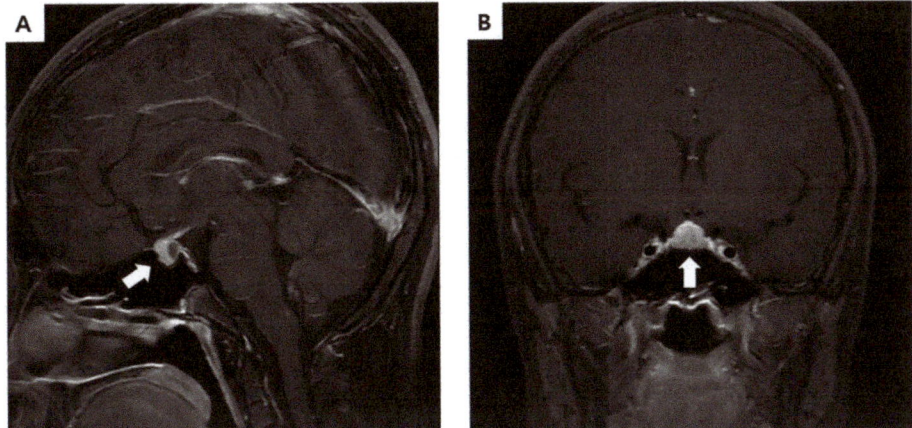

Figure 1. Sella magnetic resonance imaging (MRI) of the patient. T1 sagittal (**A**) and coronal (**B**) MRI showed a non-enhancing lesion in the posterior portion of pituitary gland measuring 8 mm in diameter with mild superior displacement of the optic chiasm (white arrow).

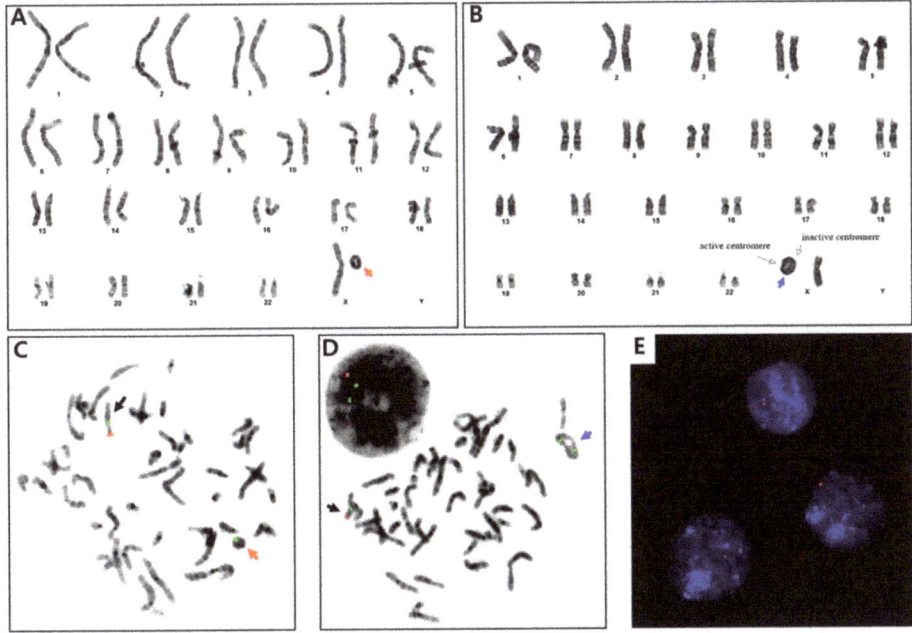

Figure 2. Chromosome study showed (**A**) a ring chromosome X (red arrow) in which breakage and reunion points are Xp22.2 and Xq23, and (**B**) a pseudodicentric ring chromosome X (blue arrow) with break and reunion at Xp22.2q27 and Xq25p11.2. Active centromere (Left white arrow) was on Xp22.2q27. (**C**,**D**) Metaphase fluorescent in situ hybridization (FISH) using an LSI KAL (on Xp22.3)/CEP X (on Xp11.1-q11.1) probe (Vysis, Dual Color Probe) showed a normal X chromosome (black arrow; one green and one red signal), a ring chromosome X with loss of the *KAL* gene (one green signal), and a pseudodicentric ring chromosome X with loss of *KAL* (two green signals). (**E**) Interphase FISH study using a TelVysion Xq/Yq probe (Vysis, Single Color probe) showed a single Xq telomere signal (red), indicating Xq telomere loss in each cell. Magnification, ×400.

The results of the renal ultrasonography and echocardiography were normal. To evaluate the possibility of other pituitary hormone deficiencies, a combined pituitary stimulation test (i.e., the cocktail test) was performed; decreased cortisol (peak cortisol 12.2 µg/dL; RR > 22 µg/dL) secretion was observed following insulin-induced hypoglycemia, which indicates adrenocorticotropic hormone (ACTH) deficiency (secondary adrenal insufficiency). The patient was administered maintenance physiologic doses of hydrocortisone, and recombinant human GH therapy was also initiated. The initiation of estrogen replacement therapy will be determined by the patient's growth velocity and emergence of secondary sexual characteristics.

3. Discussion

TS is associated with a constellation of potential abnormalities involving numerous organ systems, making it a challenging disorder for health care providers and families. Short stature, one of the common presentations that pediatricians encounter in clinical practice, is a clinical hallmark of TS. Nearly 5% of children referred for an evaluation of short stature have an identifiable pathologic cause, such as GH deficiency, chronic disease, or a genetic condition (e.g., TS) [9,10].

TS and GH deficiency are important differential diagnoses in females with short stature and are the two most frequently approved conditions for GH treatment [11]. TS can be differentiated from GH deficiency by delayed bone age, hypogonadism, characteristic phenotypic features, and peak GH levels after GH provocation tests [12]. Approximately 60% of TS may not have marked stigmata of the syndrome, such as webbed neck, wide-based nipples, and wide carrying angle to the arms, especially in girls with Turner mosaicism [13]. Short stature and delayed puberty may be the only symptoms of TS. However, other physical abnormalities may also be variably expressed. Our case showed delayed bone age and breast development, which are not common symptoms of TS. This emphasizes the importance of chromosomal analysis to rule out TS in girls with short stature [9]. Furthermore, it is important to check for GH deficiency by provocation tests in TS patients with retarded growth rates by a height of less than the 3rd percentile for their age and sex.

The coexistence of GH deficiency and TS is a very rare condition. To our knowledge, there are only a few reported cases of TS associated with GH deficiency (Table 1) [12,14–17]. Pituitary adenomas have also rarely been identified in TS patients. Review of the literature demonstrated nine case reports of women with TS who presented with pituitary adenomas during late adolescence or adulthood; six were diagnosed with functioning pituitary adenoma and three with non-functioning pituitary adenoma as in our case [8,18–25] (Table 2). Non-functioning pituitary adenomas in children and adolescents are rare; they comprise only 4 to 6% of pediatric patients, while they account for approximately 33 to 50% of adult patients with pituitary lesions [26–28]. This case presented with non-functioning pituitary adenoma associated with GH and ACTH deficiency, which is in accordance with a previous study demonstrating that non-functioning pituitary adenomas may present with GH deficiency (up to 75%), LH/FSH deficiency (~40%), or ACTH and TSH deficiency (~25%) [29].

Table 1. Comparison of clinical and laboratory features between this case and previously reported cases of TS associated with GH deficiency.

	Case in This Study	Yu et al. [12]	Yu et al. [12]	Efstathiadou et al. [14]	Gallicchino et al. [15]	Jin et al. [16]
Age at diagnosis (y) Turner syndrome	12.3	8.9	12.3	30	11	11
Age at diagnosis (y) GH deficiency	12.3	7.5	12.3	17	12	11
Height (SDS) at diagnosis Turner syndrome	−3.4	−1.89	−1.72 †	−2.35	−4.2	−3.69
Height (SDS) at diagnosis GH deficiency	−3.4	−2.30	−1.72 †	−6.0	−4.9	−3.69
Karyotype	46,X,r(X)/45,X/46,X,psu dic r(X;X)	45,X/45,X+mar	45,X/46,XX	45,X	45,X/46,XX	45,X
Peak GH on GH provocation test (ng/mL)	3.63	6.17	7.38	4.65	0.14	<5
Other pituitary hormone deficiencies	ACTH	None	None	TSH, gonadotropin	TSH, gonadotropin	None
Associated conditions	Subclinical hypothyroidism, pituitary microadenoma	Partial empty sella, horseshoe kidney	None	None	Empty sella	Chronic lymphocytic thyroiditis

GH: growth hormone, SDS: standard deviation scores, TSH: thyroid stimulating hormone, NA: not available. † Height after 2 years of growth hormone therapy.

Table 2. Comparison of clinical and laboratory features between this case and previously reported cases of TS associated with pituitary adenomas.

	Case in This Study	Yeh et al. [8]	Bolanowski et al. [18]	Gaspar et al. [19]	Mermilliod et al. [20]	Weibel et al. [21]	Dotsch et al. [22]	Willemse et al. [23]	Yamazaki et al. [24]	Gelfand et al. [25]
Age at TS diagnosis (yr)	13	16	10	16	16	43	12	19	33	26
Age at pituitary disease diagnosis (yr)	13	16	33	25	18	43	19	26	33	29
Karyotype	46,X,r(X)/45,X/46,X,psu dic r(X;X)	45,X	45,X/46,X,i(X)(q10)	45,X/46,XX	45,X	45,X/46,XX/47,XXX	45,X/46,XX	45,X	47,XXX/45,X/46,XX	45,X/47,XXX
Symptoms or labs related to pituitary disease	Short stature	Headache, vomiting, cranial nerve IV palsy	Facial changes, increased hand/foot size	Secondary amenorrhea, galactorrhea	Hypogonadotropic hypogonadism	Unexpected normalization of FSH level	Secondary amenorrhea, hyperprolactinemia	Change in appearance, enlarged feet	Dysphagia due to soft palate edema, enlarged hands/feet	Weight gain, ankle edema, acne, hirsutism
Pituitary hormone abnormalities	Deficiency in GH, ACTH	Deficiency in GnRH	GH excess	Prolactin excess	Deficiency in GnRH	Deficiency in GnRH	Prolactin excess	GH excess	GH excess	Cortisol excess

The incidental pituitary adenoma with the co-occurrence of GH deficiency and TS is very rare, and there have been no other reported cases of the co-occurrence of pituitary microadenoma, GH deficiency, and TS; the causal relationship is difficult to explain. This case demonstrates that investigating the underlying causes of short stature should be primarily based on clinical presentations and physical examination, while an accurate diagnosis is made through a combination of clinical, biochemical, and radiological evaluations.

This case was cytogenetically characterized with a unique mosaicism for three types of cells with r(X), monosomy X, and psu dic r(X), which may have occurred as a process of dynamic mosaicism. The amount of Xq deletion and r(X) has been known to associated with phenotypic severity [30]. In particular, the presence of the *XIST* gene on Xq13.2 is important. *XIST* located in the X-inactivation center is essential for the initiation and spread of X chromosome inactivation. As a general rule, when one X chromosome is structurally abnormal without involving an autosome, it is typically inactivated in a majority of cells [31,32]. However, an abnormal X chromosome that lack *XIST* fails to become inactivated, which may be associated with a more severe phenotype, including mental retardation. Fortunately, r(X) observed in our patient had intact Xq13 including *XIST*, therefore, it was expected to be inactivated. This case had a mild Turner variant phenotype, without any cardiac defect, renal malformation, and low intelligence. However, the biochemical findings revealed elevated LH and FSH levels, suggesting primary ovarian failure [33]. The patient also revealed multiple pituitary hormone deficiencies with pituitary adenoma. Given such complex phenotypes of this patient and that mosaic levels decrease with age due to the vulnerable character of r(X) [34], it is challenging to identify the effect of mosaicism on clinical phenotypes.

Recombinant human GH is a standard treatment for TS patients, although physiologically significant alterations in GH secretion have not been identified [1]. Short stature in TS is not due to hormonal deficiencies but is a consequence of haploinsufficiency of the short stature homeobox gene located on the short arm of the X chromosome (*SHOX*), a transcriptional activator in the osteogenic cell line [35]. The *SHOX* gene is located in the critical region on the X chromosome that escapes X-inactivation, and mutations or deletions are likely to exert a dosage effect [36]. When *SHOX* haploinsufficiency occurs, there is decreased chondrocyte proliferation and differentiation at the growth plate, leading not only to short stature, but also skeletal abnormalities [37]. GH stimulates linear bone growth and acts at the epiphysis to promote prechondrocyte differentiation and osteoblast expansion [1]. Promptly initiating treatment would enable the affected patients to reach an adult height within the normal population range [38,39].

In conclusion, this paper reports the first case of a unique mosaic TS patient with GH deficiency and pituitary adenoma. This case broadens and further delineates the complex genotype–phenotype of TS, and highlights the importance of performing a thorough, multidisciplinary assessment that considers numerous potential diseases and concomitant conditions when evaluating patients with short stature.

Supplementary Materials: Supplementary materials can be found at http://www.mdpi.com/2075-4418/10/10/783/s1.

Author Contributions: Conceptualization: A.Y.; data curation: A.Y.; formal analysis: E.-J.K. (Eun-Jung Kim), E.-J.K. (Eun-Jee Kim), H.-Y.K., S.-H.K.; writing—original draft: E.G.P.; writing—review and editing: A.Y. All authors have read and agreed to the published version of the manuscript.

Funding: This research received no external funding.

Acknowledgments: We sincerely appreciate our patient and her family for their participation in this study.

Conflicts of Interest: The authors declare no conflict of interest.

References

1. Sybert, V.P.; McCauley, E. Turner's syndrome. *N. Engl. J. Med.* **2004**, *351*, 1227–1238. [CrossRef] [PubMed]
2. Gravholt, C.H. Epidemiological, endocrine and metabolic features in Turner syndrome. *Eur. J. Endocrinol.* **2004**, *151*, 657–687. [CrossRef] [PubMed]

3. Bondy, C.A.; Turner Syndrome Study Group. Care of girls and women with Turner syndrome: A guideline of the Turner Syndrome Study Group. *J. Clin. Endocrinol. Metab.* **2007**, *92*, 10–25. [CrossRef] [PubMed]
4. Gravholt, C.H.; Andersen, N.H.; Conway, G.S.; Dekkers, O.M.; Geffner, M.E.; Klein, K.O.; Lin, A.E.; Mauras, N.; Quigley, C.A.; Rubin, K.; et al. Clinical practice guidelines for the care of girls and women with Turner syndrome: Proceedings from the 2016 Cincinnati International Turner Syndrome Meeting. *Eur. J. Endocrinol.* **2017**, *177*, G1–G70. [CrossRef]
5. Milbrandt, T.; Thomas, E. Turner syndrome. *Pediatr. Rev.* **2013**, *34*, 420–421. [CrossRef]
6. Jacobs, P.; Dalton, P.; James, R.; Mosse, K.; Power, M.; Robinson, D.; Skuse, D. Turner syndrome: A cytogenetic and molecular study. *Ann. Hum. Genet.* **1997**, *61*, 471–483. [CrossRef]
7. De Groote, K.; Demulier, L.; De Backer, J.; De Wolf, D.; De Schepper, J.; T'Sjoen, G.; De Backer, T. Arterial hypertension in Turner syndrome: A review of the literature and a practical approach for diagnosis and treatment. *J. Hypertens.* **2015**, *33*, 1342–1351. [CrossRef]
8. Yeh, T.; Soto, A.G.; Quintos, J.B.; Topor, L.S. Turner syndrome and pituitary adenomas: A case report and review of literature. *J. Pediatr. Endocrinol. Metab.* **2017**, *30*, 231–235. [CrossRef]
9. Barstow, C.; Rerucha, C. Evaluation of Short and Tall Stature in Children. *Am. Fam. Physician.* **2015**, *92*, 43–50.
10. Lindsay, R.; Feldkamp, M.; Harris, D.; Robertson, J.; Rallison, M. Utah Growth Study: Growth standards and the prevalence of growth hormone deficiency. *J. Pediatr.* **1994**, *125*, 29–35. [CrossRef]
11. Yavas Abali, Z.; Darendeliler, F.; Neyzi, O. A Critical Appraisal of Growth Hormone Therapy in Growth Hormone Deficiency and Turner Syndrome Patients in Turkey. *J. Clin. Res. Pediatr. Endocrinol.* **2016**, *8*, 490–495. [CrossRef]
12. Yu, J.; Shin, H.Y.; Lee, C.G.; Kim, J.H. Concomitant occurrence of Turner syndrome and growth hormone deficiency. *Korean. J. Pediatr.* **2016**, *59*, S121–S124. [CrossRef]
13. Paul Wadwa, R.; Kappy, M.S. Short stature. In *Berman's Pediatric Decision Making*, 5th ed.; Bajaj, L., Hambridge, S., Kerby, G., Nyquist, A.C., Eds.; Elsevier: Philadelphia, PA, USA, 2011.
14. Brook, C.G. Growth hormone deficiency in Turner's syndrome. *N. Engl. J. Med.* **1978**, *298*, 1203–1204. [PubMed]
15. Efstathiadou, Z.; Tsatsoulis, A. Turner's syndrome with concomitant hypopituitarism: Case report. *Hum. Reprod.* **2000**, *15*, 2388–2389. [CrossRef] [PubMed]
16. Gallicchio, C.T.; Alves, S.T.; Ramos, H.I.; Llerena, J.C.; Guimaraes, M.M. Association of Turner's syndrome and hypopituitarism: A patient report. *J. Pediatr. Endocrinol. Metab.* **2003**, *16*, 901–905. [CrossRef] [PubMed]
17. Jin, W.; Cheng, F.X.; Xiao, M.S.; Fan, Y.; Dong, W. Concurrent occurrence of chronic lymphocytic thyroiditis with hypothyroidism and growth hormone deficiency in a Turner's syndrome patient. *J. Pediatr. Endocrinol. Metab.* **2011**, *24*, 237–239. [CrossRef] [PubMed]
18. Bolanowski, M.; Lomna-Bogdanov, E.; Kosmala, W.; Malczewska, J.; Slezak, R.; Zadrozna, B.; Podgorski, J.K. Turner's syndrome followed by acromegaly in the third decade of life: An unusual coincidence of two rare conditions. *Gynecol. Endocrinol.* **2002**, *16*, 331–334. [CrossRef] [PubMed]
19. Gaspar, L.; Julesz, J.; Kocsis, J.; Pasztor, E.; Laszlo, F. Mosaic Turner's syndrome and pituitary microadenoma. *Exp. Clin. Endocrinol.* **1985**, *86*, 87–92. [CrossRef] [PubMed]
20. Mermilliod, J.A.; Gatchair-Rose, A.; Svec, F. Pituitary tumor and low gonadotropins in a patient with Turner's syndrome. *J. Louisiana. St. Med. Soc.* **1995**, *147*, 540–543. [PubMed]
21. Weibel, H.S.; Dahan, M.H. Pituitary mass and subsequent involution causing fluctuations of serum follicle-stimulating hormone levels in a Turner syndrome patient with premature ovarian failure: A case report. *J. Reprod. Med.* **2014**, *59*, 504–508. [PubMed]
22. Dotsch, J.; Schoof, E.; Hensen, J.; Dorr, H.G. Prolactinoma causing secondary amenorrhea in a woman with Ullrich-Turner syndrome. *Horm. Res.* **1999**, *51*, 256–257. [CrossRef] [PubMed]
23. Willemse, C.H. A patient suffering from Turner's syndrome and acromegaly. *Acta. Endocrinol.* **1962**, *39*, 204–212. [CrossRef] [PubMed]
24. Yamazaki, M.; Sato, A.; Nishio, S.; Takeda, T.; Miyamoto, T.; Katai, M.; Hashizume, K. Acromegaly accompanied by Turner syndrome with 47,XXX/45,X/46,XX mosaicism. *Intern. Med.* **2009**, *48*, 447–453. [CrossRef] [PubMed]
25. Gelfand, R.A. Cushing's disease associated with ovarian dysgenesis. *Am. J. Med.* **1984**, *77*, 1108–1110. [CrossRef]

26. Artese, R.; D'Osvaldo, D.H.; Molocznik, I.; Benencia, H.; Oviedo, J.; Burdman, J.A.; Basso, A. Pituitary tumors in adolescent patients. *Neurol. Res.* **1998**, *20*, 415–417. [CrossRef] [PubMed]
27. Pack, S.D.; Qin, L.; Pak, E.; Wang, Y.; Ault, D.O.; Mannan, P.; Jaikumar, S.; Stratakis, C.A.; Oldfield, E.H.; Zhuang, Z.; et al. Common genetic changes in hereditary and sporadic pituitary adenomas detected by comparative genomic hybridization. *Genes. Chromosomes. Cancer.* **2005**, *43*, 72–82. [CrossRef] [PubMed]
28. Boikos, S.A.; Stratakis, C.A. Carney complex: The first 20 years. *Curr. Opin. Oncol.* **2007**, *19*, 24–29. [CrossRef]
29. Thapar, K.; Kovacs, K.; Laws, E.R. The classification and molecular biology of pituitary adenomas. *Adv. Tech. Stand. Neurosurg.* **1995**, *22*, 3–53. [CrossRef]
30. Chauhan, P.; Jaiswal, S.K.; Lakhotia, A.R.; Rai, A.K. Molecular cytogenetic characterization of two Turner syndrome patients with mosaic ring X chromosome. *J. Assist. Reprod. Genet.* **2016**, *33*, 1161–1168. [CrossRef]
31. Leppig, K.A.; Disteche, C.M. Ring X and other structural X chromosome abnormalities: X inactivation and phenotype. *Semin. Reprod. Med.* **2001**, *19*, 147–157. [CrossRef]
32. Mazzaschi, R.L.; Taylor, J.; Robertson, S.P.; Love, D.R.; George, A.M. A turner syndrome patient carrying a mosaic distal x chromosome marker. *Case Rep. Genet.* **2014**, *2014*, 597314. [CrossRef]
33. De Moraes-Ruehsen, M.; Jones, G.S. Premature ovarian failure. *Fertil. Steril.* **1967**, *18*, 440–461. [CrossRef]
34. Atkins, L.; Sceery, R.T.; Keenan, M.E. An unstable ring chromosome in a female infant with hypotonia, seizures, and retarded development. *J. Med. Genet.* **1966**, *3*, 134–138. [CrossRef] [PubMed]
35. Rao, E.; Weiss, B.; Fukami, M.; Rump, A.; Niesler, B.; Mertz, A.; Muroya, K.; Binder, G.; Kirsch, S.; Winkelmann, M.; et al. Pseudoautosomal deletions encompassing a novel homeobox gene cause growth failure in idiopathic short stature and Turner syndrome. *Nat. Genet.* **1997**, *16*, 54–63. [CrossRef] [PubMed]
36. Ogata, T. SHOX: Pseudoautosomal homeobox containing gene for short stature and dyschondrosteosis. *Growth. Horm. IGF. Res.* **1999**, *9*, 53–57. [CrossRef]
37. Clement-Jones, M.; Schiller, S.; Rao, E.; Blaschke, R.J.; Zuniga, A.; Zeller, R.; Robson, S.C.; Binder, G.; Glass, I.; Strachan, T.; et al. The short stature homeobox gene SHOX is involved in skeletal abnormalities in Turner syndrome. *Hum. Mol. Genet.* **2000**, *9*, 695–702. [CrossRef] [PubMed]
38. Rogol, A.D.; Hayden, G.F. Etiologies and early diagnosis of short stature and growth failure in children and adolescents. *J. Pediatr.* **2014**, *164*, S1–S14.e16. [CrossRef]
39. Haymond, M.; Kappelgaard, A.M.; Czernichow, P.; Biller, B.M.; Takano, K.; Kiess, W.; The Participants in the Global Advisory Panel Meeting on the Effects of Growth Hormone. Early recognition of growth abnormalities permitting early intervention. *Acta. Paediatr.* **2013**, *102*, 787–796. [CrossRef]

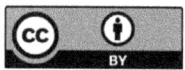

© 2020 by the authors. Licensee MDPI, Basel, Switzerland. This article is an open access article distributed under the terms and conditions of the Creative Commons Attribution (CC BY) license (http://creativecommons.org/licenses/by/4.0/).

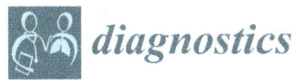

Review

Syndromic Inherited Retinal Diseases: Genetic, Clinical and Diagnostic Aspects

Yasmin Tatour and Tamar Ben-Yosef *

Ruth & Bruce Rappaport Faculty of Medicine, Technion-Israel Institute of Technology, Haifa 31096, Israel; yasmin.t.90@gmail.com
* Correspondence: benyosef@technion.ac.il; Tel.: +972-4-829-5228

Received: 9 September 2020; Accepted: 1 October 2020; Published: 2 October 2020

Abstract: Inherited retinal diseases (IRDs), which are among the most common genetic diseases in humans, define a clinically and genetically heterogeneous group of disorders. Over 80 forms of syndromic IRDs have been described. Approximately 200 genes are associated with these syndromes. The majority of syndromic IRDs are recessively inherited and rare. Many, although not all, syndromic IRDs can be classified into one of two major disease groups: inborn errors of metabolism and ciliopathies. Besides the retina, the systems and organs most commonly involved in syndromic IRDs are the central nervous system, ophthalmic extra-retinal tissues, ear, skeleton, kidney and the cardiovascular system. Due to the high degree of phenotypic variability and phenotypic overlap found in syndromic IRDs, correct diagnosis based on phenotypic features alone may be challenging and sometimes misleading. Therefore, genetic testing has become the benchmark for the diagnosis and management of patients with these conditions, as it complements the clinical findings and facilitates an accurate clinical diagnosis and treatment.

Keywords: retina; inherited retinal diseases; syndrome

1. Introduction

The retina is a multi-layered sensory tissue that lines the back of the eye. Its main function is the transduction of light energy into an electrical potential change, via a process known as phototransduction. The light-sensitive elements of the retina are the photoreceptor cells. The retina contains two types of photoreceptors, rods and cones. Rods (approximately 120 million in the human eye) are in charge of night vision, while cones (6 to 7 million in the human eye) are in charge of visual acuity and color vision. The highest cone concentration is found in the central region of the retina, known as the macula. Photoreceptors are highly compartmentalized cells, with the nucleus and other cellular organs located in the inner segment (IS), while the entire phototransduction machinery is included in the outer segment (OS).

Inherited retinal diseases (IRDs), which are among the most common genetic diseases in humans, define a clinically heterogeneous group of disorders, which cause visual loss due to improper development, dysfunction or premature death of the retinal photoreceptors [1]. IRDs are distinguished by several factors, including the type and location of affected cells and the timing of disease onset. The most common form of IRD is retinitis pigmentosa (RP) (also known as rod–cone dystrophy) [2]. Other IRD forms include cone/cone–rod dystrophy (CD/CRD) [3]; Leber congenital amaurosis (LCA) [4]; macular dystrophy (MD); and achromatopsia (rod monochromatism) [5], among others.

IRD is also one of the most genetically heterogeneous groups of disorders in humans, with over 260 genes identified to date (RetNet at https://sph.uth.edu/retnet/). It can be inherited as autosomal recessive (AR), autosomal dominant (AD) or X-linked (XL). Mitochondrial and digenic modes of inheritance have also been described. While in most cases of IRD the disease is limited to the eye (non-syndromic), over 80 forms of syndromic IRD have been described. Approximately 200 genes are associated with these syndromes (Table 1). In some cases of syndromic IRD, the retinal disease may be the presenting symptom and other systemic findings evolve during childhood, puberty or later on in life. In other cases, the first identifiable symptom of the syndrome is non-ocular and the retinal phenotype is revealed only later in life.

The topic of systemic diseases associated with IRDs has been reviewed before, including the description of some of these syndromes [6]. In the current review, we provide a comprehensive summary of the vast majority of syndromic IRD forms reported to date, for which the underlying gene/s have been identified (as listed in OMIM-Online Mendelian Inheritance in Man, https://www.ncbi.nlm.nih.gov/omim, and reported in the literature). We discuss different aspects, including the marked genetic heterogeneity of some of these syndromes, phenotypic overlap and diagnostic approaches.

Table 1. Syndromic inherited retinal diseases (IRDs).

Syndrome (MIM/Reference)	Gene	Inheritance *	Main Ocular Phenotypes #	Main Extra-Ocular Phenotypes ¶
Abetalipoproteinemia; ABL (#200100)	MTTP	AR	RP	Fat malabsorption, neurodegeneration, acanthocytosis
Aicardi Syndrome; AIC (#304050)	Xp22 abnormalities	XLD	Chorioretinopathy, OA, microphthalmia, optic nerve coloboma, cataract	Callosal agenesis, PGR, microcephaly, ID, skeletal anomalies, neoplasia
Alagille Syndrome 1; ALGS1 (#118450)	JAG1	AD	Iris stromal hypoplasia, posterior embryotoxon, microcornea, anomalous optic disc, peripapillary retinal depigmentation, chorioretinopathy	Liver disease, skeletal and renal involvement, characteristic facial features, ID, FTT
Alport Syndrome 1; ATS1 (#3010150)	COL4A5	XLD	Fleck retinopathy, cataract, myopia, corneal abnormalities	HL, renal disease
Alstrom Syndrome; ALMS (#203800)	ALMS1	AR	CRD, MD, cataract	DD, SS, obesity, HL, cardiac, skeletal, hepatic, renal and endocrine involvement
Alpha-Methylacyl-CoA Racemase Deficiency; AMACRD (#614307)	AMACR	AR	RP	Neurodegeneration
Autoimmune Polyendocrine Syndrome, Type I, with or without Reversible Metaphyseal Dysplasia; APS1 (#240300)	AIRE	AD, AR	RP, keratopathy, keratoconjunctivitis	Multiple autoantibodies, anemia, hepatic, gastrointestinal, dental, skin, hair and endocrine involvement, hypogonadism
Bardet–Biedl Syndrome; BBS (#209900, #615981, #600151, #615982, #615983, #605231, #615984, #615985, #615986, #615987, #615988, #615989, #615990, #615991, 615992, #615993, #615994, #615995, #615996, #617119, #617406) [7]	BBS1, BBS2, ARL6, BBS4, BBS5, MKKS, BBS7, TTC8, PTHB1, BBS10, TRIM32, BBS12, MKS1, CEP290, WDPCP, SDCCAG8, LZTFL1, BBIP1, IFT27, IFT74, C8ORF37, CEP164	AR	RP, strabismus, cataract	ID, SS, obesity, hypogonadism, renal disease, polydactyly
Cerebellar Atrophy with Pigmentary Retinopathy [8]	MSTO1	AR	RD	Cerebellar atrophy, ID, PGR
Congenital Disorder of Glycosylation; CDG (#212065, #617082, #613861, #608799, #300896)	PMM2, NUS1, DHDDS, DPM1, SLC35A2	AR	RP	FTT, microcephaly, ID, neurodegeneration, cardiac, hepatic, gastrointestinal, renal and hematological involvement

Table 1. Cont.

Syndrome (MIM/Reference)	Gene	Inheritance *	Main Ocular Phenotypes #	Main Extra-Ocular Phenotypes ¶
Congenital Disorder of Glycosylation with Defective Fucosylation 2; CDGF2 (#618324)	FCSK	AR	MD, OA, strabismus	FTT, ID, hypotonia, neurodegeneration, gastrointestinal anomalies
Cranioectodermal Dysplasia 4; CED4 (#614378)	WDR19	AR	RP	Skeletal anomalies, SS, respiratory, hepatic and renal involvement
Ceroid Lipofuscinosis, Neuronal; CLN (#256730, #204500, #204200, #256731, #601780, #610951, #600143, #610127, #614706)	PPT1, TPP1, CLN3, CLN5, CLN6, MFSD8, CLN8, CTSD, GRN	AR	RP, CRD, OA	Microcephaly, ID, neurodegeneration
Cohen Syndrome; COH1 (#216550)	VPS13B	AR	RD, OA, strabismus, high myopia	ID, DD, microcephaly, SS, obesity, skeletal, cardiac, hematological and endocrine involvement
Coenzyme Q10 Deficiency, Primary, 1; COQ10D1 (#607426)	COQ2	AR	RP	ID, cerebellar atrophy, HL, cardiac, hepatic, renal and muscular involvement
Combined Oxidative Phosphorylation Deficiency 29; COXPD29 (#616811)	TXN2	AR	RD, OA	Microcephaly, hypotonia, DD, ID, neurodegeneration
Charcot–Marie–Tooth Disease, X-linked recessive, 5; CMTX5 (#311070)	PRPS1	XLR	RP, OA	Peripheral neuropathy, HL
Cone–Rod Dystrophy and Hearing Loss 1; CRDHL1 (#617236)	CEP78	AR	CRD	HL
Cockayne Syndrome; CS (#216400, #133540)	ERCC8, ERCC6	AR	RD, OA, cataract, strabismus	IUGR, PGR, microcephaly, ID, neurodegeneration, HL, renal, skeletal and skin involvement
Cystinosis, Nephropathic; CTNS (#219800, #219900)	CTNS	AR	RD, corneal crystals	Renal disease, neurodegeneration, skeletal and endocrine anomalies
Danon Disease (#300257)	LAMP2	XLD	RD	Cardiac disease, myopathy, ID
Diabetes and Deafness, Maternally Inherited; MIDD (#520000)	MTTL1, MTTE, MTTK, mitochondrial DNA rearrangements	Mi	RD, MD, ophthalmoplegia	HL, cardiac and neurological anomalies, diabetes mellitus
Dyskeratosis Congenita, Autosomal Dominant 3; DKCA3 (#613990)	TINF2	AD	RD, blockage of lacrimal ducts	IUGR, SS, microcephaly, ID, HL, respiratory, skin, skeletal and hematological involvement, neoplasia
Hypobetalipoproteinemia, Familial, 1; FHBL1 (#615558)	APOB	AR	RP	Fat malabsorption, neurodegeneration, acanthocytosis
Hypobetalipoproteinemia, Acanthocytosis, Retinitis Pigmentosa and Pallidal Degeneration; HARP (#607236)	PANK2	AR	RP	Fat malabsorption, neurodegeneration, acanthocytosis
Hypotrichosis, Congenital, with Juvenile Macular Dystrophy; HJMD (#601553)	CDH3	AR	MD	Hypotrichosis
Hermansky–Pudlak Syndrome; HPS (#614072, #614073, #614077)	HPS3, HPS4, BLOC1S3	AR	Hypopigmentation of retina and choroid, foveal hypoplasia, nystagmus, iris transillumination	Skin and hair hypopigmentation, bleeding diathesis

Table 1. Cont.

Syndrome (MIM/Reference)	Gene	Inheritance *	Main Ocular Phenotypes #	Main Extra-Ocular Phenotypes ¶
Hyper-IgD Syndrome; HIDS (#260920)	MVK	AR	RP	Hematological anomalies, gastrointestinal and skeletal involvement, periodic fever
Hyperoxaluria, Primary, Type I; HP1 (#259900)	AGXT	AR	RD, OA	Renal disease, dental, cardiovascular and skin involvement, peripheral neuropathy
Intellectual Developmental Disorder and Retinitis Pigmentosa; IDDRP (#618195)	SCAPER	AR	RP, MD, cataract	ID, skeletal abnormalities, male sterility
Jalili Syndrome (#217080)	CNNM4	AR	CRD	Amelogenesis imperfecta
Joubert Syndrome; JBTS (#213300, #608091, #608629, #610188, #610688, #611560, #612291, #612285, #614464, #614465, #614844, #614970, #615636, #615665, #616781, #617121, #617562, #617622, #618161, #300804)	INPP5E, TMEM216, AHI1, CEP290, TMEM67, RPGRIP1L, ARL13B, CC2D2A, CEP41, TMEM138, ZNF423, TMEM231, CSPP1, PDE6D, CEP104, MKS1, TMEM107, ARMC9, ARL3	AR	RD, chorioretinal coloboma, optic nerve coloboma, microphthalmia, oculomotor apraxia, esotropia, ptosis	Brain structural anomalies, FTT, macrocephaly, ID, neurodegeneration, genitourinary, hepatic, respiratory and skeletal involvement
	OFD1	XLR		
Kearns–Sayre Syndrome; KSS (#530000)	Mitochondrial DNA deletions	Mi	RD, ophthalmoplegia	SS, microcephaly, neurodegeneration, cardiac, renal and endocrine involvement
Laurence–Moon Syndrome; LNMS (#245800)	PNPLA6	AR	Chorioretinal degeneration	ID, neurodegeneration, genitourinary abnormalities
Leber Congenital Amaurosis with Early-Onset Deafness; LCAEOD (#617879)	TUBB4B	AD	LCA	HL
Lipodystrophy, familial partial, type7; FPLD7 (#606721)	CAV1	AD	RD, cataract	Lack of facial fat, orthostatic hypotension, neurological and skin involvement
Methylmalonic Aciduria and Homocystinuria, cblC type; MAHCC (#277400)	MMACHC	AR	RP, CRD	FTT, microcephaly, ID, neurodegeneration, renal and hematological involvement
Mevalonic Aciduria; MEVA (#610377)	MVK	AR	RP, OA, cataract	FTT, DD, neurodegeneration, spleen, hepatic, skeletal, skin and hematological involvement
Microcephaly and Chorioretinopathy, autosomal recessive; MCCRP (#251270, #616171, #616335)	TUBGCP6, PLK4, TUBGCP4	AR	Chorioretinopathy, OA, microphthalmia, microcornea, cataract	IUGR, microcephaly, brain structural anomalies, DD, ID, neurodegeneration, SS
Microcephaly with or without Chorioretinopathy, Lymphedema or Mental Retardation; MCLMR (#152950)	KIF11	AD	Chorioretinopathy, myopia, hypermetropia, corneal opacity, microcornea, microphthalmia, cataract	Microcephaly, ID, neurodegeneration, lymphedema
Microphthalmia, Syndromic 5; MCOPS5 (#610125)	OTX2	AD	RD, microphthalmia, anophthalmia, optic nerve hypoplasia or agenesis, microcornea, cataract	Brain structural anomalies, hypotonia, pituitary dysfunction, DD, SS, cleft palate, abnormal genitalia, joint laxity

Table 1. Cont.

Syndrome (MIM/Reference)	Gene	Inheritance *	Main Ocular Phenotypes #	Main Extra-Ocular Phenotypes ¶
Mitochondrial Complex II Deficiency (#252011)	SDHA, SDHD, SDHAF1	AR	RD, OA, ptosis, ophthalmoplegia	SS, cardiac, skeletal, muscular and neurological involvement
Mitochondrial Complex IV Deficiency (#220110)	APOPT1, COA3, COX6A2, COX6B1, COX8A, COX10, COX14, COX20, PET100, TACO1	AR	RD, OA, ptosis	FTT, brain structural anomalies, ID, HL, cardiac, respiratory, hepatic, renal and muscular involvement
Mucolipidosis III alpha/beta; MLIII A/B (#252600)	GNPTAB	AR	RD, corneal clouding	Neurodegeneration, ID, SS, coarse facies, skeletal, cardiac and skin involvement
Mucolipidosis IV; ML4 (#252650)	MCOLN1	AR	RD, OA, corneal disease, strabismus	Microcephaly, ID, neurodegeneration
Mucopolysaccharidosis; MPS (#309900, #252930, #607014, #253000, #253010)	IDS	XLR	RP, ptosis, corneal clouding	Neurodegeneration, ID, SS, coarse facies, HL, skeletal, cardiac, respiratory, hepatic, gastrointestinal and skin involvement
	HGSNAT, IDUA, GALN5, GLB1	AR		
Nephronophthisis 15; NPHP15 (#614845)	CEP164	AR	LCA	Renal disease
Neurodegeneration with Brain Iron Accumulation 1; NBIA1 (#234200)	PANK2	AR	RD, OA, eyelid apraxia	Neurodegeneration, gastrointestinal, skeletal, skin and muscular involvement
Neuropathy, Ataxia and Retinitis Pigmentosa; NARP (#551500)	MTATP6	Mi	RP	Neurodegeneration, ataxia
Norrie Disease; ND (#310600)	NDP	XLR	Retinal dysgenesis, retinal dysplasia, OA, microphthalmia, vitreous atrophy, corneal opacities, iris atrophy, cataract	HL, ID, neurodegeneration
Oculoauricular Syndrome; OCACS (#612109)	HMX1	AR	RP, microphthalmia, microcornea, cataract, microphakia, sclerocornea, increased intraocular pressure	External ear abnormalities
Orofaciodigital Syndrome XVI; OFD16 (#617563)	TMEM107	AR	RD, oculomotor apraxia, ptosis	Facial anomalies, breathing abnormalities, polydactyly, hypotonia, ID, neurological anomalies
Oliver–McFarlane Syndrome; OMCS (#275400)	PNPLA6	AR	Chorioretinopathy, OA	SS, ID, neurodegeneration, obesity, male external genitalia abnormalities, endocrine anomalies
Peroxisomal Acyl-CoA Oxidase Deficiency (#264470)	ACOX1	AR	RD, OA, strabismus	Neurodegeneration, ID, HL, liver disease
Peroxisome Biogenesis Disorder; PBD (#214100, #614866, #601539, #234580, #614879, #266510)	PEX1, PEX2, PEX5, PEX6, PEX7, PEX12	AR	RD, OA, corneal clouding, cataract	FTT, neurodegeneration, ID, HL, dental, cardiac, hepatic, genitourinary and skeletal involvement
Posterior Column Ataxia with Retinitis Pigmentosa; AXPC1 (#609033)	FLVCR1	AR	RP, OA	Posterior column ataxia, neurodegeneration, gastrointestinal and skeletal involvement
Polyneuropathy, Hearing Loss, Ataxia, Retinitis Pigmentosa and Cataract; PHARC (#612674)	ABHD12	AR	RP, OA, cataract	Ataxia, neurodegeneration, HL

Table 1. Cont.

Syndrome (MIM/Reference)	Gene	Inheritance *	Main Ocular Phenotypes #	Main Extra-Ocular Phenotypes ¶
Pseudoxanthoma Elasticum; PXE (#264800)	ABCC6	AR	RD, MD, choroidal neovascularization	Skin lesions, cardiovascular disease, gastrointestinal and genitourinary involvement
Refsum Disease, classic (#266500)	PHYH	AR	RP	Neurodegeneration, ataxia, HL, anosmia, cardiac, skeletal and skin involvement
Retinal Dystrophy, Iris Coloboma and Comedogenic Acne Syndrome; RDCCAS (#615147)	RPB4	AR	RD, coloboma of the iris, displacement of the pupil, microcornea, cataract	Comedogenic acne
Retinal Dystrophy and Iris Coloboma with or without Cataract; RDICC (#616722)	MIR204	AD	RD, coloboma of the iris, congenital cataract	
Retinal Dystrophy, Juvenile Cataracts and Short Stature Syndrome; RDJCSS (#616108)	RDH11	AR	RD, juvenile cataracts	SS, DD, ID, dental anomalies
Retinal Dystrophy and Obesity; RDOB (#616188)	TUB	AR	RD	Obesity
Revesz Syndrome (#268130)	TINF2	AD	RD	IUGR, brain structural anomalies, neurodegeneration, ID, aplastic anemia, skin, hair and nail abnormalities
Retinitis Pigmentosa–Deafness Syndrome (#500004)	MTTS2	Mi	RP	HL
Retinitis Pigmentosa and Erythrocytic Microcytosis; RPEM (#616959)	TRNT1	AR	RP	Erythrocytic microcytosis and additional hematologic abnormalities
Retinitis Pigmentosa, Hypopituitarism, Nephronophtisis and mild Skeletal Dysplasia; RHYNS (#602152)	TMEM67	AR	RP	Hypopituitarism, renal disease, skeletal anomalies, HL
Retinitis Pigmentosa 82 with or without Situs Inversus; RP82 (#615434)	ARL2BP	AR	RP	Situs inversus, male infertility
Retinitis Pigmentosa with or without Skeletal Anomalies; RPSKA (#250410)	CWC27	AR	RP	SS, skeletal anomalies, ID
Retinitis Pigmentosa, X-linked and Sinorespiratory Infections, with or without Deafness (#300455)	RPGR	XL	RP	Recurrent respiratory infections, HL
Senior–Løken Syndrome; SLSN (#266900, #606996, #609254, #610189, #613615, #616307, #616629)	NPHP1, NPHP4, IQCB1, CEP290, SDCCAG8, WDR19, TRAF3IP1	AR	RP, LCA	Renal disease
Short Stature, Hearing Loss, Retinitis Pigmentosa and Distinctive Facies; SHRF (#617763)	EXOSC2	AR	RP, corneal dystrophy, glaucoma, strabismus	SS, facial anomalies, HL, neurodegeneration, DD, ID
Sideroblastic Anemia with B-cell Immunodeficiency, Periodic Fevers and Developmental Delay; SIFD (#616084)	TRNT1	AR	RP	Sideroblastic anemia, immunodeficiency, growth retardation, DD, periodic fever, HL, neurological, cardiac and renal involvement

Table 1. Cont.

Syndrome (MIM/Reference)	Gene	Inheritance *	Main Ocular Phenotypes #	Main Extra-Ocular Phenotypes ¶
Spondylometaphyseal Dysplasia with Cone–Rod Dystrophy; SMDCRD (#608940)	PCYT1A	AR	CRD	Skeletal anomalies, PGR
Spondylometaphyseal Dysplasia, Axial; SMDAX (#602271)	CFAP410	AR	RP, CRD, OA	Skeletal anomalies, respiratory disease, reduced sperm motility
Short-Rib Thoracic Dysplasia 9 with or without Polydactyly; SRTD9 (#266920)	IFT140	AR	RP	Skeletal anomalies, renal disease, ID
Thiamine-Responsive Megaloblastic Anemia Syndrome; TRMA (#249270)	SLC19A2	AR	OA, RD	Megaloblastic anemia, diabetes mellitus, HL
Usher Syndrome; USH (#276900, #276904, #601067, #602083, #606943, #614869, #276901, #605472, #611383, #276902, #614504)	MYO7A, USH1C, CDH23, PCDH15, USH1G, CIB2, USH2A, ADGRV1, WHRN, CLRN1, HARS1	AR	RP	HL, vestibular dysfunction
Wolfram Syndrome 1, WFS1 (#222300)	WFS1	AR	OA, RD	Diabetes mellitus, diabetes insipidus, HL, neurodegeneration, genitourinary and neurologic involvement
White–Sutton Syndrome, WHSUS (#616364)	POGZ	AD	RP, OA, cortical blindness	DD, characteristic facial features, hypotonia, HL, joint laxity, gastrointestinal anomalies
Xeroderma Pigmentosum, group B; XPB (#610651)	ERCC3	AR	RD, OA, micropathalmia	Neoplasia, skin anomalies, CC, microcephaly, IIL, ID, brain structural anomalies, neurodegeneration

* AD, autosomal dominant; AR, autosomal recessive; Mi, mitochondrial; XL, X-linked; XLD, X-linked dominant; XLR, X-linked recessive. # CRD, cone–rod dystrophy; LCA, Leber congenital amaurosis; MD, macular dystrophy; OA, optic atrophy; RD, retinal dystrophy; RP, retinitis pigmentosa. ¶ DD, developmental delay; FTT, failure to thrive; HL, hearing loss; ID, intellectual disability; IUGR, intrauterine growth restriction; PGR, postnatal growth retardation; SS, short stature.

2. Syndromic IRD Types

The majority of syndromic IRDs are recessively inherited and rare. Many, although not all, syndromic IRDs can be classified into one of two major disease groups: inborn errors of metabolism (IEM) and ciliopathies.

IEMs are genetic disorders leading to failure of carbohydrate metabolism, protein metabolism, fatty acid oxidation or glycogen storage. Many IEMs present with neurologic symptoms [9]. The retina develops from an embryonic forebrain pouch and is considered an extension of the brain. Therefore, neurodegeneration resulting from IEMs often involves retinal degeneration (RD) as well. Major forms of syndromic IRD that belong to the IEM group include congenital disorders of glycosylation (CDG) [10], neuronal ceroid lipofuscinoses (CLNs) [11], mucopolysaccharidoses (MPSs) [12], peroxisomal diseases [13] and more (Table 1).

Ciliopathies are a group of genetic diseases caused by mutations in genes associated with the structure and function of primary cilia. Primary cilia function as signaling hubs that sense environmental cues and are pivotal for organ development and function, and for tissue homeostasis. By their nature, cilia defects are usually pleiotropic, affecting more than one system [14]. Photoreceptor OSs are highly modified primary sensory cilia. The proximal end of the OS is linked to the cell body (i.e., the IS) via a connecting cilium which is structurally homologous to the transition zone of primary cilia [15]. Consequently, retinal pathogenesis is a common finding in ciliopathies. Other organs which are commonly affected in ciliopathies are the central nervous system (CNS), kidney, liver, skeleton and inner ear. Major forms of syndromic IRD that belong to the ciliopathy group include Bardet–Biedl

Syndrome (BBS) [16], Joubert Syndrome (JBTS) [17], Usher Syndrome (USH) [18], Senior–Løken Syndrome (SLN) [19] and Alstrom Syndrome (ALMS) [20] (Table 1).

3. Genetic Heterogeneity in Syndromic IRDs

Over 80 forms of syndromic IRD have been described (Table 1). Most of these syndromes are caused by a single gene. However, 14 of 81 (17%) of the syndromes listed in Table 1 are genetically heterogeneous, and some of them are associated with multiple causative genes. The most genetically heterogeneous forms of syndromic IRD are three recessively inherited ciliopathies: BBS, JBTS and USH. The protein products of the genes associated with each one of these ciliopathies tend to form multi-protein complexes in the retina and in additional tissues, thus explaining the similar phenotypes caused by mutations in each of these genes.

BBS (prevalence of about 1/125,000) is characterized by a combination of RP, postaxial polydactyly (and other skeletal abnormalities), hypogonadism, renal disease, intellectual disability (ID) and truncal obesity [16]. Twenty-one causative genes have been reported to date (OMIM) (Table 1). Their protein products are involved in lipid homeostasis, intraflagellar transport, establishing planar cell polarity, regulation of intracellular trafficking and centrosomal functions. Eight of these genes encode for subunits of a protein complex, the BBSome, which is integral in ciliary as well as intracellular trafficking [21]. In the retina, the BBSome is required for photoreceptor OS formation and maintenance [22], as well as for retinal synaptogenesis [23].

JBTS (prevalence of 1/55,000–1/200,000) is characterized by a peculiar midbrain–hindbrain malformation, known as the molar tooth sign. The neurological presentation of JBTS includes hypotonia that evolves into ataxia, developmental delay, abnormal eye movements and neonatal breathing abnormalities. This picture is often associated with variable multiorgan involvement, mainly of the retina, kidney and liver [17]. RD has been reported in 38% of patients [24]. To date, 36 causative genes have been identified, all encoding for proteins expressed in the primary cilium or its apparatus (OMIM). Mutations in 20 of these genes (listed in Table 1) have been specifically associated with RD and additional ocular abnormalities (such as nystagmus and oculomotor apraxia). Ocular abnormalities have also been reported in patients with mutations in most other JBTS genes. However, since RD was not specifically reported in these patients, these genes are not listed in Table 1. Given the marked phenotypic heterogeneity found in JBTS patients, it is very likely that a retinal phenotype will be associated with these genes in the future, as additional patients are discovered.

USH (prevalence of 1–4/25,000) is characterized by the combination of RP and sensorineural hearing loss (HL). Based on the severity and progression of HL, age at onset of RP and the presence or absence of vestibular impairment, the majority of USH cases can be classified into one of three clinical subtypes (USH1-3). Eleven USH genes have been identified to date (OMIM) (Table 1). Their protein products are associated with a wide range of functions, including actin-binding molecular motors, cell adhesion, scaffolding and cellular trafficking. USH proteins form complexes and function cooperatively in neurosensory cells of both the retina and the inner ear (reviewed in [18,25]).

4. Phenotypic Overlap in Syndromic IRDs

When referring to syndromic IRD, phenotypic overlap is a common phenomenon, which can be divided into three groups, as detailed below:

4.1. Phenotypic Overlap between Different IRD Syndromes

Many types of syndromic IRD have a multi-systemic nature. Certain organs are commonly involved in syndromic IRDs. Specifically, CNS involvement (usually manifested as ID) is found in 68% of IRD syndromes (Table 1 and Figure 1), and over 80 genes are associated with the combination of IRD and ID [26] (Table 1). In addition to ID, the most common findings in syndromic IRD are extra-retinal eye abnormalities and ear, skeletal, renal and cardiovascular involvement (Figure 1). Most of these syndromes are phenotypically heterogeneous, with many patients exhibiting only some of the phenotypic features. These factors lead to a marked phenotypic overlap between different syndromes, and to a diagnostic challenge. For example, the combination of RD, ID, renal disease and skeletal abnormalities is found in numerous forms of syndromic IRD, including BBS, JBTS and ALMS, among others (Table 1). The combination of retinal abnormalities and HL as prominent symptoms is found in USH, as well as in CRD and HL 1 syndrome [27], Leber congenital amaurosis with early-onset deafness syndrome [28], Norrie disease [29], peroxisome biogenesis disorders, Refsum disease [30] and more (Table 1). These overlaps may often lead to diagnostic mistakes [27,31,32].

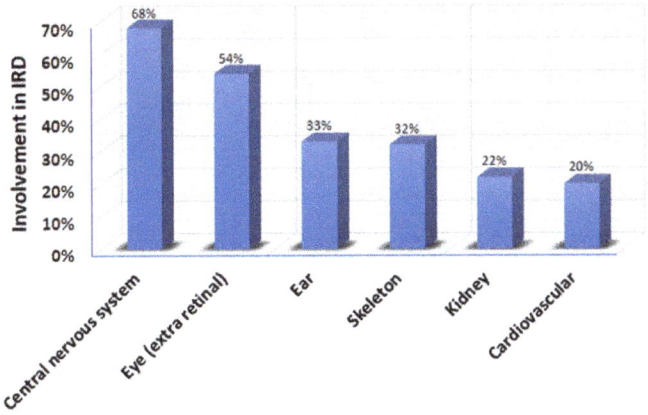

Figure 1. Systems and organs most commonly involved in syndromic IRDs.

4.2. Syndromic Versus Non-Syndromic IRD Caused by the Same Genes

Twenty-eight of the genes listed in Table 1 can cause both syndromic and non-syndromic IRD (Table 2 and Figure 2). In general, milder hypomorphic mutations in these genes are associated with non-syndromic IRD, while null mutations lead to the involvement of additional tissues. In addition, the involvement of additional genetic and environmental factors in the determination of the final phenotypic outcome cannot be excluded. A prominent example is the *USH2A* gene. Mutations in this gene are the most common cause of USH, and specifically of USH2 (RP with congenital, mild to moderate sensorineural HL) [33]. Moreover, *USH2A* variants are also one of the commonest causes of AR non-syndromic RP worldwide [34–36]. It appears that the specific combination of *USH2A* variants determines whether one has USH2 or non-syndromic RP [37–39]. In addition, RD is more severe in patients with *USH2A*-related USH2 than in patients with *USH2A*-related non-syndromic RP. However, the reason is not completely understood [38].

Table 2. Genes underlying both syndromic and non-syndromic IRDs.

Gene	Syndromic IRD	Non-Syndromic IRD (MIM)	Reference
ABHD12	PHARC	arRP	[40]
AHI1	JBTS3	arRP	[41]
ALMS1	ALMS	arCRD, arEORD	[42]
ARL2BP	RP with situs inversus	arRP (#615434)	[43,44]
ARL3	JBTS35	adRP (#618173)	[45]
ARL6	BBS3	arRP (#613575)	[46]
BBS2	BBS2	arRP (#616562)	[47]
C8ORF37	BBS21	arCRD, arRP (#614500)	[48]
CC2D2A	JBTS9, MKS6	arRP	[49]
CEP290	BBS14, JBTS5, MKS4, SLSN6	arLCA (#611755)	[50]
CFAP410	SMDAX	arRD with or without macular staphyloma (#617547)	[51,52]

Table 2. Cont.

Gene	Syndromic IRD	Non-Syndromic IRD (MIM)	Reference
CLN3	CLN3	arRP	[53]
CLRN1	USH3A	arRP (#614180)	[54]
CWC27	RPSKA	arRP (#250410)	[55]
DHDDS	CDG1BB	arRP (#613861)	[56,57]
FLVCR1	PCARP	arRP	[58]
HGSNAT	MPS3C	arRP (#616544)	[59]
IFT140	SRTD9 with/without polydactyly	arRP (#617781)	[60]
IQCB1	SLSN5	arLCA	[61]
MFSD8	CLN7	arMD (#616170), arRD	[62]
MMACHC	MAHCC	arMD	[63]
MVK	HIDS, MEVA	arRP	[64]
NDP	ND	XL EVR (#305390)	[65]
OFD1	JBTS10	XL RP (#300424)	[66]
OTX2	RD with pituitary dysfunction	adPD (#610125)	[67]
RPGR	RP, sinorespiratory infections and deafness	XL CRD (#304020), XL MD (#300834), XL RP (#300029)	[68]
TTC8	BBS8	arRP (#613464)	[69]
USH2A	USH2A	arRP (#613809)	[70]

ALMS: Alstrom syndrome; ar: autosomal recessive; ad: autosomal dominant; BBS: Bardet–Biedl syndrome; CDG: congenital disorder of glycosylation; CLN: ceroid lipofuscinosis neuronal; CRD: cone–rod dystrophy; EORD: early-onset retinal degeneration; EVR: exudative vitreoretinopathy; HIDS: hyper-IgD syndrome; JBTS: Joubert syndrome; LCA: Leber congenital amaurosis; MAHCC: methylmalonic aciduria and homocystinuria, cblC type; MD: macular dystrophy; MEVA: mevalonic aciduria; MKS: Meckel syndrome; MPS: mucopolysaccharidosis; ND: Norrie disease; PCARP: posterior column ataxia with retinitis pigmentosa; PD: pattern dystrophy; PHARC: polyneuropathy, hearing loss, ataxia, retinitis pigmentosa and cataract; RD: retinal dystrophy; RP: retinitis pigmentosa; RPSKA: retinitis pigmentosa with skeletal anomalies; SLSN: Senior–Løken syndrome; SMDAX: spondylometaphyseal dysplasia axial; SRTD: short-rib thoracic dysplasia; USH: Usher syndrome; XL: X-linked.

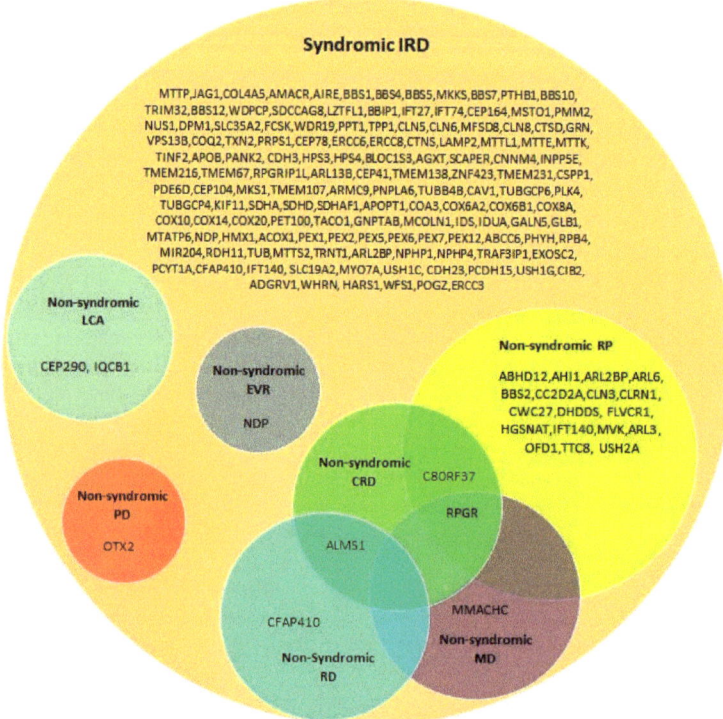

Figure 2. A Venn diagram showing the involvement of syndromic IRD genes in non-syndromic IRD phenotypes. CRD: cone–rod dystrophy; EVR: exudative vitreoretinopathy; LCA: Leber congenital amaurosis; MD: macular dystrophy; PD: pattern dystrophy; RD: retinal dystrophy; RP: retinitis pigmentosa.

4.3. Co-Existence of Non-Syndromic IRD and Additional Non-Ocular Diseases

IRD is one of the most genetically heterogeneous groups of disorders in humans, and most cases of IRD are non-syndromic. Non-syndromic IRD may coincide with other genetic (and non-genetic) rare conditions, leading to a clinical suspicion or diagnosis of a syndrome. For example, co-occurrence of non-syndromic RP and non-syndromic HL in a family may appear as USH [71].

5. Diagnostic Challenges

Due to the high degree of phenotypic variability and phenotypic overlap found in syndromic IRD, as described above, correct diagnosis based on phenotypic features alone may be challenging and sometimes misleading. Therefore, genetic testing has become the benchmark for the diagnosis and management of patients with these conditions, as it complements the clinical findings and facilitates an accurate clinical diagnosis. Establishing a correct diagnosis is important for both the patients and their family members, for multiple reasons: it enables the understanding of the natural history course, and the prediction of disease prognosis; it aids in tailoring correct follow-up and treatment, including potential gene-targeted therapies [72]; it leads to a reduction in disease prevalence, by genetic screening and counseling in high-risk populations; it allows the patients to pursue prenatal counseling and reproductive planning; and it enables identification of novel disease genes and mechanisms.

The existence of common founder mutations in certain populations allows for quick and efficient mutation screening in affected individuals, based on the relevant phenotype and ethnic background. This is performed by PCR-based DNA amplification and Sanger sequencing, or by specifically designed assays. Some examples are common USH3A-, USH1F-, ML4- and BBS2-causative mutations found in the Ashkenazi Jewish population [73–76]; and USH3A- and MKS1-causative mutations found in the Finnish population [77,78]. Nevertheless, for most syndromic IRD patients worldwide, this strategy is not effective.

Currently, the most efficient approach for genetic diagnosis in monogenic diseases, including IRDs, is next-generation sequencing (NGS). NGS technologies facilitate the screening of the entire genome (whole genome sequencing, WGS); of all protein-coding regions (whole exome sequencing, WES); or of protein-coding regions of pre-determined panels of genes (targeted NGS, T-NGS) [79,80]. Since protein-coding regions comprise only 1–2% of the entire genome while harboring over 85% of variants causing Mendelian disorders, WES is still considered as the method of choice for genetic analysis, in both clinical and research settings. However, worldwide diagnostic yields of IRD patients by WES only range between 60% and 70% [36,81,82]. The missing mutations can be divided into four groups: (1) mutations located within exons, but missed due to technical issues, e.g., lack of coverage; (2) mutations located within covered exons, but missed due to limitations in data analysis and interpretation; (3) non-coding variants that may affect gene expression, mRNA stability, splicing and more; and (4) structural variants, such as large deletions, duplications and inversions, which are missed by WES. The latter two may be identified by WGS [34].

6. Summary and Conclusions

Over 80 forms of syndromic IRDs have been described, and approximately 200 causative genes identified. Due to the high degree of phenotypic variability and phenotypic overlap found in syndromic IRD, correct diagnosis based on phenotypic features alone is insufficient, and genetic testing has become the benchmark for the diagnosis and management of patients with these conditions. For most patients, molecular diagnosis should be based on NGS technologies. Currently, WES is the most popular approach for genetic analysis in patients with monogenic diseases, including IRDs. However, the continuous progress in both technical and bioinformatic aspects, as well as the reduction of costs, is already leading to a shift towards WGS as the method of choice.

Author Contributions: Conceptualization, T.B.-Y.; methodology, T.B.-Y.; validation, Y.T. and T.B.-Y.; formal analysis, Y.T.; investigation, Y.T. and T.B.-Y.; resources, T.B.-Y.; data curation, Y.T. and T.B.-Y.; writing—original draft preparation, T.B.-Y.; writing—review and editing, T.B.-Y.; supervision, T.B.-Y.; funding acquisition, T.B.-Y. All authors have read and agreed to the published version of the manuscript.

Funding: This research was funded by the Israel Science Foundation (grant number 525/19).

Conflicts of Interest: The authors declare no conflict of interest. The funders had no role in the design of the study; in the collection, analyses, or interpretation of data; in the writing of the manuscript, or in the decision to publish the results.

References

1. Duncan, J.L.; Pierce, E.A.; Laster, A.M.; Daiger, S.P.; Birch, D.G.; Ash, J.D.; Iannaccone, A.; Flannery, J.G.; Sahel, J.A.; Zack, D.J.; et al. Inherited Retinal Degenerations: Current Landscape and Knowledge Gaps. *Transl. Vis. Sci. Technol.* **2018**, *7*, 6. [CrossRef] [PubMed]
2. Verbakel, S.K.; van Huet, R.A.C.; Boon, C.J.F.; den Hollander, A.I.; Collin, R.W.J.; Klaver, C.C.W.; Hoyng, C.B.; Roepman, R.; Klevering, B.J. Non-syndromic retinitis pigmentosa. *Prog. Retin. Eye Res.* **2018**, *66*, 157–186. [CrossRef] [PubMed]
3. Thiadens, A.A.; Phan, T.M.; Zekveld-Vroon, R.C.; Leroy, B.P.; van den Born, L.I.; Hoyng, C.B.; Klaver, C.C.; Roosing, S.; Pott, J.W.; van Schooneveld, M.J.; et al. Clinical course, genetic etiology, and visual outcome in cone and cone-rod dystrophy. *Ophthalmology* **2012**, *119*, 819–826. [CrossRef] [PubMed]
4. Kumaran, N.; Moore, A.T.; Weleber, R.G.; Michaelides, M. Leber congenital amaurosis/early-onset severe retinal dystrophy: Clinical features, molecular genetics and therapeutic interventions. *Br. J. Ophthalmol.* **2017**, *101*, 1147–1154. [CrossRef] [PubMed]
5. Tsang, S.H.; Sharma, T. Rod Monochromatism (Achromatopsia). *Adv. Exp. Med. Biol.* **2018**, *1085*, 119–123.
6. Werdich, X.Q.; Place, E.M.; Pierce, E.A. Systemic diseases associated with retinal dystrophies. *Semin. Ophthalmol.* **2014**, *29*, 319–328. [CrossRef]
7. Shamseldin, H.E.; Shaheen, R.; Ewida, N.; Bubshait, D.K.; Alkuraya, H.; Almardawi, E.; Howaidi, A.; Sabr, Y.; Abdalla, E.M.; Alfaifi, A.Y.; et al. The morbid genome of ciliopathies: An update. *Genet. Med.* **2020**, *22*, 1051–1060. [CrossRef]
8. Iwama, K.; Takaori, T.; Fukushima, A.; Tohyama, J.; Ishiyama, A.; Ohba, C.; Mitsuhashi, S.; Miyatake, S.; Takata, A.; Miyake, N.; et al. Novel recessive mutations in MSTO1 cause cerebellar atrophy with pigmentary retinopathy. *J. Hum. Genet.* **2018**, *63*, 263–270. [CrossRef]
9. Ferreira, C.R.; van Karnebeek, C.D.M. Inborn errors of metabolism. *Handb. Clin. Neurol.* **2019**, *162*, 449–481.
10. Freeze, H.H.; Schachter, H.; Kinoshita, T. Genetic Disorders of Glycosylation. In *Essentials of Glycobiology*, 3rd ed.; Varki, A., Cummings, R.D., Esko, J.D., Stanley, P., Hart, G.W., Aebi, M., Darvill, A.G., Kinoshita, T., Packer, N.H., Prestegard, J.H., et al., Eds.; Cold Spring Harbor Laboratory Press: New York, NY, USA, 2017; Chapter 45.
11. Nita, D.A.; Mole, S.E.; Minassian, B.A. Neuronal ceroid lipofuscinoses. *Epileptic Disord.* **2016**, *18*, 73–88. [CrossRef]
12. Muenzer, J. Overview of the mucopolysaccharidoses. *Rheumatology (Oxford)* **2011**, *50* (Suppl. 5), v4–v12. [CrossRef]
13. Imanaka, T. Biogenesis and Function of Peroxisomes in Human Disease with a Focus on the ABC Transporter. *Biol. Pharm. Bull.* **2019**, *42*, 649–665. [CrossRef] [PubMed]
14. Sreekumar, V.; Norris, D.P. Cilia and development. *Curr. Opin. Genet. Dev.* **2019**, *56*, 15–21. [CrossRef] [PubMed]
15. May-Simera, H.; Nagel-Wolfrum, K.; Wolfrum, U. Cilia—The sensory antennae in the eye. *Prog. Retin. Eye Res.* **2017**, *60*, 144–180. [CrossRef]
16. Tsang, S.H.; Aycinena, A.R.P.; Sharma, T. Ciliopathy: Bardet-Biedl Syndrome. *Adv. Exp. Med. Biol.* **2018**, *1085*, 171–174. [PubMed]
17. Valente, E.M.; Dallapiccola, B.; Bertini, E. Joubert syndrome and related disorders. *Handb. Clin. Neurol.* **2013**, *113*, 1879–1888. [PubMed]
18. Geleoc, G.G.S.; El-Amraoui, A. Disease mechanisms and gene therapy for Usher syndrome. *Hear. Res.* **2020**, *394*, 107932. [CrossRef] [PubMed]

19. Tsang, S.H.; Aycinena, A.R.P.; Sharma, T. Ciliopathy: Senior-Loken Syndrome. *Adv. Exp. Med. Biol.* **2018**, *1085*, 175–178. [PubMed]
20. Tsang, S.H.; Aycinena, A.R.P.; Sharma, T. Ciliopathy: Alstrom Syndrome. *Adv. Exp. Med. Biol.* **2018**, *1085*, 179–180. [PubMed]
21. Petriman, N.A.; Lorentzen, E. Moving proteins along in the cilium. *Elife* **2020**, *9*, e55254. [CrossRef]
22. Hsu, Y.; Garrison, J.E.; Kim, G.; Schmitz, A.R.; Searby, C.C.; Zhang, Q.; Datta, P.; Nishimura, D.Y.; Seo, S.; Sheffield, V.C. BBSome function is required for both the morphogenesis and maintenance of the photoreceptor outer segment. *PLoS Genet.* **2017**, *13*, e1007057. [CrossRef]
23. Hsu, Y.; Garrison, J.E.; Seo, S.; Sheffield, V.C. The absence of BBSome function decreases synaptogenesis and causes ectopic synapse formation in the retina. *Sci. Rep.* **2020**, *10*, 8321. [CrossRef]
24. Wang, S.F.; Kowal, T.J.; Ning, K.; Koo, E.B.; Wu, A.Y.; Mahajan, V.B.; Sun, Y. Review of Ocular Manifestations of Joubert Syndrome. *Genes* **2018**, *9*, 605. [CrossRef] [PubMed]
25. El-Amraoui, A.; Petit, C. The retinal phenotype of Usher syndrome: Pathophysiological insights from animal models. *Comptes Rendus Biol.* **2014**, *337*, 167–177. [CrossRef] [PubMed]
26. Yang, X.R.; Benson, M.D.; MacDonald, I.M.; Innes, A.M. A diagnostic approach to syndromic retinal dystrophies with intellectual disability. *Am. J. Med. Genet. C Semin. Med. Genet.* **2020**, *184*, 538–570. [CrossRef] [PubMed]
27. Namburi, P.; Ratnapriya, R.; Khateb, S.; Lazar, C.H.; Kinarty, Y.; Obolensky, A.; Erdinest, I.; Marks-Ohana, D.; Pras, E.; Ben-Yosef, T.; et al. Bi-allelic Truncating Mutations in CEP78, Encoding Centrosomal Protein 78, Cause Cone-Rod Degeneration with Sensorineural Hearing Loss. *Am. J. Hum. Genet.* **2016**, *99*, 777–784. [CrossRef]
28. Luscan, R.; Mechaussier, S.; Paul, A.; Tian, G.; Gerard, X.; Defoort-Dellhemmes, S.; Loundon, N.; Audo, I.; Bonnin, S.; LeGargasson, J.F.; et al. Mutations in TUBB4B Cause a Distinctive Sensorineural Disease. *Am. J. Hum. Genet.* **2017**, *101*, 1006–1012. [CrossRef]
29. Sims, K.B. NDP-Related Retinopathies. In *GeneReviews®*; Adam, M.P., Ardinger, H.H., Pagon, R.A., Wallace, S.E., Bean, L.J., Stephens, K., Amemiya, A., Eds.; University of Washington: Seattle, WA, USA, 2014.
30. Tsang, S.H.; Sharma, T. Inborn Errors of Metabolism: Refsum Disease. *Adv. Exp. Med. Biol.* **2018**, *1085*, 191–192.
31. Raas-Rothschild, A.; Wanders, R.J.; Mooijer, P.A.; Gootjes, J.; Waterham, H.R.; Gutman, A.; Suzuki, Y.; Shimozawa, N.; Kondo, N.; Eshel, G.; et al. A PEX6-defective peroxisomal biogenesis disorder with severe phenotype in an infant, versus mild phenotype resembling Usher syndrome in the affected parents. *Am. J. Hum. Genet.* **2002**, *70*, 1062–1068. [CrossRef]
32. Smith, C.E.; Poulter, J.A.; Levin, A.V.; Capasso, J.E.; Price, S.; Ben-Yosef, T.; Sharony, R.; Newman, W.G.; Shore, R.C.; Brookes, S.J.; et al. Spectrum of PEX1 and PEX6 variants in Heimler syndrome. *Eur. J. Hum. Genet.* **2016**, *24*, 1565–1571. [CrossRef]
33. Le Quesne Stabej, P.; Saihan, Z.; Rangesh, N.; Steele-Stallard, H.B.; Ambrose, J.; Coffey, A.; Emmerson, J.; Haralambous, E.; Hughes, Y.; Steel, K.P.; et al. Comprehensive sequence analysis of nine Usher syndrome genes in the UK National Collaborative Usher Study. *J. Med. Genet.* **2012**, *49*, 27–36. [CrossRef] [PubMed]
34. Carss, K.J.; Arno, G.; Erwood, M.; Stephens, J.; Sanchis-Juan, A.; Hull, S.; Megy, K.; Grozeva, D.; Dewhurst, E.; Malka, S.; et al. Comprehensive Rare Variant Analysis via Whole-Genome Sequencing to Determine the Molecular Pathology of Inherited Retinal Disease. *Am. J. Hum. Genet.* **2017**, *100*, 75–90. [CrossRef] [PubMed]
35. Dockery, A.; Stephenson, K.; Keegan, D.; Wynne, N.; Silvestri, G.; Humphries, P.; Kenna, P.F.; Carrigan, M.; Farrar, G.J. Target 5000: Target Capture Sequencing for Inherited Retinal Degenerations. *Genes* **2017**, *8*, 304. [CrossRef] [PubMed]
36. Sharon, D.; Ben-Yosef, T.; Goldenberg-Cohen, N.; Pras, E.; Gradstein, L.; Soudry, S.; Mezer, E.; Zur, D.; Abbasi, A.H.; Zeitz, C.; et al. A nationwide genetic analysis of inherited retinal diseases in Israel as assessed by the Israeli inherited retinal disease consortium (IIRDC). *Hum. Mutat.* **2019**, *41*, 140–149. [CrossRef] [PubMed]
37. Lenassi, E.; Vincent, A.; Li, Z.; Saihan, Z.; Coffey, A.J.; Steele-Stallard, H.B.; Moore, A.T.; Steel, K.P.; Luxon, L.M.; Heon, E.; et al. A detailed clinical and molecular survey of subjects with nonsyndromic USH2A retinopathy reveals an allelic hierarchy of disease-causing variants. *Eur. J. Hum. Genet.* **2015**, *23*, 1318–1327. [CrossRef] [PubMed]

38. Pierrache, L.H.; Hartel, B.P.; van Wijk, E.; Meester-Smoor, M.A.; Cremers, F.P.; de Baere, E.; de Zaeytijd, J.; van Schooneveld, M.J.; Cremers, C.W.; Dagnelie, G.; et al. Visual Prognosis in USH2A-Associated Retinitis Pigmentosa Is Worse for Patients with Usher Syndrome Type IIa Than for Those with Nonsyndromic Retinitis Pigmentosa. *Ophthalmology* **2016**, *123*, 1151–1160. [CrossRef] [PubMed]
39. Sengillo, J.D.; Cabral, T.; Schuerch, K.; Duong, J.; Lee, W.; Boudreault, K.; Xu, Y.; Justus, S.; Sparrow, J.R.; Mahajan, V.B.; et al. Electroretinography Reveals Difference in Cone Function between Syndromic and Nonsyndromic USH2A Patients. *Sci. Rep.* **2017**, *7*, 11170. [CrossRef]
40. Nishiguchi, K.M.; Avila-Fernandez, A.; van Huet, R.A.; Corton, M.; Perez-Carro, R.; Martin-Garrido, E.; Lopez-Molina, M.I.; Blanco-Kelly, F.; Hoefsloot, L.H.; van Zelst-Stams, W.A.; et al. Exome sequencing extends the phenotypic spectrum for ABHD12 mutations: From syndromic to nonsyndromic retinal degeneration. *Ophthalmology* **2014**, *121*, 1620–1627. [CrossRef]
41. Nguyen, T.T.; Hull, S.; Roepman, R.; van den Born, L.I.; Oud, M.M.; de Vrieze, E.; Hetterschijt, L.; Letteboer, S.J.F.; van Beersum, S.E.C.; Blokland, E.A.; et al. Missense mutations in the WD40 domain of AHI1 cause non-syndromic retinitis pigmentosa. *J. Med. Genet.* **2017**, *54*, 624–632. [CrossRef]
42. Aldrees, A.; Abdelkader, E.; Al-Habboubi, H.; Alrwebah, H.; Rahbeeni, Z.; Schatz, P. Non-syndromic retinal dystrophy associated with homozygous mutations in the ALMS1 gene. *Ophthalmic Genet.* **2019**, *40*, 77–79. [CrossRef]
43. Audo, I.; El Shamieh, S.; Mejecase, C.; Michiels, C.; Demontant, V.; Antonio, A.; Condroyer, C.; Boyard, F.; Letexier, M.; Saraiva, J.P.; et al. ARL2BP mutations account for 0.1% of autosomal recessive rod-cone dystrophies with the report of a novel splice variant. *Clin. Genet.* **2017**, *92*, 109–111. [PubMed]
44. Davidson, A.E.; Schwarz, N.; Zelinger, L.; Stern-Schneider, G.; Shoemark, A.; Spitzbarth, B.; Gross, M.; Laxer, U.; Sosna, J.; Sergouniotis, P.I.; et al. Mutations in ARL2BP, encoding ADP-ribosylation-factor-like 2 binding protein, cause autosomal-recessive retinitis pigmentosa. *Am. J. Hum. Genet.* **2013**, *93*, 321–329. [CrossRef] [PubMed]
45. Holtan, J.P.; Teigen, K.; Aukrust, I.; Bragadottir, R.; Houge, G. Dominant ARL3-related retinitis pigmentosa. *Ophthalmic Genet.* **2019**, *40*, 124–128. [CrossRef] [PubMed]
46. Aldahmesh, M.A.; Safieh, L.A.; Alkuraya, H.; Al-Rajhi, A.; Shamseldin, H.; Hashem, M.; Alzahrani, F.; Khan, A.O.; Alqahtani, F.; Rahbeeni, Z.; et al. Molecular characterization of retinitis pigmentosa in Saudi Arabia. *Mol. Vis.* **2009**, *15*, 2464–2469.
47. Shevach, E.; Ali, M.; Mizrahi-Meissonnier, L.; McKibbin, M.; El-Asrag, M.; Watson, C.M.; Inglehearn, C.F.; Ben-Yosef, T.; Blumenfeld, A.; Jalas, C.; et al. Association Between Missense Mutations in the BBS2 Gene and Nonsyndromic Retinitis Pigmentosa. *JAMA Ophthalmol.* **2015**, *133*, 312–318. [CrossRef]
48. Khan, A.O.; Decker, E.; Bachmann, N.; Bolz, H.J.; Bergmann, C. C8orf37 is mutated in Bardet-Biedl syndrome and constitutes a locus allelic to non-syndromic retinal dystrophies. *Ophthalmic Genet.* **2016**, *37*, 290–293. [CrossRef]
49. Mejecase, C.; Hummel, A.; Mohand-Said, S.; Andrieu, C.; El Shamieh, S.; Antonio, A.; Condroyer, C.; Boyard, F.; Foussard, M.; Blanchard, S.; et al. Whole exome sequencing resolves complex phenotype and identifies CC2D2A mutations underlying non-syndromic rod-cone dystrophy. *Clin. Genet.* **2019**, *95*, 329–333. [CrossRef]
50. den Hollander, A.I.; Koenekoop, R.K.; Yzer, S.; Lopez, I.; Arends, M.L.; Voesenek, K.E.; Zonneveld, M.N.; Strom, T.M.; Meitinger, T.; Brunner, H.G.; et al. Mutations in the CEP290 (NPHP6) gene are a frequent cause of Leber congenital amaurosis. *Am. J. Hum. Genet.* **2006**, *79*, 556–561. [CrossRef]
51. Khan, A.O.; Eisenberger, T.; Nagel-Wolfrum, K.; Wolfrum, U.; Bolz, H.J. C21orf2 is mutated in recessive early-onset retinal dystrophy with macular staphyloma and encodes a protein that localises to the photoreceptor primary cilium. *Br. J. Ophthalmol.* **2015**, *99*, 1725–1731. [CrossRef]
52. Suga, A.; Mizota, A.; Kato, M.; Kuniyoshi, K.; Yoshitake, K.; Sultan, W.; Yamazaki, M.; Shimomura, Y.; Ikeo, K.; Tsunoda, K.; et al. Identification of Novel Mutations in the LRR-Cap Domain of C21orf2 in Japanese Patients With Retinitis Pigmentosa and Cone-Rod Dystrophy. *Investig. Ophthalmol. Vis. Sci.* **2016**, *57*, 4255–4263. [CrossRef]
53. Ku, C.A.; Hull, S.; Arno, G.; Vincent, A.; Carss, K.; Kayton, R.; Weeks, D.; Anderson, G.W.; Geraets, R.; Parker, C.; et al. Detailed Clinical Phenotype and Molecular Genetic Findings in CLN3-Associated Isolated Retinal Degeneration. *JAMA Ophthalmol.* **2017**, *135*, 749–760. [CrossRef] [PubMed]

54. Khan, M.I.; Kersten, F.F.; Azam, M.; Collin, R.W.; Hussain, A.; Shah, S.T.; Keunen, J.E.; Kremer, H.; Cremers, F.P.; Qamar, R.; et al. CLRN1 mutations cause nonsyndromic retinitis pigmentosa. *Ophthalmology* **2011**, *118*, 1444–1448. [CrossRef] [PubMed]
55. Xu, M.; Xie, Y.A.; Abouzeid, H.; Gordon, C.T.; Fiorentino, A.; Sun, Z.; Lehman, A.; Osman, I.S.; Dharmat, R.; Riveiro-Alvarez, R.; et al. Mutations in the Spliceosome Component CWC27 Cause Retinal Degeneration with or without Additional Developmental Anomalies. *Am. J. Hum. Genet.* **2017**, *100*, 592–604. [CrossRef] [PubMed]
56. Lam, B.L.; Zuchner, S.L.; Dallman, J.; Wen, R.; Alfonso, E.C.; Vance, J.M.; Pericak-Vance, M.A. Mutation K42E in dehydrodolichol diphosphate synthase (DHDDS) causes recessive retinitis pigmentosa. *Adv. Exp. Med. Biol.* **2014**, *801*, 165–170.
57. Zelinger, L.; Banin, E.; Obolensky, A.; Mizrahi-Meissonnier, L.; Beryozkin, A.; Bandah-Rozenfeld, D.; Frenkel, S.; Ben-Yosef, T.; Merin, S.; Schwartz, S.B.; et al. A missense mutation in DHDDS, encoding dehydrodolichyl diphosphate synthase, is associated with autosomal-recessive retinitis pigmentosa in Ashkenazi Jews. *Am. J. Hum. Genet.* **2011**, *88*, 207–215. [CrossRef]
58. Kuehlewein, L.; Schols, L.; Llavona, P.; Grimm, A.; Biskup, S.; Zrenner, E.; Kohl, S. Phenotypic spectrum of autosomal recessive retinitis pigmentosa without posterior column ataxia caused by mutations in the FLVCR1 gene. *Graefes Arch. Clin. Exp. Ophthalmol.* **2019**, *257*, 629–638. [CrossRef]
59. Haer-Wigman, L.; Newman, H.; Leibu, R.; Bax, N.M.; Baris, H.N.; Rizel, L.; Banin, E.; Massarweh, A.; Roosing, S.; Lefeber, D.J.; et al. Non-syndromic retinitis pigmentosa due to mutations in the mucopolysaccharidosis type IIIC gene, heparan-alpha-glucosaminide N-acetyltransferase (HGSNAT). *Hum. Mol. Genet.* **2015**, *24*, 3742–3751. [CrossRef]
60. Xu, M.; Yang, L.; Wang, F.; Li, H.; Wang, X.; Wang, W.; Ge, Z.; Wang, K.; Zhao, L.; Li, H.; et al. Mutations in human IFT140 cause non-syndromic retinal degeneration. *Hum. Genet.* **2015**, *134*, 1069–1078. [CrossRef]
61. Stone, E.M.; Cideciyan, A.V.; Aleman, T.S.; Scheetz, T.E.; Sumaroka, A.; Ehlinger, M.A.; Schwartz, S.B.; Fishman, G.A.; Traboulsi, E.I.; Lam, B.L.; et al. Variations in NPHP5 in patients with nonsyndromic leber congenital amaurosis and Senior-Loken syndrome. *Arch. Ophthalmol.* **2011**, *129*, 81–87. [CrossRef]
62. Khan, K.N.; El-Asrag, M.E.; Ku, C.A.; Holder, G.E.; McKibbin, M.; Arno, G.; Poulter, J.A.; Carss, K.; Bommireddy, T.; Bagheri, S.; et al. Specific Alleles of CLN7/MFSD8, a Protein That Localizes to Photoreceptor Synaptic Terminals, Cause a Spectrum of Nonsyndromic Retinal Dystrophy. *Investig. Ophthalmol. Vis. Sci.* **2017**, *58*, 2906–2914. [CrossRef]
63. Collison, F.T.; Xie, Y.A.; Gambin, T.; Jhangiani, S.; Muzny, D.; Gibbs, R.; Lupski, J.R.; Fishman, G.A.; Allikmets, R. Whole Exome Sequencing Identifies an Adult-Onset Case of Methylmalonic Aciduria and Homocystinuria Type C (cblC) with Non-Syndromic Bull's Eye Maculopathy. *Ophthalmic Genet.* **2015**, *36*, 270–275. [CrossRef] [PubMed]
64. Siemiatkowska, A.M.; van den Born, L.I.; van Hagen, P.M.; Stoffels, M.; Neveling, K.; Henkes, A.; Kipping-Geertsema, M.; Hoefsloot, L.H.; Hoyng, C.B.; Simon, A.; et al. Mutations in the mevalonate kinase (MVK) gene cause nonsyndromic retinitis pigmentosa. *Ophthalmology* **2013**, *120*, 2697–2705. [CrossRef] [PubMed]
65. Chen, Z.Y.; Battinelli, E.M.; Fielder, A.; Bundey, S.; Sims, K.; Breakefield, X.O.; Craig, I.W. A mutation in the Norrie disease gene (NDP) associated with X-linked familial exudative vitreoretinopathy. *Nat. Genet.* **1993**, *5*, 180–183. [CrossRef] [PubMed]
66. Webb, T.R.; Parfitt, D.A.; Gardner, J.C.; Martinez, A.; Bevilacqua, D.; Davidson, A.E.; Zito, I.; Thiselton, D.L.; Ressa, J.H.; Apergi, M.; et al. Deep intronic mutation in OFD1, identified by targeted genomic next-generation sequencing, causes a severe form of X-linked retinitis pigmentosa (RP23). *Hum. Mol. Genet.* **2012**, *21*, 3647–3654. [CrossRef]
67. Vincent, A.; Forster, N.; Maynes, J.T.; Paton, T.A.; Billingsley, G.; Roslin, N.M.; Ali, A.; Sutherland, J.; Wright, T.; Westall, C.A.; et al. OTX2 mutations cause autosomal dominant pattern dystrophy of the retinal pigment epithelium. *J. Med. Genet.* **2014**, *51*, 797–805. [CrossRef]
68. Tee, J.J.; Smith, A.J.; Hardcastle, A.J.; Michaelides, M. RPGR-associated retinopathy: Clinical features, molecular genetics, animal models and therapeutic options. *Br. J. Ophthalmol.* **2016**, *100*, 1022–1027. [CrossRef]

69. Riazuddin, S.A.; Iqbal, M.; Wang, Y.; Masuda, T.; Chen, Y.; Bowne, S.; Sullivan, L.S.; Waseem, N.H.; Bhattacharya, S.; Daiger, S.P.; et al. A splice-site mutation in a retina-specific exon of BBS8 causes nonsyndromic retinitis pigmentosa. *Am. J. Hum. Genet.* **2010**, *86*, 805–812. [CrossRef]
70. Rivolta, C.; Sweklo, E.A.; Berson, E.L.; Dryja, T.P. Missense mutation in the USH2A gene: Association with recessive retinitis pigmentosa without hearing loss. *Am. J. Hum. Genet.* **2000**, *66*, 1975–1978. [CrossRef]
71. Ehrenberg, M.; Weiss, S.; Orenstein, N.; Goldenberg-Cohen, N.; Ben-Yosef, T. The co-occurrence of rare non-ocular phenotypes in patients with inherited retinal degenerations. *Mol. Vis.* **2019**, *25*, 691–702.
72. Ku, C.A.; Pennesi, M.E. The new landscape of retinal gene therapy. *Am. J. Med. Genet. C Semin. Med. Genet.* **2020**, *184*, 846–859. [CrossRef]
73. Bach, G.; Webb, M.B.; Bargal, R.; Zeigler, M.; Ekstein, J. The frequency of mucolipidosis type IV in the Ashkenazi Jewish population and the identification of 3 novel MCOLN1 mutations. *Hum. Mutat.* **2005**, *26*, 591. [CrossRef] [PubMed]
74. Ben-Yosef, T.; Ness, S.L.; Madeo, A.C.; Bar-Lev, A.; Wolfman, J.H.; Ahmed, Z.M.; Desnick, R.J.; Willner, J.P.; Avraham, K.B.; Ostrer, H.; et al. A mutation of PCDH15 among Ashkenazi Jews with the type 1 Usher syndrome. *N. Engl. J. Med.* **2003**, *348*, 1664–1670. [CrossRef] [PubMed]
75. Fedick, A.; Jalas, C.; Abeliovich, D.; Krakinovsky, Y.; Ekstein, J.; Ekstein, A.; Treff, N.R. Carrier frequency of two BBS2 mutations in the Ashkenazi population. *Clin. Genet.* **2014**, *85*, 578–582. [CrossRef] [PubMed]
76. Ness, S.L.; Ben-Yosef, T.; Bar-Lev, A.; Madeo, A.C.; Brewer, C.C.; Avraham, K.B.; Kornreich, R.; Desnick, R.J.; Willner, J.P.; Friedman, T.B.; et al. Genetic homogeneity and phenotypic variability among Ashkenazi Jews with Usher syndrome type III. *J. Med. Genet.* **2003**, *40*, 767–772. [CrossRef] [PubMed]
77. Joensuu, T.; Hamalainen, R.; Yuan, B.; Johnson, C.; Tegelberg, S.; Gasparini, P.; Zelante, L.; Pirvola, U.; Pakarinen, L.; Lehesjoki, A.E.; et al. Mutations in a novel gene with transmembrane domains underlie Usher syndrome type 3. *Am. J. Hum. Genet.* **2001**, *69*, 673–684. [CrossRef]
78. Kyttala, M.; Tallila, J.; Salonen, R.; Kopra, O.; Kohlschmidt, N.; Paavola-Sakki, P.; Peltonen, L.; Kestila, M. MKS1, encoding a component of the flagellar apparatus basal body proteome, is mutated in Meckel syndrome. *Nat. Genet.* **2006**, *38*, 155–157. [CrossRef]
79. Branham, K.; Schlegel, D.; Fahim, A.T.; Jayasundera, K.T. Genetic testing for inherited retinal degenerations: Triumphs and tribulations. *Am. J. Med. Genet. C Semin. Med. Genet.* **2020**, *184*, 571–577. [CrossRef]
80. Mansfield, B.C.; Yerxa, B.R.; Branham, K.H. Implementation of a registry and open access genetic testing program for inherited retinal diseases within a non-profit foundation. *Am. J. Med. Genet. C Semin. Med. Genet.* **2020**, *184*, 838–845. [CrossRef]
81. Stone, E.M.; Andorf, J.L.; Whitmore, S.S.; DeLuca, A.P.; Giacalone, J.C.; Streb, L.M.; Braun, T.A.; Mullins, R.F.; Scheetz, T.E.; Sheffield, V.C.; et al. Clinically Focused Molecular Investigation of 1000 Consecutive Families with Inherited Retinal Disease. *Ophthalmology* **2017**, *124*, 1314–1331. [CrossRef]
82. Haer-Wigman, L.; van Zelst-Stams, W.A.; Pfundt, R.; van den Born, L.I.; Klaver, C.C.; Verheij, J.B.; Hoyng, C.B.; Breuning, M.H.; Boon, C.J.; Kievit, A.J.; et al. Diagnostic exome sequencing in 266 Dutch patients with visual impairment. *Eur. J. Hum. Genet.* **2017**, *25*, 591–599. [CrossRef]

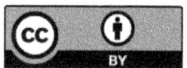

© 2020 by the authors. Licensee MDPI, Basel, Switzerland. This article is an open access article distributed under the terms and conditions of the Creative Commons Attribution (CC BY) license (http://creativecommons.org/licenses/by/4.0/).

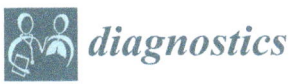

Review

Current Status of Genetic Counselling for Rare Diseases in Spain

Sara Álvaro-Sánchez [1], Irene Abreu-Rodríguez [2], Anna Abulí [3,4], Clara Serra-Juhé [5,6] and Maria del Carmen Garrido-Navas [1,7,*]

1. CONGEN, Genetic Counselling Services, C/Albahaca 4, 18006 Granada, Spain; info@congen.es
2. Genetics Service, Hospital del Mar Research Institute, IMIM, 08003 Barcelona, Spain; abreuire@gmail.com
3. Department of Clinical and Molecular Genetics, Hospital Vall d'Hebron, 08035 Barcelona, Spain; anna.abuli@gmail.com
4. Medicine Genetics Group, Vall d'Hebron Research Institute (VHIR), 08035 Barcelona, Spain
5. U705 CIBERER, Genetics Department, Hospital de la Santa Creu i Sant Pau, Universitat Autònoma de Barcelona, 08193 Barcelona, Spain; clara.seju@gmail.com
6. Centro de Investigación Biomédica en Red en Enfermedades Raras (CIBERER), 28029 Madrid, Spain
7. Genetics Department, Faculty of Sciences, Universidad de Granada, 18071 Granada, Spain
* Correspondence: carmen.garrido@genyo.es; Tel.: +34-958-071-196

Abstract: Genetic Counselling is essential for providing personalised information and support to patients with Rare Diseases (RD). Unlike most other developed countries, Spain does not recognize geneticists or genetic counsellors as healthcare professionals Thus, patients with RD face not only challenges associated with their own disease but also deal with lack of knowledge, uncertainty, and other psychosocial issues arising as a consequence of diagnostic delay. In this review, we highlight the importance of genetic counsellors in the field of RD as well as evaluate the current situation in which rare disease patients receive genetic services in Spain. We describe the main units and strategies at the national level assisting patients with RD and we conclude with a series of future perspectives and unmet needs that Spain should overcome to improve the management of patients with RD.

Keywords: genetic counselling; rare diseases; professional recognition

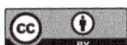

1. The Role of Genetic Counselling for Rare Diseases

Rare Diseases (RD) are defined as such by their low prevalence although their frequency changes depending on the continent. For instance, the European definition of a rare disease is that affecting less than 1/2000 individuals whereas, in the US, this frequency is even lower, affecting only 1/5000 individuals [1,2]. It is worth mentioning at this point the especially challenging cases of ultra-rare disorders, defined as those affecting less than 1/2,000,000 individuals [3]. It is mainly their uncommonness that makes RD so difficult to diagnose producing a diagnostic delay of more than 5 years [4]. Particularly, diagnosis of a rare disease was greater than 10 years in one in five patients in Spain according to a study by the *Spanish Federation of Rare Diseases* (FEDER) [5]. Furthermore, complexity of the symptoms, overlap of phenotypes and increasing number of gene/phenotype relationships extremely difficult diagnosis of these patients [6]. To overcome this complexity, different approaches using algorithms and artificial intelligence are being developed [7,8]. It is estimated that around 80% of RD have genetic aetiology [1,2,9,10] implying that genetic testing might be needed at some point of a patient's lifetime either to effectively reach a genetic diagnosis or to evaluate familial implications, such as recurrence risk of the disorder and identification of other family members at risk [11].

Diagnosis of RD (either clinical, genetic, or both) is not the end of the journey for patients and their families but rather the beginning. Once a genetic diagnosis is achieved, patients need support to understand not only the implications of this verdict and the real meaning of carrying a genetic abnormality but also, and sometimes more importantly, to grief and to adapt to all psychosocial aspects involved [9,12,13]. Furthermore, genetics is shared among the family having implications for the closer relatives accounting for their risk of carrying a disease-causing variant [14]. These disease-causing genetic changes might be passed from one generation to the next, although for rare disorders they also might occur de novo, with the patient being the first affected person in the family [15–17]. Inheritance of these variants increases the risk of passing the disease to the next generation, and thus, some relatives who might be carriers will need support, help and guidance to manage and plan a future pregnancy trying to reduce risks of having an affected child [18,19]. However, there are still challenges for the application of cascade genetic testing, such as cost, cultural and social issues, communication (including reduced access to genetic counsellors) and logistic issues (including lack of genetic specialists or the geographical location). For example, living in a different region than the patient testing positive might make family screening of relatives difficult and unequal access to genetics services will also complicate cascade testing [13,14,20]. Furthermore, for some genetic diseases, inheritance patterns and mechanisms of disease are complex and require genetic specialists enriched with communication skills to help families understand the genetic cause and implications for the family [21].

From the patients' (and their families') perspective, having a rare disease encompasses a series of milestones that need to be accomplished to reach a final diagnosis and satisfactory disease management. First of all, when a child is born with a rare disease, the roles of the whole family are turned upside down because they now need to cope with a variety of symptoms together with many social, emotional and economical challenges [10,22]. Secondly, the unceasing visits to a long list of specialists not only affects the whole family psychologically and emotionally but also might, in some cases, be detrimental for the diagnosis [23,24]. Since not all specialists work within the same team/setting, clinical information from one specialty might not be correctly (or timely) communicated to others producing a delay in the diagnosis. This is especially important in Spain that is a fragmented country with 17 autonomous regions. Even though economically the Spanish National Health System (SNS) is centralized, access to medical records from different autonomous regions is sometimes challenging, having 15/17 of them access to electronic medical records [25]. Subsequently, parents usually share their situation with other parents and search on the Internet [26] and social media [27] to finally approach some patients with similar clinical characteristics or patient organizations providing support and information [28]. At some point, genetic testing is performed (may be ordered by a clinician with a suspicion of a disease that needs confirmation or as a suggestion from a patient's advocacy group that shares some knowledge with the parents). More than one genetic testing might be needed to reach a genetic diagnosis and genetic testing will not always be the answer for the parents or the patient [23]; however, there is no doubt that at this point of the journey, patients and their families have already struggled a lot with the healthcare system and received very little (if any) support from it.

Genetic Counselling, either provided by clinical geneticists or genetic counsellors is the communicative process for helping people understand the implications of a genetic variant in their life and health as well as adapting to the medical, psychological and familial consequences of genetic disease [29,30]. The role of a genetic counsellor involves many tasks (see Supplementary Table S1 for core competencies) that are expected to accomplish in order to ensure an individual has enough personalized information and support to be able to deal not only with their genetic disease as well as to make informed decisions [31–33]. Ideally, from the very first visit to a specialist, patients should receive support from a genetic counsellor (in coordination with multidisciplinary genetics units) being able to dig around the clinical and family data and offer an adequate clinical letter to patients. This might help identification of potential inheritance patterns, but more importantly, will assist families to cope with difficulties along the way by empowering them with knowledge and referring them to specialists (neurologist, ophthalmologist, nephrologist, social services, etc.) for their follow-up [12,34]. In fact, a study evaluating the economic impact of using genomic sequencing to diagnose RD highlighted that parents find genetic counsellors to be a valuable resource facilitating complex decisions [11] and some others highlight the cost-effectiveness of providing Genetic Counselling [35,36]. Finally, it is worth mentioning the harm produced when no appropriate Genetic Counselling is provided to RD patients, impacting at many levels [37]. This negative outcome might be traduced into psychosocial effects, inappropriate genetic tests, misinterpretation of results, or even inadequate disease management that consequently bring distress and discomfort to patients [38]. Despite all of this, the state of this profession globally varies widely among continents and even countries [39].

Unfortunately, the situation is particularly difficult in Spain which is, at the moment, the only European country not legally recognizing clinical geneticists as healthcare professionals and thus impeding patients to have access to these specialists [30]. Reaching legal recognition will have a profound impact not only on clinical geneticists (as they will be considered part of the healthcare community, facilitating access to promotion, specific training, equality on the salary and conditions, etc.) but also will tremendously impact patients. Once clinical geneticists are recognized as part of the healthcare team, referral to those specialists will be easier, faster, and more efficient so patients with RD will benefit from receiving more integrative clinical supervision.

Due to this circumstance, each hospital delivers genetic services in a unique way, existing as highly specialized centres or others with scarce or even absence of this service. The main objective of this paper was to evaluate the current state of Genetic Counselling in Spain particularly focusing on the management of RD. To do so, we will describe the main units and strategies at the national level aiding patients with RD and we will highlight the main future trends and unmet needs that Spain needs to overcome to improve the management of patients with RD.

2. Genetic Services (Including Genetic Counselling) for Rare Diseases in Spain

Despite the lack of recognition in Spain of Clinical Genetics as a healthcare specialty, the current legislation for biomedical research states that any specialist with sufficient genetics background and communication skills can provide Genetic Counselling [40]. According to the current records, specific Spanish hospitals provided Genetic Counselling since the 1970s. As recommended by the European Society for Medical Oncology (ESMO) and the American Society of Clinical Oncology (ASCO), an oncologist should be able to identify inheritance patterns predisposing to hereditary cancers [41] and this statement has driven an improper use of Genetic Counselling in oncological settings. Thus, historically, Genetic Counselling Units in Spain primarily were associated with Cancer Genetic Counselling. In fact, the Spanish Society of Medical Oncology (SEOM) has in its website (https://seom.org/informacion-sobre-el-cancer/consejo-genetico/unidades-consejo-genetico (accessed on 5 December 2021) an updated list of specialized centres providing Genetic Counselling in the country (most of them providing Genetic Counselling in the oncological field but also in other areas, such as reproduction, neurology or cardiology among others). According to the most updated version, Spain counts with 85 public and 20 private units which include genetic counselling among their services, as well as 49 public and 27 private laboratories dedicated mainly to performing genetic studies but most of which have specialists offering Genetic Counselling (in this case mainly focussed to the specialists ordering the tests) (Figure 1). However, in most cases, professionals providing Genetic Counselling do not have specific training. In fact, it is important to highlight that there are only 29 European registered genetic counsellors in Spain, which contrasts with the number of genetic services. The realization that genetics has a strong impact not only on preventing but also treating cancer has led to the implementation of genetic studies, such as multi-gene panels [42] to identify high-risk individuals allowing family screening studies. Furthermore, the increasing use of genetic variants identification (either in the tumour itself or at the circulating level) for targeted treatments in cancer [2,43] supports the implementation of Genetic Counselling in this area. However, no such effort has been made regarding other genetic diseases, such as RD to clearly assess the advantages of implementing Genetic Counselling to improve current care provided to affected patients and their families in Spain.

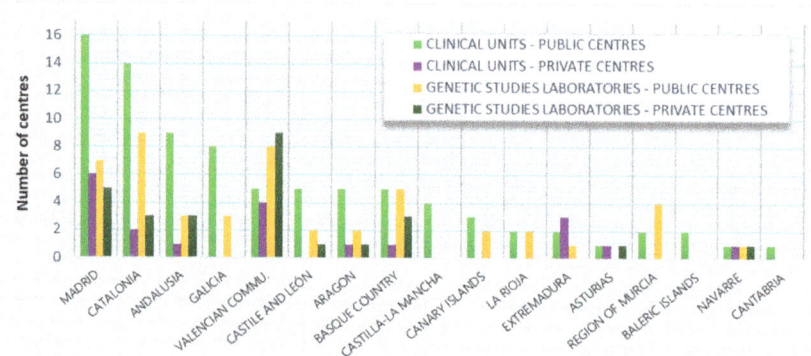

Figure 1. Number of public and private centres in Spain providing Genetic Counselling services by region. Source: Spanish Society of Medical Oncology (SEOM), 2021.

Another clinical area being historically related to Genetic Counselling with a special interest for RD is reproductive medicine. According to the *European Society of Human Genetics* (ESHG) and the *European Society of Human Reproduction and Embryology* (ESHRE), Genetic Counselling should always be provided to any patient showing infertility as well as for prenatal genetic diagnosis (PND) [44]. In fact, genetic services in the area of reproductive medicine in Spain have been largely provided by gynaecologists and they ordered genetic tests after positive prenatal screening or upon advanced maternal age to confirm the presence of chromosomal anomalies [45] without the inclusion of a genetic specialist in the process. With the implementation of carrier screening tests [19], a gynaecologist can also evaluate the risk of a couple (or even gamete donors) of carrying genetic variants responsible for autosomal recessive or an X-linked genetic disease. Thus, they might be able to reduce the risks of having an affected child with diseases, such as cystic fibrosis [46] or X-fragile by the use of preimplantation genetic diagnosis (PGD) [47]. Also, prenatal genetic testing (either non-invasive as a screening method or invasive as a diagnostic tool) might allow early detection of genetic abnormalities. Finally, in neonatal care, newborn screening can also reduce diagnosis time for a genetic disease allowing rapid actions to be taken [18,24]. Thus, as methodology and genetic information become more complex and options in the reproductive field are increasing, other professionals, such as biologists, embryologists, clinical geneticists, genetic counsellors, and clinical laboratory geneticists need also to be involved from a clinical care perspective. For example, regarding foetal anomalies that eventually led to pregnancy termination, a recent study evaluated the importance of providing personalized counselling and support facilitating the grieving process [48] and in this case, it was a duty of obstetric-gynaecologic nurses, mainly.

Regardless of the efforts described above and even though Genetic Counselling is well defined in the Spanish law for Biomedical Research [40], recognition of clinical geneticists, genetic counsellors and clinical laboratory geneticists as healthcare specialists is still an unsatisfied demand. Although with different competencies for each specialty (see Supplementary Table S2), they all perform complementary tasks that eventually improve patient management. Whereas one professional profile is focused on clinical diagnosis (clinical geneticist), another is centred on emotional support to the patient (genetic counsellor) and the third one is responsible for providing adequate tools to perform genetic testing (laboratory geneticist). Several attempts tried to develop a certification for the training of these professionals although there is not a national strategy that establishes a roadmap for this educational path. For example, the Spanish Association for Human Genetics (AEGH) developed an accreditation system open to graduates in medicine, biology, biochemistry, pharmacy and chemistry [49]. Regarding Master's education, the University Pompeu Fabra successfully achieved four graduations for a master's degree training future genetic counsellors. Students from the first promotion of this Master founded the Spanish Association of Genetic Counselling (SEAGen) creating awareness about the need for professionalization. More recently (2019–2021) the Autonomous University of Barcelona also promoted an MSc in Healthcare Genetics with three paths: clinical genetics, clinical laboratory genetics and Genetic Counselling. Currently, the only itinerary accredited by the European Board of Medical Genetics (EBMG) is the one for Genetic Counselling. However, none of these efforts have been legally recognized as official training and professionals specialized in Medical Genetics (Clinical Geneticists, Genetic Counsellors and Clinical laboratory Geneticists) still have difficult access to work as healthcare specialists in Spain [30,34], with the detriment that this causes to patients.

In contrast with the lack of specific Genetic Counselling Services for RD in Spain, highly specialized multidisciplinary units and/or centres (CSUR, *Reference Centres, Services and Units*) for particular diseases (some of them of low prevalence) are being created since 2008. Currently, there are 71 specific disease groups that are covered by up to 297 CSUR in the country. However, one of the main objectives of these units is not necessarily medical assistance but to become a reference contact for disease management strategies definition as well as support for both, patients and clinicians dealing with a particular disease [50]. In fact, these centres or units belong to public hospitals that agglutinate a series of clinical specialists who are experts in specific disease groups (but they are not a genetic service itself). Clinicians join creating multidisciplinary groups to serve as reference centres for the whole country, but as genetic counsellors are not usually incorporated in these groups, patients lack this service. Clinicians in these CSUR might be specialized in specific methodologies and are able to define therapeutic strategies or function as consultants for the general practitioner of the patients with these pathologies but do not necessarily deal with the patient directly offering genetic counselling. Regarding these CSUR, there are three main regions in Spain accumulating most of these centres: Catalonia (97/297), Madrid (89/297) and Andalusia (39/297) (Figure 2), implying that most patients need to move from their region to a different one to receive specialized disease management. Despite being specialized in some genetic diseases, this CSUR does not provide Genetic Counselling as a service, neither do other centres offering genetic testing to their patients.

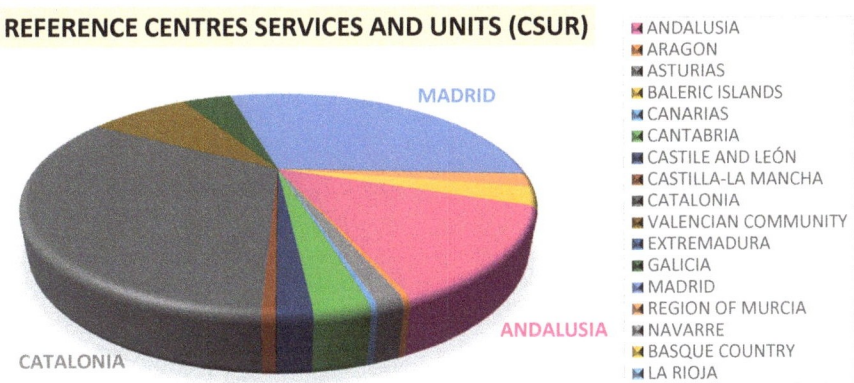

Figure 2. CSUR distribution. Most of these *Reference Centres, Services* and *Units* (CSUR) are in the regions of Catalonia, Madrid, and Andalusia. Source: Listado CSUR, 2021.

Since the establishment of the first 36 CSUR in 2008, there has been a great expansion of these centres, reaching a total of 297 in 2021 (Figure 3). In addition, as new CSURs are established, the range of RD to which they give support is rising (see list of https://www.mscbs.gob.es/profesionales/CentrosDeReferencia/docs/ListaCSUR.pdf) CSURs (accessed on 5 December 2021). Of the 71 groups of diseases, the most prevalent are those treating childhood eye disorders, congenital and/or family heart diseases, metabolic and neuromuscular diseases, neurocutaneous disorders, epidermolysis bullosa, rare hereditary anaemias and congenital coagulopathies, among others. These CSUR allow continuous patient care independently of their age. Currently, there are 74 paediatric CSUR, 109 specialized in adult diseases and 114 attending both children and adults.

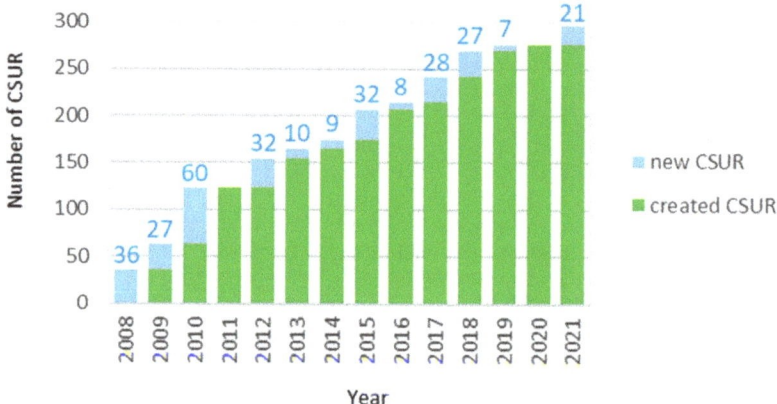

Figure 3. Number of *Reference Centres, Services* and *Units* (CSUR) along the time. Source: Listado CSUR, 2021.

Contrarily to the difficulties encountered for the recognition of the profession that impedes in many cases access to these specialists, Spain has made a significant effort for several years to create national strategies and documents supporting patients with RD.

One example is a compendium created in conjunction with the *Institute for Research of Rare Diseases* (IIER) and the *Institute of Health Carlos III* (ISCIII) summarizing the main RD by organs and giving a brief introduction about orphan drugs, social services and other aspects of interest [51]. Also, since 2008 collaboration between National Alliances and EURORDIS implemented the National Plans and Strategies for RD with several joint actions to integrate policy measures [3,52]. In 2011 the ISCIII and the *Rare Diseases Network Biomedical Research Consortium* (CIBERER) created a national registry for patients with RD to be used in research [53]. In fact, lots of investments and actions were made to promote research in the RD field, neglecting improvements in the clinical, daily life of patients that need continuous support and advice regarding their disease. Collaborations between research centres and hospitals allowed concentrating efforts in particular diseases, such as neuromuscular [54,55], retinal [56,57] and cardiovascular [58] rare diseases among others, to provide the most comprehensive management, including Genetic Counselling, although this effort should be extended to ideally all RD.

3. Current Needs and Future Directions of Genetic Counselling for Rare Diseases

The so-called "diagnostic odyssey" is the process during which most patients with a rare disease and their families try to find the cause, name, prognostic and treatment of their disease [20,59]. This long journey usually begins with the first symptoms and hopefully (but not always) ends a few years later, with the diagnosis of the disease [9]. The future of RD envisions a faster diagnosis thanks to high-throughput Next Generation Sequencing (NGS) technologies as well as artificial intelligence [60] with the intention of helping clinicians to shorten the time to diagnosis. Several studies demonstrate the utility of whole-exome (WES) [61,62] or whole-genome (WGS) [63,64] sequencing, as well as including other omics, such as RNA-seq or methylation profiles, increasing the diagnostic yield particularly on undiagnosed individuals with a suspected genetic condition [65,66]. Nevertheless, the improvement in diagnostic efficiency comes with several shortcomings, such as cost and time/analysis load [24,67] that are expected to be solved in the near future as technology improves in efficiency. However, it is important to recognise diagnostic limitations for each technology and it is at this point at which genetic (or genomic) counsellors provide an added value. In addition, there are other limitations from the ethical point of view that might have a stronger impact on patients and are not so easy to tackle. Some of these are identification and interpretation of variants of uncertain significance (VUS), secondary and incidental findings, or equal access to genetic information, among others [66,68,69]. Furthermore, the fact that some patients have multiple disease-causing variants (polygenic diseases) and also several genetic diagnoses complicate the interpretation of genetic data, and thus, require expert geneticists (all three specialties: clinical geneticists, genetic counsellors and clinical laboratory geneticists) to provide enough information and support to patients [34,70].

Following the recommendations of the American College of Medical Genetics (ACMG) and the European Board of Medical Genetics (EBMG), three Spanish scientific societies (AEGH, SEQC-ML and SEOM) elaborated a consensus document for the implementation of NGS multigene panels in the evaluation of hereditary cancer predisposition in which Genetic Counselling takes place both before and after genetic testing [71]. However, no such document is produced specifically for RD, and thus, not all patients undergoing a genetic test for diagnostic purposes receive a Genetic Counselling pre-test and/or post-test session. In fact, this service should be of greater importance when accounting for WES/WGS as the possibility of identifying secondary findings and/or VUS is greater [65,66,72,73]

Shortening the diagnostic process and providing adequate management to patients with a rare disease in Spain necessarily implies a series of changes both in the SNS and in the Spanish society. The 2014 update of the Strategy for Rare Diseases of the Spanish National Health System proposed a series of Action Strategies for the prevention and early detection of RD [74]. One of them claims that patients should have better access to diagnostic tests and Genetic Counselling services. In fact, most patients in Spain are unable to reach an early diagnosis mainly due to inadequate approach as a consequence of a deficiency in the training of clinicians as specialized training for Clinical Genetics does not exist [5,29]. This, together with the lack of recognition of genetic counsellors to support patients, is translated into inappropriate genetic tests lengthening the diagnostic process, increasing clinical expenses, and adding anxiety to patients. Another of the needs highlighted in this strategy is to provide continuous training to specialists who make up these multidisciplinary teams, with emphasis on Primary Care professionals. Particularly, in the context of Primary Care, an online tool (DICE-APER protocol) was developed to speed up the diagnosis of RD [74,75]. However, many patients refer to the lack of knowledge about RD by the general practitioner taking care of them [76]. This situation is shown in the studies by Ramalle-Gómara et al. and Bueno et al. in which even clinicians are aware of the lack of knowledge and specific training they have regarding RD [59,77]. In addition, adequate training of these specialists will improve the emotional state and well-being of patients and their families, as many perceive a feeling of abandonment that forces them to turn to patient organizations for support [78].

4. Conclusions

The main goal of this paper was to provide a comprehensive overview of the current situation of Genetic Counselling in Spain, particularly focussed on RD. To introduce the matter, we started by describing the importance of providing Genetic Counselling to patients with RD. Then, we continued by describing the main genetic services providing Genetic Counselling in Spain with special interest to those highly specialized for RD. We also made a brief description of some of the research initiatives in which Spain is involved regarding RD and we finished by highlighting some of the current needs and future directions in Genetic Counselling for RD.

We emphasised that the current situation of Genetic Counselling for RD in Spain is jeopardised by the lack of recognition of Clinical Genetics as a healthcare specialty within the SNS. This must include three professional profiles: clinical genetics, genetic counselling, and clinical laboratory genetics. Currently, there are more than 3 million people in Spain affected by a rare disease and the implementation of next generation sequencing technologies is improving diagnostic yield. By understanding this reality, we ought to take advantage of these technologies to improve patient management. However, it is necessary to solve the lack of access to specialized professionals who are capable of analysing and interpreting this information. Thus, it is necessary to create multidisciplinary teams providing integrative solutions for the needs of patients with RD. Ideally, these clinical genetics services would include a team of specialist physicians, nurses, psychologists, as well as new professional profiles, such as bioinformatics.

Clinical guidelines and management strategies must be implemented at the national level allowing better coordination between different centres to make society/professionals aware of the existence of CSURs and to create new ones capable of correctly managing patients regardless of their residence location. Furthermore, the incorporation of specialists providing Genetic Counselling into multidisciplinary groups dealing with RD patients is essential to provide personal and familial information and support accompanying them throughout this uncertain and unpredictable journey. Furthermore, the actualization of the current registries at the national level to estimate the prevalence of RD, to understand their distribution is needed to develop appropriate action strategies.

Finally, updated and continuous training of health professionals on the new advances for diagnosis and treatment of RD will be necessary to guarantee equal access of patients to quality health services, thus improving the management of their disease and consequently, improving their quality of life.

Supplementary Materials: The following are available online at https://www.mdpi.com/article/10.3390/diagnostics11122320/s1. Table S1. Core competences of Genetic Counsellors adapted from the European Board of Medical Genetics (EBMG) recommendations; Table S2. Summary of the main tasks performed by the different healthcare professionals that should be involved in RD patients' management.

Author Contributions: All authors have read and agreed to the published version of the manuscript.

Funding: This research received no external funding.

Institutional Review Board Statement: Not applicable.

Informed Consent Statement: Not applicable.

Data Availability Statement: Data from this review was extracted from the following links: https://seom.org/informacion-sobre-el-cancer/consejo-genetico/unidades-consejo-genetico (accessed on 5 December 2021); https://www.mscbs.gob.es/profesionales/CentrosDeReferencia/docs/ListaCSUR.pdf (accessed on 5 December 2021).

Conflicts of Interest: The authors declare no conflict of interest.

References

1. Nguengang Wakap, S.; Lambert, D.M.; Olry, A.; Rodwell, C.; Gueydan, C.; Lanneau, V.; Murphy, D.; Le Cam, Y.; Rath, A. Estimating cumulative point prevalence of rare diseases: Analysis of the Orphanet database. *Eur. J. Hum. Genet.* **2020**, *28*, 165–173. [CrossRef] [PubMed]
2. Brittain, H.K.; Scott, R.; Thomas, E. The rise of the genome and personalised medicine. *Clin. Med. J. R. Coll. Physicians Lond.* **2017**, *17*, 545–551. [CrossRef]
3. Hennekam, R.C.M. Care for patients with ultra-rare disorders. *Eur. J. Med. Genet.* **2011**, *54*, 220–224. [CrossRef] [PubMed]
4. Macnamara, E.F.; Schoch, K.; Kelley, E.G.; Fieg, E.; Brokamp, E.; Signer, R.; LeBlanc, K.; McConkie-Rosell, A.; Palmer, C.G.S. Cases from the Undiagnosed Diseases Network: The continued value of counseling skills in a new genomic era. *J. Genet. Couns.* **2019**, *28*, 194–201. [CrossRef]

5. Huete, A.; Díaz, E. FEDER Estudio sobre situación de necesidades Sociosanitarias de las personas con Enfermedades Raras en España. Estudio ENSERio. Available online: Enfermedades-raras.org/images/stories/documentos/Estudio_ENSERio.pdf (accessed on 5 December 2021).
6. Groza, T.; Köhler, S.; Moldenhauer, D.; Vasilevsky, N.; Baynam, G.; Zemojtel, T.; Schriml, L.M.; Kibbe, W.A.; Schofield, P.N.; Beck, T.; et al. The Human Phenotype Ontology: Semantic Unification of Common and Rare Disease. *Am. J. Hum. Genet.* **2015**, *97*, 111–124. [CrossRef] [PubMed]
7. Faviez, C.; Chen, X.; Garcelon, N.; Neuraz, A.; Knebelmann, B.; Salomon, R.; Lyonnet, S.; Saunier, S.; Burgun, A. Diagnosis support systems for rare diseases: A scoping review. *Orphanet J. Rare Dis.* **2020**, *15*, 94. [CrossRef]
8. Yang, J.; Dong, C.; Duan, H.; Shu, Q.; Li, H. RDmap: A map for exploring rare diseases. *Orphanet J. Rare Dis.* **2021**, *16*, 101. [CrossRef] [PubMed]
9. Merker, V.L.; Plotkin, S.R.; Charns, M.P.; Meterko, M.; Jordan, J.T.; Elwy, A.R. Effective provider-patient communication of a rare disease diagnosis: A qualitative study of people diagnosed with schwannomatosis. *Patient Educ. Couns.* **2021**, *104*, 808–814. [CrossRef]
10. Dos Santos Luz, G.; Da Silva, M.R.S.; De Montigny, F. Rare diseases: Diagnostic and therapeutic journey of the families of affected people. *ACTA Paul. Enferm.* **2015**, *28*, 395–400. [CrossRef]
11. Pollard, S.; Weymann, D.; Dunne, J.; Mayanloo, F.; Buckell, J.; Buchanan, J.; Wordsworth, S.; Friedman, J.M.; Stockler-Ipsiroglu, S.; Dragojlovic, N.; et al. Toward the diagnosis of rare childhood genetic diseases: What do parents value most? *Eur. J. Hum. Genet.* **2021**, *29*, 1491–1501. [CrossRef]
12. Helm, B.M. Exploring the Genetic Counselor's Role in Facilitating Meaning-Making: Rare Disease Diagnoses. *J. Genet. Couns.* **2015**, *24*, 205–212. [CrossRef]
13. Ormondroyd, E.; Mackley, M.P.; Blair, E.; Craft, J.; Knight, J.C.; Taylor, J.; Taylor, J.C.; Wilkie, A.O.M.; Watkins, H. Insights from early experience of a Rare Disease Genomic Medicine Multidisciplinary Team: A qualitative study. *Eur. J. Hum. Genet.* **2017**, *25*, 680–686. [CrossRef]
14. Germain, D.P.; Moiseev, S.; Suárez-Obando, F.; Al Ismaili, F.; Al Khawaja, H.; Altarescu, G.; Barreto, F.C.; Haddoum, F.; Hadipour, F.; Maksimova, I.; et al. The benefits and challenges of family genetic testing in rare genetic diseases—Lessons from Fabry disease. *Mol. Genet. Genom. Med.* **2021**, *9*, e1666. [CrossRef] [PubMed]
15. Veltman, J.A.; Brunner, H.G. De novo mutations in human genetic disease. *Nat. Rev. Genet.* **2012**, *13*, 565–575. [CrossRef] [PubMed]
16. Alonso-Gonzalez, A.; Rodriguez-Fontenla, C.; Carracedo, A. De novo Mutations (DNMs) in Autism Spectrum Disorder (ASD): Pathway and Network Analysis. *Front. Genet.* **2018**, *9*, 406. [CrossRef]
17. Boycott, K.M.; Vanstone, M.R.; Bulman, D.E.; MacKenzie, A.E. Rare-disease genetics in the era of next-generation sequencing: Discovery to translation. *Nat. Rev. Genet.* **2013**, *14*, 681–691. [CrossRef]
18. Cornel, M.C.; Rigter, T.; Jansen, M.E.; Henneman, L. Neonatal and carrier screening for rare diseases: How innovation challenges screening criteria worldwide. *J. Community Genet.* **2020**, *12*, 257–265. [CrossRef]
19. Abulí, A.; Boada, M.; Rodríguez-Santiago, B.; Coroleu, B.; Veiga, A.; Armengol, L.; Barri, P.N.; Pérez-Jurado, L.A.; Estivill, X. NGS-Based Assay for the Identification of Individuals Carrying Recessive Genetic Mutations in Reproductive Medicine. *Hum. Mutat.* **2016**, *37*, 516–523. [CrossRef] [PubMed]
20. Qian, E.; Thong, M.-K.; Flodman, P.; Gargus, J. A comparative study of patients' perceptions of genetic and genomic medicine services in California and Malaysia. *J. Community Genet.* **2019**, *10*, 351–361. [CrossRef]
21. Eggermann, T. Prenatal Detection of Uniparental Disomies (UPD): Intended and Incidental Finding in the Era of Next Generation Genomics. *Genes* **2020**, *11*, 1454. [CrossRef]
22. Pelentsov, L.J.; Fielder, A.L.; Laws, T.A.; Esterman, A.J. The supportive care needs of parents with a child with a rare disease: Results of an online survey. *BMC Fam. Pract.* **2016**, *17*, 88. [CrossRef]
23. Hartley, T.; Lemire, G.; Kernohan, K.D.; Howley, H.E.; Adams, D.R.; Boycott, K.M. New Diagnostic Approaches for Undiagnosed Rare Genetic Diseases. *Annu. Rev. Genom. Hum. Genet.* **2020**, *21*, 351–372. [CrossRef]
24. Garcia-Herrero, S.; Simon, B.; Garcia-Planells, J. The Reproductive Journey in the Genomic Era: From Preconception to Childhood. *Genes* **2020**, *11*, 1521. [CrossRef]
25. Bernal, E.; Sandra, D.; Juan, G.-A.; Fernando, O.; Sánchez Martínez, I.; Ramón, J.; Luz, R.; Peña-Longobardo, M.; Ridao-López, M.; Hernández-Quevedo, C. Spain Health system review. *Health Syst. Transit.* **2018**, *20*, 1–179.
26. Honor, N.; Tracey, C.; Begley, T.; King, C.; Lynch, A.M. Internet Use by Parents of Children with Rare Conditions: Findings from a Study on Parents' Web Information Needs. *J. Med. Internet. Res.* **2017**, *19*, e51. [CrossRef]
27. Pemmaraju, N.; Utengen, A.; Gupta, V.; Kiladjian, J.J.; Mesa, R.; Thompson, M.A. Rare Cancers and Social Media: Analysis of Twitter Metrics in the First 2 Years of a Rare-Disease Community for Myeloproliferative Neoplasms on Social Media—#MPNSM. *Curr. Hematol. Malig. Rep.* **2017**, *12*, 598–604.
28. Pinto, D.; Martin, D.; Chenhall, R. The involvement of patient organisations in rare disease research: A mixed methods study in Australia. *Orphanet J. Rare Dis.* **2016**, *11*, 2. [CrossRef]
29. López-Fernández, A.; Serra-Juhé, C.; Balmaña, J.; Tizzano, E.F. Genetic counsellors in a multidisciplinary model of clinical genetics and hereditary cancer. *Med. Clín. (Engl. Ed.)* **2020**, *155*, 77–81. [CrossRef]

30. Abacan, M.; Alsubaie, L.; Barlow-Stewart, K.; Caanen, B.; Cordier, C.; Courtney, E.; Davoine, E.; Edwards, J.; Elackatt, N.; Gardiner, K.; et al. The Global State of the Genetic Counseling Profession. *Eur. J. Hum. Genet.* **2019**, *27*, 183–197. [CrossRef] [PubMed]
31. Ayres, S.; Gallacher, L.; Stark, Z.; Brett, G.R. Genetic counseling in pediatric acute care: Reflections on ultra-rapid genomic diagnoses in neonates. *J. Genet. Couns.* **2019**, *28*, 273–282. [CrossRef] [PubMed]
32. Peron, A.; Au, K.S.; Northrup, H. Genetics, genomics, and genotype–phenotype correlations of TSC: Insights for clinical practice. *Am. J. Med. Genet. Part C Semin. Med. Genet.* **2018**, *178*, 281–290. [CrossRef] [PubMed]
33. Bamshad, M.J.; Magoulas, P.L.; Dent, K.M. Genetic counselors on the frontline of precision health. *Am. J. Med. Genet. Part C Semin. Med. Genet.* **2018**, *178*, 5–9. [CrossRef]
34. Cordier, C.; McAllister, M.; Serra-Juhe, C.; Bengoa, J.; Pasalodos, S.; Bjornevoll, I.; Feroce, I.; Moldovan, R.; Paneque, M.; Lambert, D. The recognition of the profession of Genetic Counsellors in Europe. *Eur. J. Hum. Genet.* **2018**, *26*, 1719–1720. [CrossRef] [PubMed]
35. Payne, K.; Eden, M. Measuring the economic value of genetic counselling. *Eur. J. Med. Genet.* **2019**, *62*, 385–389. [CrossRef] [PubMed]
36. Willcocks, D.; Soulodre, C.; Zierler, A.; Cowan, K.; Smitko, E.; Schwarz, K.; Mcdowell, S.; Ng, V.; Mitchell, A.; Lang, A.; et al. Genome-Wide Sequencing for Unexplained Developmental Disabilities or Multiple Congenital Anomalies: A Health Technology Assessment. *Ont. Health Technol. Assess. Ser.* **2020**, *20*, 1–178.
37. Raspa, M.; Moultrie, R.; Toth, D.; Haque, S.N. Barriers and Facilitators to Genetic Service Delivery Models: Scoping Review. *Interact. J. Med. Res.* **2021**, *10*, e23523. [CrossRef]
38. Bensend, T.A.; Veach, P.M.C.; Niendorf, K.B. What's the Harm? Genetic Counselor Perceptions of Adverse Effects of Genetics Service Provision by Non-Genetics Professionals. *J. Genet. Couns.* **2014**, *23*, 48–63. [CrossRef]
39. Ormond, K.E.; Laurino, M.Y.; Barlow-Stewart, K.; Wessels, T.M.; Macaulay, S.; Austin, J.; Middleton, A. Genetic counseling globally: Where are we now? *Am. J. Med. Genet. Part C Semin. Med. Genet.* **2018**, *178*, 98–107. [CrossRef]
40. BOE.es. BOE-A-2007-12945 Ley 14/2007, de 3 de Julio, de Investigación Biomédica. 2007. Available online: https://www.boe.es/buscar/act.php?id=BOE-A-2007-12945&p=20110602&tn=2 (accessed on 5 December 2021).
41. Dittrich, C.; Kosty, M.; Jezdic, S.; Pyle, D.; Berardi, R.; Bergh, J.; El-Saghir, N.; Lotz, J.-P.; Österlund, P.; Pavlidis, N.; et al. ESMO/ASCO Recommendations for a Global Curriculum in Medical Oncology Edition 2016. *ESMO Open* **2016**, *1*, 97. [CrossRef]
42. Richardson, M.; Min, H.J.; Hong, Q.; Compton, K.; Mung, S.W.; Lohn, Z.; Nuk, J.; McCullum, M.; Portigal-Todd, C.; Karsan, A.; et al. Oncology Clinic-Based Hereditary Cancer Genetic Testing in a Population-Based Health Care System. *Cancers* **2020**, *12*, 338. [CrossRef]
43. Morganti, S.; Tarantino, P.; Ferraro, E.; D'Amico, P.; Duso, B.A.; Curigliano, G. Next generation sequencing (NGS): A revolutionary technology in pharmacogenomics and personalized medicine in cancer. In *Advances in Experimental Medicine and Biology*; Springer: Cham, Switzerland, 2019; Volume 1168, pp. 9–30.
44. Harper, J.; Geraedts, J.; Borry, P.; Cornel, M.C.; Dondorp, W.J.; Gianaroli, L.; Harton, G.; Milachich, T.; Kääriäinen, H.; Liebaers, I.; et al. Current issues in medically assisted reproduction and genetics in Europe: Research, clinical practice, ethics, legal issues and policy. *Hum. Reprod.* **2014**, *29*, 1603–1609. [CrossRef] [PubMed]
45. Mademont-Soler, I.; Morales, C.; Clusellas, N.; Soler, A.; Sánchez, A. Prenatal cytogenetic diagnosis in Spain: Analysis and evaluation of the results obtained from amniotic fluid samples during the last decade. *Eur. J. Obstet. Gynecol. Reprod. Biol.* **2011**, *157*, 156–160. [CrossRef] [PubMed]
46. Bienvenu, T.; Lopez, M.; Girodon, E. Molecular Diagnosis and Genetic Counseling of Cystic Fibrosis and Related Disorders: New Challenges. *Genes* **2020**, *11*, 619. [CrossRef] [PubMed]
47. Alfaro Arenas, R.; Rosell Andreo, J.; Heine Suñer, D.; Pía Cordero, M.; Fernández Yagüe, C.; Cerdá, C.; Amengual, M.; Lladó, M.; de Juan, E.P.; Mariscal, T.; et al. Fragile X syndrome screening in pregnant women and women planning pregnancy shows a remarkably high FMR1 premutation prevalence in the Balearic Islands. *Am. J. Med. Genet. Part B Neuropsychiatr. Genet.* **2016**, *171*, 1023–1031. [CrossRef]
48. Atienza-Carrasco, J.; Linares-Abad, M.; Padilla-Ruiz, M.; Morales-Gil, I.M. Experiences and outcomes following diagnosis of congenital foetal anomaly and medical termination of pregnancy: A phenomenological study. *J. Clin. Nurs.* **2020**, *29*, 1220–1237. [CrossRef] [PubMed]
49. Abad-Perotín, R.; Barco, Á.A.-D.; Silva-Mato, A. A Survey of Ethical and Professional Challenges Experienced by Spanish Health-Care Professionals that Provide Genetic Counseling Services. *J. Genet. Couns.* **2012**, *21*, 85–100. [CrossRef] [PubMed]
50. BOE.es. BOE-A-2006-19626 Real Decreto 1302/2006, de 10 de Noviembre. Por el que se Establecen las BASES del procedimiento para la Designación y Acreditación de los Centros, Servicios y Unidades de Referencia del Sistema Nacional de Salud. 2006. Available online: https://www.boe.es/buscar/doc.php?id=BOE-A-2006-19626 (accessed on 5 December 2021).
51. Izquierdo Martínez, M.; Avellaneda Fernandez, A. *Enfermedades Raras un Enfoque Práctico*; ISCIII: Madrid, Spain, 2004; ISBN 8495463210.
52. EURORDIS. The Voice of Rare Disease Patients in Europe. Available online: https://www.eurordis.org/nationalplans/spain (accessed on 31 August 2021).
53. ISCIII. RPER v.17.0. Available online: https://registroraras.isciii.es/Comun/Inicio.aspx (accessed on 26 August 2021).

54. Martorell, L.; Cobo, A.M.; Baiget, M.; Naudó, M.; Poza, J.J.; Parra, J. Prenatal diagnosis in myotonic dystrophy type 1. Thirteen years of experience: Implications for reproductive counselling in DM1 families. *Prenat. Diagn.* **2007**, *27*, 68–72. [CrossRef]
55. Yubero, D.; Benito, D.N.; Pijuan, J.; Armstrong, J.; Martorell, L.; Fernàndez, G.; Maynou, J.; Jou, C.; Roldan, M.; Ortez, C.; et al. The Increasing Impact of Translational Research in the Molecular Diagnostics of Neuromuscular Diseases. *Int. J. Mol. Sci.* **2021**, *22*, 4274. [CrossRef]
56. Blanco-Kelly, F.; García Hoyos, M.; Lopez Martinez, M.; Lopez-Molina, M.; Riveiro-Alvarez, R.; Fernandez-San Jose, P.; Avila-Fernandez, A.; Corton, M.; Millan, J.; García Sandoval, B.; et al. Dominant Retinitis Pigmentosa, p.Gly56Arg Mutation in NR2E3: Phenotype in a Large Cohort of 24 Cases. *PLoS ONE* **2016**, *11*, e0149473. [CrossRef]
57. Bravo-Gil, N.; Méndez-Vidal, C.; Romero-Pérez, L.; González-del Pozo, M.; Rodríguez-de la Rúa, E.; Dopazo, J.; Borrego, S.; Antiñolo, G. Improving the management of Inherited Retinal Dystrophies by targeted sequencing of a population-specific gene panel. *Sci. Rep.* **2016**, *6*, 23910. [CrossRef] [PubMed]
58. van de Laar, I.; Arbustini, E.; Loeys, B.; Björck, E.; Murphy, L.; Groenink, M.; Kempers, M.; Timmermans, J.; Roos-Hesselink, J.; Benke, K.; et al. European reference network for rare vascular diseases (VASCERN) consensus statement for the screening and management of patients with pathogenic ACTA2 variants. *Orphanet J. Rare Dis.* **2019**, *14*, 264. [CrossRef]
59. Ramalle-Gómara, E.; Domínguez-Garrido, E.; Gómez-Eguílaz, M.; Marzo-Sola, M.E.; Ramón-Trapero, J.L.; Gil-de-Gómez, J. Education and information needs for physicians about rare diseases in Spain. *Orphanet J. Rare Dis.* **2020**, *15*, 18. [CrossRef] [PubMed]
60. Christian Hirsch, M.; Ronicke, S.; Krusche, M.; Doris Wagner, A. Rare diseases 2030: How augmented AI will support diagnosis and treatment of rare diseases in the future. *Ann. Rheum. Dis.* **2020**, *79*, 740–743. [CrossRef] [PubMed]
61. Yang, Y.; Muzny, D.; Reid, J.; Bainbridge, M.; Willis, A.; Ward, P.; Braxton, A.; Beuten, J.; Xia, F.; Niu, Z.; et al. Clinical whole-exome sequencing for the diagnosis of mendelian disorders. *N. Engl. J. Med.* **2013**, *369*, 1502–1511. [CrossRef]
62. Yang, Y.; Muzny, D.; Xia, F.; Niu, Z.; Person, R.; Ding, Y.; Ward, P.; Braxton, A.; Wang, M.; Buhay, C.; et al. Molecular findings among patients referred for clinical whole-exome sequencing. *JAMA* **2014**, *312*, 1870–1879. [CrossRef]
63. Stavropoulos, D.; Merico, D.; Jobling, R.; Bowdin, S.; Monfared, N.; Thiruvahindrapuram, B.; Nalpathamkalam, T.; Pellecchia, G.; Yuen, R.; Szego, M.; et al. Whole Genome Sequencing Expands Diagnostic Utility and Improves Clinical Management in Pediatric Medicine. *NPJ Genom. Med.* **2016**, *1*, 15012. [CrossRef] [PubMed]
64. Palmer, E.; Sachdev, R.; Macintosh, R.; Melo, U.; Mundlos, S.; Righetti, S.; Kandula, T.; Minoche, A.; Puttick, C.; Gayevskiy, V.; et al. Diagnostic Yield of Whole Genome Sequencing after Nondiagnostic Exome Sequencing or Gene Panel in Developmental and Epileptic Encephalopathies. *Neurology* **2021**, *96*, e1770–e1782. [CrossRef]
65. Bhatia, N.S.; Lim, J.Y.; Bonnard, C.; Kuan, J.L.; Brett, M.; Wei, H.; Cham, B.; Chin, H.; Bosso-Lefevre, C.; Dharuman, P.; et al. Singapore Undiagnosed Disease Program: Genomic Analysis aids Diagnosis and Clinical Management. *Arch. Dis. Child.* **2021**, *106*, 31–37. [CrossRef]
66. Tibben, A.; Dondorp, W.; Cornelis, C.; Knoers, N.; Brilstra, E.; van Summeren, M.; Bolt, I. Parents, their children, whole exome sequencing and unsolicited findings: Growing towards the child's future autonomy. *Eur. J. Hum. Genet.* **2021**, *29*, 911–919. [CrossRef]
67. Abbott, M.; McKenzie, L.; Moran, B.V.G.; Heidenreich, S.; Hernández, R.; Hocking-Mennie, L.; Clark, C.; Gomes, J.; Lampe, A.; Baty, D.; et al. Continuing the sequence? Towards an economic evaluation of whole genome sequencing for the diagnosis of rare diseases in Scotland. *J. Community Genet.* **2021**, *1*, 1–15. [CrossRef]
68. Wouters, R.H.P.; Bijlsma, R.M.; Frederix, G.W.J.; Ausems, M.G.E.M.; van Delden, J.J.M.; Voest, E.E.; Bredenoord, A.L. Is It Our Duty to Hunt for Pathogenic Mutations? *Trends Mol. Med.* **2018**, *24*, 3–6. [CrossRef]
69. Fraiman, Y.S.; Wojcik, M.H. The influence of social determinants of health on the genetic diagnostic odyssey: Who remains undiagnosed, why, and to what effect? *Pediatr. Res.* **2020**, *89*, 295–300. [CrossRef]
70. Narayanan, D.; Udyawar, D.; Kaur, P.; Sharma, S.; Suresh, N.; Nampoothiri, S.; do Rosario, M.; Somashekar, P.; Rao, L.; Kausthubham, N.; et al. Multilocus disease-causing genomic variations for Mendelian disorders: Role of systematic phenotyping and implications on genetic counselling. *Eur. J. Hum. Genet.* **2021**, *29*, 1774–1780. [CrossRef]
71. Luis Soto, J.; Blanco, I.; Díez, O.; García Planells, J.; Lorda, I.; Matthijs, G.; Robledo, M.; Souche, E.; Lázaro, C. Documento de consenso sobre la implementación de la secuenciación masiva de nueva generación en el diagnóstico genético de la predisposición hereditaria al cáncer. *Med. Clin.* **2017**, *151*, 80.e1–80.e10. [CrossRef]
72. Elliott, A.M.; Dragojlovic, N.; Campbell, T.; Adam, S.; du Souich, C.; Fryer, M.; Lehman, A.; van Karnebeek, C.; Lynd, L.D.; Friedman, J.M. Utilization of telehealth in paediatric genome-wide sequencing: Health services implementation issues in the CAUSES Study. *J. Telemed. Telecare* **2021**, 1357633X20982737. [CrossRef]
73. Elliott, A.M. Genetic counseling and genome sequencing in pediatric rare disease. *Cold Spring Harb. Perspect. Med.* **2020**, *10*, a036632. [CrossRef]
74. Consejo Interterritorial del Sistema Nacional de Salud. *Estrategia en Enfermedades Raras del Sistema Nacional de Salud SANIDAD 2013 Ministerio de Sanidad, Servicios Sociales E Igualdad*; SANIDAD: Madrid, Spain, 2014.
75. Enfermedades Raras. Enfermedades Raras. Available online: https://dice-aper.semfyc.es/?page_id=37&lang=en (accessed on 24 August 2021).
76. Zurynski, Y.; Deverell, M.; Dalkeith, T.; Johnson, S.; Christodoulou, J.; Leonard, H.; Elliott, E.J. Australian children living with rare diseases: Experiences of diagnosis and perceived consequences of diagnostic delays. *Orphanet J. Rare Dis.* **2017**, *12*, 68. [CrossRef]

77. Bueno, E.G.; Ruano García, M.; Guerra de los Santos, J.M.; Montero Vásquez, I. Conocimientos médicos sobre enfermedades raras por parte de los profesionales de la salud. *Salud Ciencia* **2015**, *21*, 604–609.
78. Alfaro, T.M.; Wijsenbeek, M.S.; Powell, P.; Stolz, D.; Hurst, J.R.; Kreuter, M.; Moor, C.C. Educational aspects of rare and orphan lung diseases. *Respir. Res.* **2021**, *22*, 92. [CrossRef] [PubMed]

MDPI
St. Alban-Anlage 66
4052 Basel
Switzerland
Tel. +41 61 683 77 34
Fax +41 61 302 89 18
www.mdpi.com

Diagnostics Editorial Office
E-mail: diagnostics@mdpi.com
www.mdpi.com/journal/diagnostics

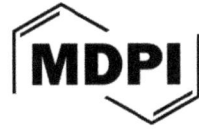

www.ingramcontent.com/pod-product-compliance
Lightning Source LLC
LaVergne TN
LVHW070606100526
838202LV00012B/580